Social Capital and Health

T0140445

Social Capital and Health

Edited by

Ichiro Kawachi

Harvard University
Boston, Massachusetts, USA

S.V. Subramanian

Harvard University
Boston, Massachusetts, USA

Daniel Kim

Harvard University
Boston, Massachusetts, USA

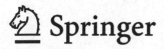 Springer

Ichiro Kawachi
Department of Society, Human
   Development and Health
Harvard School of Public Health
Kresge Buliding, 7th Floor
677 Huntington Avenue
Boston, MA 02115
USA

S.V. Subramanian
Department of Society, Human
   Developmnt, and Health
Harvard School of Public Health
Kresge Buliding, 7th Floor
677 Huntington Avenue
Boston, MA 02115
USA

Daniel Kim
Department of Society, Human
   Development, and Health
Harvard School of Public Health
Kresge Buliding, 7th Floor
677 Huntington Avenue
Boston, MA 02115

ISBN 978-1-4419-2435-3   e-ISBN 978-0-387-71311-3

Printed on acid-free paper.

© 2010 Springer Science + Business Media, LLC
All rights reserved. This work may not be translated or copied in whole or in part without the written permission of the publisher (Springer Science+Business Media, LLC, 233 Spring Street, New York, NY 10013, USA), except for brief excerpts in connection with reviews or scholarly analysis. Use in connection with any form of information storage and retrieval, electronic adaptation, computer software, or by similar or dissimilar methodology now known or hereafter developed is forbidden.
The use in this publication of trade names, trademarks, service marks and similar terms, even if they are not identified as such, is not to be taken as an expression of opinion as to whether or not they are subject to proprietary rights.

9 8 7 6 5 4 3 2 1

springer.com

Acknowledgments

Professor Trudy Harpham (chapter 3) would like to thank her mother, Constance Harpham, for enabling so many good things in life to happen.

The authors of chapter 2 (Cynthia Lakon, Dionne Godette and John Hipp) acknowledge the support provided in part by the National Institute on Drug Abuse (NIDA) grant number DA16094 administered through the Transdisciplinary Drug Abuse Prevention Research Center (TPRC) at the University of Southern California. The chapter was also supported by the W.K. Kellogg Foundation Scholars in Health Disparities Program at the Harvard School of Public Health and the National Institute on Alcohol Abuse and Alcoholism grant number P60 AA013759–02s2 administered through the Boston University Youth Alcohol Prevention Center. Finally, the authors would also like to express their gratitude to Dr. Tom Valente.

Richard Carpiano authored chapter 5 while he was a Robert Wood Johnson Foundation Health & Society Scholar at the University of Wisconsin-Madison. Some of the empirical findings detailed within are drawn from a study supported through a pilot grant from the University of Wisconsin Health & Society Scholars Program. Quantitative findings are based on data from the Los Angeles Family and Neighborhood Survey, which is funded by a grant R01 HD35944 from the United States National Institute of Child Health and Human Development to RAND in Santa Monica, California. He also wishes to thank Stephanie Robert for helpful comments, as well as many colleagues who have helped to facilitate the theoretical and empirical studies detailed here.

The research described in chapter 7 (the economic approach to studying cooperation and trust) was funded by the National Science Foundation (SES-0094800) and the Schroeder Center for Health Care Policy at the Thomas Jefferson Program in Public Policy at the College of William and Mary. Lisa Anderson and Jennifer Mellor would like to thank Jeff Milyo for valuable comments on their work.

Astier Almedom (chapter 9) was supported by the Henry R. Luce Program in Science and Humanitarianism at Tufts University.

Kathleen Cagney and Ming Wen (chapter 11) would like to thank their colleague, Dr. Christopher Browning (Ohio State University). Ming Wen thanks her mother, Hua Wen, for her support.

Vish Viswanath (chapter 12) would like to acknowledge the assistance of Shoba Ramanadhan on his chapter.

Ichiro Kawachi acknowledges the generous support of the MacArthur Network on Socioeconomic Status and Health, and the always helpful advice of his colleagues in the Network: Nancy Adler, Teresa Seeman, Bruce McEwen, Sheldon Cohen, Mark Cullen, Ana Diez Roux, David Williams, Karen Matthews, Michael Marmot, and Judith Stewart.

S V Subramanian would like to acknowledge the support of the National Institutes of Health via a Career Development Award (NHLBI 1 K25 HL081275). He also thanks his wife, Nithya, and two children, Maya and Swara, and his mother. He dedicates this effort of his to his father.

Daniel Kim wishes to thank his parents, Sung Gyum Kim and Hae Ja Kim, for their enduring support.

Contents

List of Contributors

Astier M. Almedom, PhD, Tufts University, Boston, MA.

Lisa R. Anderson. PhD, College of William and Mary, Williamsburg, VA.

Rebecca O. Cadigan, MS, Harvard School of Public Health, Boston, MA.

Kathleen A. Cagney, PhD, University of Chicago, Chicago, IL.

Richard M. Carpiano, PhD, MPH, University of British Columbia, Vancouver, Canada.

Douglas Glandon, PhD, Tufts University, Boston, MA.

Dionne C. Godette, PhD, University of Georgia, Athens, GA.

Trudy Harpham, PhD, London South Bank University, London, U.K.

John R. Hipp, MS, PhD, University of California, Irvine, Irvine, CA.

Ichiro Kawachi, MD, PhD, Harvard School of Public Health, Boston, MA.

Daniel Kim, MD, MPH, MSc, Harvard School of Public Health, Boston, MA.

Howard K. Koh, MD, MPH, FACP, Harvard School of Public Health, Boston, MA.

Cynthia M. Lakon, PhD, Keck School of Medicine, University of Southern California, Alhambra, CA.

Martin Lindström, PhD, Malmö University Hospital/Lund University, Malmö, Sweden.

Jennifer M. Mellor, PhD, College of William and Mary, Williamsburg, VA.

S.V. Subramanian, PhD, Harvard School of Public Health, Boston, MA.

Martin Van Der Gaag, PhD, Department of Public Administration and Communication Sciences, Faculty of Social Sciences, Vrije Universiteit Amsterdam, The Netherlands

K. Viswanath, PhD, Dana Farber Cancer Institute & Harvard School of Public Health, Boston, MA.

Martin Webber, MSc, Institute of Psychiatry, Kings College London, London, U.K.

Ming Wen, PhD, University of Utah, Salt Lake City, UT.

Rob Whitley, PhD, Dartmouth Medical School/Dartmouth Psychiatric Research Center, Lebanon, NH.

1
Social Capital and Health
A Decade of Progress and Beyond

ICHIRO KAWACHI, S.V. SUBRAMANIAN, AND DANIEL KIM

Pick any current issue of a journal such as *Social Science & Medicine* or the *Journal of Epidemiology and Community Health* and one is bound to see a featured article about social capital and health. Search on Pubmed for "social capital and health", and one sees over 27,500 articles listed (as of December 2006). Enter the same search term in Google, and you get over 9 million hits. Yet wind the clock back to circa 1996 and one would be hard pressed to find an article in the public health literature that even mentioned this concept. In other words, within a short span of a decade, social capital has entered the mainstream of public health discourse, where it is now the theme of professional conferences, as well as the topic of white papers put out by government health agencies worldwide. For sure social capital was talked about in fields outside public health prior to 1996 – in sociology (Bourdieu, 1986; Coleman, 1990), economics (Loury, 1992), and political science (Putnam, 1993) – but the explosion of interest in applying the concept to public health is a comparatively recent phenomenon (Figure 1.1).

The purpose of this book is to take stock of what we have learned during the first decade of research on social capital and health. What *is* social capital? How do we measure it? What have we learned so far about the empirical relationships between social capital and specific health outcomes? What is the potential utility of the concept for designing interventions to improve population health? These are some of the questions that individual chapters will address.

As one would expect, whenever a new and important concept is introduced to a field, it is critically scrutinized and debated. Social capital is no exception. As Szreter and Woolcock (2004) declared, social capital has become one of the "essentially contested concepts" in the social sciences, like "class", "race", and "gender". There are skeptics who maintain that in its most benign versions, social capital represents old ideas dressed up in fancy economic language while at its worst the concept represents a dangerous distraction from more pressing public health agendas such as the political struggle for justice and equality (more about this later). The chapters gathered in this book seek to present a picture of the state of the art in the field of social capital research, warts and all. Individual scholars provide different – and

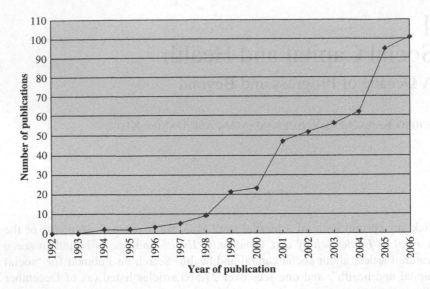

FIGURE 1.1. Papers on social capital and health indexed in MEDLINE 1992–2006

occasionally conflicting – points of view about the definitions and measurement of social capital, which we (the editors) take to be a healthy reflection of the debates in the field. There is no single definition of social capital that everyone would agree upon; nor is there a standardized approach to measuring it – at least not so far. Instead, we have endeavored to provide a survey of the field "from 30,000 feet", making sure that a diversity of approaches and opinions has been represented by a group of leading scholars working at the intersection of social capital and population health.

1.1. Definitions of Social Capital – One or Many?

One of the most confusing and frustrating aspects of social capital, at least in the public health field, has been the lack of consensus concerning its definition. Vagueness in defining the concept reaches back to Coleman who devoted an entire chapter to social capital in his 1990 textbook *The Foundations of Social Theory*. In it, Coleman defined social capital as "not a single entity, but a variety of different entities having two characteristics in common: They all consist of some aspect of social structure, and they facilitate certain actions of individuals who are within the structure" (Coleman, 1990. p. 302). Alas, like the parable of the blind Indian sages who reached radically different conclusions concerning the nature of the elephant after each had touched a different part of the animal's anatomy, public health researchers have often been guilty of lumping all sorts of disparate social phenomena under the label of "social capital". As the term has entered everyday political discourse, it seems to have become further debased, to the extent that some have bemoaned that social capital has become devoid of all meaning.

We are obviously not so pessimistic (else we would not have agreed to edit this book!). In fact, we believe that a survey of the uses of the term social capital in public health research reveals two distinct conceptions (Kawachi, 2006). On the one hand, social capital has been conceptualized as the resources – for example, trust, norms, and the exercise of sanctions – available to members of social groups. The social group can take different forms, such as a work place, a voluntary organization, or a tightly-knit residential community. We refer to this definition as the "social cohesion" school of social capital.[1] The salient feature of this approach is that social capital is conceptualized as a group attribute, i.e. as a property of the organization or the community, as opposed to a description of the individual members who belong to the group. Hence, a given member of a group may be an uncooperative, mistrusting individual, but he or she may reside in a community where others are trusting and helpful toward each other. The uncooperative individual may then end up benefiting from (or free-riding on) the generosity of his neighbors – for example, by refusing to participate in the annual community drive to pick up rubbish off the streets, but nonetheless benefiting from the voluntary labor of his neighbors. Alternatively, the individual may feel pressured to take part in the activities organized by his Pollyannaish neighbors, and begin to feel put upon and stressed. In both scenarios, what the social cohesion school of social capital emphasizes are the so-called "contextual" influences of the collective exerted on the individual (Kawachi & Berkman, 2000). Empirically demonstrating the existence of contextual influences on health requires special study designs and analytical techniques, a point we shall return to later.

Distinct from the social cohesion school, the "network" theory of social capital defines the concept in terms of the resources – for example, social support, information channels, social credentials – that are embedded within an individual's social networks (Lin, 1999). In contrast to the social cohesion approach, network analysts conceptualize and measure social capital as both an individual attribute as well as a property of the collective (the social network). Most network analysts do not simultaneously assess social capital at both the individual and group levels, but rather they have tended to assess one or the other depending on their method of measurement. Methodological individualists, like van der Gaag and Webber (chapter 2) have developed instruments (e.g. the Resource Generator) to assess individual social capital, conceptualized as valued resources that individuals can access through their social networks. These valued resources can be accessed in several domains of life (at work, in private life), and spans across a range of goods from the material (e.g. borrowing money) to the symbolic (e.g. prestige and influence). An alternative network-based approach to measuring individual social

---

[1] Moore et al.(2005) have also labeled this the "communitarian" definition of social capital

capital is exemplified by Nan Lin's Position Generator (Lin, 2001), which relies upon asking individuals (the egos) to nominate others in their network (the alters) who hold valuable occupations (e.g. doctor, lawyer, lobbyist), and who could provide the egos with access to resources such as advice, prestige, and political connections.

In contrast to the mapping of ego-centered network resources just described, other network analysts have approached the measurement of social capital by mapping whole social networks (see chapter 4 by Lakon, Godette and Hipp). This method involves approaching every member within a defined social structure (e.g. members of an organization, or a network of organizations within a city) to establish the existence and characteristics of connections between them. The resulting sociogram is amenable to mathematical manipulation, from which it is possible to derive structural properties of the group. In turn, some of these group properties have direct relevance to health promotion. Thus, for example, the introduction of an innovation – say a campaign to encourage smoking cessation in the work place – would be predicted to diffuse more quickly within a more structurally dense network.[2] Although it would be a mistake to equate social capital with every structural network property derived from sociometric analysis, several of the concepts described by this approach – such as centrality, and network bridges – are directly relevant to social capital, if not actual measurements of it (see chapter 4 for a more rigorous defense of this thesis).

To summarize, empirical research on social capital has stimulated a vigorous debate regarding its conceptualization and definition. A fundamental point of contention is whether social capital ought to be considered as an individual or as a group attribute. Our tentative answer to this question is that it is both. Although the social cohesion approach to social capital conceptualizes it as a group attribute, the network-based definition embraces both the individual (ego-centered) and group (sociometric) levels of analysis. A second fundamental point of contention is whether social capital ought to be conceptualized as social cohesion or as resources embedded in networks. Again, our tentative answer is yes to both, although a citation network analysis of the public health literature on social capital found that researchers have given far more emphasis to the social cohesion definition of social capital (Moore, Shiell, Hawe, & Haines, 2005), a point that is also made by Richard Carpiano in chapter 5. Of course, we cannot reject the possibility that at some future date, an international consensus conference of scholars might agree to reserve the use of the term "social capital" only to refer to network-based resources, and to expel social cohesion from the umbrella of the label (just as Pluto was demoted from the status of a planet in the solar system at a recent conference of astronomers!). We, however, do not find cogent arguments to be dogmatic on this issue. Both the social cohesion and the network definitions of social capital have merit in pointing to the existence of valued resources (capital) that inhere within, and are by-products of, social relationships.

---

[2] See chapter 4 for a precise definition of network density.

1.2. Bonding Versus Bridging Social Capital

Regardless of whether one subscribes to the social cohesion school of social capital or the network school, consensus now exists about the importance of distinguishing between bonding and bridging social capital (Gittell & Vidal, 1998; Kawachi, 2006; Szreter & Woolcock, 2004). Bonding capital refers to resources that are accessed within social groups whose members are alike ("homophilous") in terms of their social identity, such as class or race. By contrast, bridging capital refers to the resources accessed by individuals and groups through connections that cross class, race/ethnicity, and other boundaries of social identity.[3] Although few empirical studies so far have actually measured both bonding and bridging capital, growing evidence suggests that distinguishing between these types will help us to understand how social capital promotes – or harms – the health of individuals.

One of the early criticisms of the public health literature on social capital has been that researchers have tended to emphasize social capital's salutary impacts on health whilst neglecting or downplaying its damaging effects. This bias no doubt stemmed from earlier attempts at defining social capital ("version 1.0") in which the concept was defined according to its *functions* (e.g. "facilitating desirable outcomes") rather than by its forms (as in "resources available through social connections"). Most researchers now acknowledge the inherent circularity in defining a cause based on its consequences – i.e. "if a community has poor outcomes (for example, high rates of crime or infant mortality), it must be because it is lacking in social capital." Portes (1998) in an influential article drew attention to the so called dark sides of social capital, which include: (a) excessive demands placed upon members of cohesive groups to provide support to others; (b) expectations of conformity that may result in restrictions on individual freedom as well as intolerance of diversity; (c) the exercise of in-group solidarity to exclude members of out-groups, or in some cases, even to oppress them; and (d) the down-leveling of norms within a tightly-knit group that can hold back the prospects of upward social mobility (for example, in Jay MacLeod's (1987) ethnographic study of a disadvantaged high school in Clarendon Heights, the peer group of "Hallway Hangers" devalues conventional success which serves to level its members' aspirations for educational achievement).

As these examples make clear, social capital – like any form of capital (for example, money) – can translate into both good ends and bad ends. Church soup kitchens provide social capital, but so do the Ku Klux Klan and the mafia (at least to its members, though not for society at large). Accordingly current definitions of social capital (version 2.0 and beyond) are agnostic with regard to the consequences

---

[3] Some scholars refer to an additional category, "linking" social capital, to refer to connections between individuals and groups who interact across explicit power or authority gradients in society (Szreter & Woolcock, 2004). We treat linking capital as a special case of bridging social capital.

of the uses to which network-based resources are put. However, distinguishing between bonding and bridging capital may help to explain the sometimes conflicting effects associated with social capital. To give an example, strong bonding capital often promotes strong within-group identity. In India, membership in the local branch of the Bharatiya Janata Party (BJP) no doubt encourages a person's sense of Hindu nationalism, while conversely belonging to the Muslim League does the same for Muslims. Both are forms of bonding capital. One might further predict that the stronger the bonding capital within religious groups in a given locality, the higher the levels of between-group tensions. Ashutosh Varshney (2002) at Michigan University conducted an empirical examination of outbreaks of sectarian violence in India. One of the puzzles uncovered by this study was the observation that there are marked variations in the history of ethnic conflict across cities in India that on the surface had roughly the same proportion of Hindu and Muslim residents. According to Varshney, the difference (i.e. why some cities were successful in maintaining the peace while others were racked by violence and conflict) was attributable to the presence of bridging social capital within the peaceful cities. Bridging capital in this case took the form of integrated civic organizations – business groups, trade unions, professional groups, and even reading circles – that included among its members both Muslims and Hindus. Such organizations, Varshney argues, have proved extremely effective at preventing the outbreak of violence, for example by maintaining channels of communication across the religious groups, and by being efficient at killing rumors that trouble-makers attempted to spread within the community in order to incite riots.

Bonding capital represents an important survival mechanism for residents of disadvantaged communities. As Carol Stack's (1974) ethnographic study of a poor African-American community revealed, high levels of mutual support through kinship networks are the primary mechanism for "getting by" in such communities. At the same time, bonding capital often extracts a cost to the providers of support in terms of the mental and financial strain of caring for others in need. Consistent with this notion, in a small study of a disadvantaged minority community in Birmingham, Alabama, Mitchell and LaGory (2002) reported that high bonding social capital (measured by the strength of trust and associational ties with others of a similar racial and educational background as the respondent) was paradoxically associated with higher levels of mental distress. In the same study, however, individuals who reported social ties to others who were unlike them with respect to race and class (i.e. who had access to bridging capital) were less likely to report mental distress.

Additional studies from Baltimore, Maryland (Caughy, O'Campo, & Muntaner C, 2003), and Adelaide, Australia (Ziersch & Baum, 2004), suggest that stronger bonding ties within disadvantaged communities may be a detriment to the health of residents. In a low-income neighborhood of Baltimore, children of mothers who reported lower levels of attachment to their community reported fewer behavioral and mental health problems (Caughy et al., 2003), while in a study of a working class suburb in Adelaide, Ziersch and Baum (2004) found that involvement in community groups was associated with worse physical health as measured by the

SF-12 health status survey. Qualitative interviews with residents in the same study found that respondents were more apt to link their participation in local community groups with negative mental and physical health outcomes.

The emerging picture from these studies seems to be that bonding capital within disadvantaged communities may be a health liability rather than a force for health promotion that it is often assumed to be. The key to improving health therefore appears to lie in residents' ability to access resources outside their immediate social milieu, i.e. access to bridging social capital. More refined tests of this hypothesis would be made possible by incorporating explicit measures of bridging capital into future studies, exemplified by network-based concepts such as heterogeneity and "upper reachability" (see chapter 4 for a more detailed exposition).

1.3. Social Capital Research within a Muli-Level Analytical Framework

As will become evident in Part II of this book summarizing the empirical evidence on social capital and health (chapters 8 through 11), a growing number of studies in public health have adopted a multi-level framework to analyze the relationship between social cohesion and specific outcomes.[4] Multi-level approaches have proved useful in two fundamental ways: (a) by enabling researchers to demonstrate whether social cohesion has an independent "contextual" effect on individual health outcomes, over and above the characteristics of individuals belonging to the social group; and (b) by permitting researchers to explicitly test for cross-level interactions between community social cohesion and individual characteristics, such as socioeconomic status, race/ethnicity, and gender. A third way in which multilevel models are of substantial relevance (even though this aspect remains under-utilized in social capital research) is by enabling researchers to develop unconfounded measures of social cohesion from survey data aggregated up to the group level. Before we elaborate on the above functions of multilevel models, we discuss the intrinsic relevance of the multilevel study approach for social capital and health research.

Figure 1.2 identifies a typology of designs for data collection and analyses (Blakely & Subramanian, 2006; Blakely & Woodward, 2000; Subramanian, Glymour, & Kawachi, 2007) where the rows indicate the level or unit at which the outcome variable is being measured (i.e. at the individual level (y) or the aggregate, or ecological, level (Y)), and the columns indicate whether the exposure is being measured at the individual level (x) or the ecological level (X). Study-type $\{y,x\}$ is most commonly encountered when the researcher aims to link exposures measured at the individual level (e.g. diet) to individual health

---

[4] Social capital research from a network perspective has either analyzed individual level data (from ego-centered assessment) or group level data (via sociometric analyses).

	Exposure	
	x	X
y	{y, x} **Traditional risk factor study**	{y, X} **Contextual study**
Y	{Y, x}[(A)]	{Y, X} **Ecological study**

(Left axis label: **Outcome**)

FIGURE 1.2. A typology of studies (adapted from Blakely TA & Woodward AJ (2000); and Blakely T & Subramanian SV (2006))

Note: [(A)] This type of study is impossible to specify as it stands. Practically speaking, it will either take the form of Y,X}, i.e. ecological study, where will now simply be central tendency of x. Or, if dis-aggregation of y is possible, so that we can observe y, then it will be equivalent to y,x}.

outcomes (e.g. obesity). By ignoring ecological effects (whether implicitly or explicitly), study-type {y,x} assumes that health is primarily determined by individual choices and actions (Moon et al., 2005). By contrast, study-type{Y,X} – referred to as the "ecological study" – may seem intuitively suited to research on ecological exposures, such as social capital, and population health. However, study-type{Y,X} conflates the genuinely ecological with "aggregate" or compositional effects (Moon et al., 2005), and precludes the possibility of testing heterogeneous contextual effects on different types of individuals. An association between community social capital and health could simultaneously reflect both contextual and aggregate (or compositional) influences. In this situation the interpretative question becomes particularly relevant. If common membership of a community by a set of individuals influences their health over and above individual characteristics, then there may indeed be an ecological effect (i.e. the whole may be more than the sum of its parts). Alternatively, an association between a community level exposure and average community health status may simply reflect the underlying individual-level relationships between x and y. For example, if we find that average levels of obesity tend to be higher in neighborhoods with lower levels of social capital, such an observation need not, by itself, provide insight into the causal question of interest: i.e. does living in high social capital neighborhoods increase individual residents' risk of obesity compared to living in a low-social capital neighborhood?

Answering the above question requires a study of the type $\{y,X\}$, i.e. in which an ecological exposure (e.g. the proportion of community members reporting trust) is linked to an individual outcome (obesity). A more complete representation would be type $\{y,x,X\}$ whereby we have an individual outcome (y), individual covariates (x) and ecologic exposure (X) reflecting a multilevel structure of individuals nested within ecologies. When the ecological exposure is an aggregate measure of individual characteristics, such as percent trust, it is obvious that information on both individual trust and average neighborhood trust is required to test for a contextual effect (Kawachi & Subramanian, 2006; Subramanian, Kim, & Kawachi, 2002).

A fundamental motivation for study-type $\{y,x,X\}$ is to distinguish "neighborhood differences in health" from "the difference a neighborhood makes to individual health outcomes" (Moon et al., 2005). Stated differently, contextual effects on the individual outcome can only be ascertained after individual factors that reflect the composition of the neighborhood have been controlled. Indeed, compositional explanations for ecological variations in health are common, to paraphrase the methodologist Gary King, "if we really understood [health variations], we would not need to know much of contextual effects"(King, 1997). This is an important challenge for researchers interested in understanding the effects of social capital on health.

The multilevel framework with its simultaneous examination of the characteristics of the individuals at one level and the context or ecologies in which they are located at another level offers a comprehensive framework for understanding the ways in which places can affect people (contextual effect) or, alternatively, people can affect places (composition). Adopting a multilevel framework implies that variations in health outcomes are determined by both individual risk and protective factors, *as well as* by community risk and resilience factors. As such, interventions to mitigate adverse health outcomes can be offered at both the individual and community levels.

1.4. Multilevel Models in Social Capital and Health Research

In the presence of a multilevel data, as described above, there are substantive as well as technical reasons to use multilevel statistical models to analyze such data (Goldstein, 2003; Raudenbush & Bryk, 2002). We will not review the basic principles of multilevel modeling here as they have been described elsewhere in the context of health research (Blakely & Subramanian, 2006; Moon et al., 2005; Subramanian, 2004; Subramanian, Jones, & Duncan, 2003b; Subramanian et al., 2007); but we provide a brief overview of the relevance of multilevel models for social capital and health research.

1.4.1. Evaluating the Independent Contribution
of Community Social Capital

A fundamental application of multilevel methods for social capital and health research is evaluating the independent contribution of community social capital on individual health outcomes, net of individual covariates (including those social capital dimensions that may have been measured at the level of individuals) (Kawachi & Subramanian, 2006; Subramanian et al., 2002). We provide a hypothetical example of a study to investigate the influence of community social capital on individual body mass index (BMI).

For the purposes of the worked example, we shall assume that our indicator of social capital is a measure of perceived trust. At the individual level, social capital is measured by each individual's level of trust of others in the community. At the neighborhood level, we can construct a measure of social capital based upon aggregating individual responses to survey items about trust (e.g. the proportion reporting that they trust their neighbors). Following this, we can have a two-level structure where the outcome is the BMI, y for individual i (level-1) in neighborhood j (level-2). For simplicity, we will restrict this example to a single social capital indicator, trust. Trust can be measured as whether the subject reports a high or low level of trust (x_{1ij}) for every individual i in neighborhood j and coded 1 if the subject reports mistrust, 0 otherwise; and one neighborhood-level exposure, $\bar{X}_{1j}$, the proportion of subjects reporting mistrust in neighborhood j. With few exceptions (Subramanian et al., 2002), researchers have *not* considered individual analogues of social capital, and individual measures have been limited to demographic and socioeconomic characteristics of the individual. We consider the example of individual perception of trust to emphasize the substantive relevance of controlling for this individual (compositional) measure while evaluating the contextual influence of community social capital.

Multilevel models operate by developing regression equations at each level of analysis. Thus, models are specified at two levels. The level-1 model can be:

$$y_{ij} = \beta_{0j} + \beta_1 x_{1ij} + e_{0ij} \tag{1}$$

where, β_{0j} (the intercept) is the mean BMI for the jth neighborhood for the group reporting high trust (the reference group); β_1 is the average differential in the BMI for individuals who report mistrust (x_{1ij}), across all neighborhoods. Meanwhile, e_{0ij} is the individual or the level-1 residual term. We can elaborate β_{0j} in the following manner:

$$\beta_{0j} = \beta_0 + u_{0j} \tag{2}$$

where, u_{0j}, estimates the differential contribution (positive or negative) that a neighborhood makes to the prediction of the individual BMI, independent of the individual's report of mistrust.

The neighborhood effect, u_{0j}, can be treated in one of two ways. One option is to estimate each one separately (i.e. treat them as any categorical variable in the fixed part of a single level regression model). We can then adopt the usual OLS regression to obtain the parameter estimates (the fixed-effect approach). On the other hand, if neighborhoods are treated as a (random) sample from a population of neighborhoods (which might include neighborhoods in future studies if one has complete population data), and the interest is in making inferences about the variation between neighborhoods (as compared to making inferences only about the sampled neighborhoods) that would constitute a multilevel statistical approach (the random-effect approach). Just as a sample of individuals is used to make inferences about the population rather than about each individual, the neighborhoods are instruments for making inferences about the relevant population of neighborhoods.

The choice of whether to use a fixed or random approach is a substantive one: are neighborhood differences a nuisance (in which case one would perform a fixed-effects single-level regression) or do neighborhood differences represent important processes that predict individual outcomes (in which case, one would perform a random-effects multilevel regression)? Indeed, a fixed effects approach is *not* an option for the typical multilevel research with intrinsic interest in estimating the effect of neighborhood-level exposures on the individual outcome, because the fixed effects of each neighborhood and neighborhood exposure (e.g. mistrust) are entirely confounded and, therefore, the latter are not identifiable (Fielding, 2004). As such, the fixed effects approach to modeling neighborhood differences is unsuitable for the sort of complex questions to which multilevel modeling has been addressed.

An attractive feature of multilevel models is their utility in modeling neighborhood and individual characteristics simultaneously. The model specified in equation (2) can be extended to include a neighborhood exposure, $\bar{X}_{1j}$, the proportion of individuals reporting mistrust in neighborhood j:

$$y_{ij} = \beta_{0j} + \beta_1 x_{1ij} + e_{0ij} \tag{3}$$

Note that the separate specification of micro (equation 2) and macro (equation 4) models correctly recognizes that the contextual variables ($\bar{X}_{1j}$) are predictors of between-neighborhood differences, as specified in equation (3). Substituting equation (3) into the micro model (1) yields:

$$\beta_{0j} = \beta_0 + u_{0j} \tag{4}$$

Specifically, α_1 estimates the marginal change in BMI for a unit change in level of neighborhood social capital ($\bar{X}_{1j}$), and is the parameter that quantifies the contextual effect of neighborhood social capital on individual BMI, conditional on individual characteristics (e.g. individual trust, but also age, sex, race/ethnicity, socioeconomic status, etc.).

The classic formulation of a contextual model in equation (4), however, is susceptible to high collinearity between the individual and neighborhood exposures of social capital, leading to poor precision (Aitkin & Longford, 1986). One solution is to reformulate equation (4) with x_{1ij} (individual trust coded as 1 for subjects who report low trust, 0 for those who report high trust) centered around its neighborhood mean, $\bar{X}_{1j}$ (neighborhood mistrust). For individuals who report mistrust, $(1 - \bar{X}_{1j})$ then equals the proportion not reporting mistrust in neighborhood j; for individuals not reporting mistrust, $(0 - \bar{X}_{1j})$ equals minus the proportion individuals who report mistrust in neighborhood j. The reformulated model is then:

$$y_{ij} = \beta_0 + \beta_1(x_{1ij} - \bar{X}_{1j}) + \alpha_1\bar{X}_{1j} + (u_{0j} + e_{0ij}) \tag{5}$$

Equation (5) is simply a re-parameterization of equation (4) with the contextual effect of mistrust, α_1 of equation (4) being equivalent to $\alpha_1 - \beta_1$ of equation (5) (Raudenbush, 1989). However, in equation (5) the individual level mistrust, $x_{1ij} - \bar{X}_{1j}$, is orthogonal to its neighborhood analogue $\bar{X}_{1j}$, thus overcoming the problem of collinearity. Substantively, centering the individual mistrust at its neighborhood average allows us to disentangle the pure individual and contextual effects of social capital on BMI. Thus, β_1 now measures the pure individual effect of mistrust on BMI, *within* a neighborhood, while α_1 measures the contextual effect of mistrust on BMI *between* neighborhoods. Such a formulation is useful in evaluating the clustering of individual exposures by neighborhoods.

1.4.2. Considering Cross-Level Interactions Between Community Social Capital and Individual Characteristics

Equation (5) can be further extended to evaluate whether the effect of neighborhood social capital on individual BMI is different for individuals reporting high or low trust. This can be achieved by introducing a "cross-level interaction" in the fixed part of the multilevel regression model between the "group-centered" individual mistrust $(x_{1ij} - \bar{X}_{1j})$ and neighborhood mistrust $(\bar{X}_{1j})$, given as $((x_{1ij} - \bar{X}_{1j})(\bar{X}_{1j}))$, referred to as X_{2ij} in the following equation:

$$y_{ij} = \beta_0 + \beta_1(x_{1ij} - \bar{X}_{1j}) + \alpha_1\bar{X}_{1j} + \alpha_2\bar{X}_{2j}$$
$$(u_{0j} + u_{1j}(x_{1ij} - \bar{X}_{1j}) + e_{0ij}) \tag{6}$$

The above formulation tests for the presence of interaction between a level-2 (neighborhood mistrust) and level-1 exposure (individual trust), represented by the fixed parameter, α_2. Specifically, α_1 estimates the marginal change in BMI for a unit change in the neighborhood mistrust for individuals reporting high trust; while α_2 estimates the extent to which the marginal change in BMI for a unit change in the neighborhood mistrust is different for individuals reporting mistrust. Note that the random part of the model has an additional random term, u_{1j}, associated with $x_{1ij} - \bar{X}_{1j}$. Underlying the test of a cross-level interaction is the anticipation that the neighborhood variation in BMI is different for individuals who report high or low trust that can then be explained in differential quantities (cross-level interactions effects) by levels of neighborhood social capital.

While the example considered here is a single normally distributed response variable (BMI) for illustration, multilevel models are capable of handling binary outcomes, proportions (as logit, log-log, and probit models); multiple categories (as ordered and unordered multinomial models); and counts (as poisson and negative binomial distribution models). These models essentially work by assuming a specific, non-Gaussian distribution for the random part at level-1, while maintaining the normality assumptions for random parts at higher levels. Consequently, the discussion presented in this paper focusing at the community level would continue to hold regardless of the nature of the response variable, with some important exceptions (Browne et al., 2005; Goldstein, Browne, & Rasbash, 2002).

1.4.3. Refining Survey-Based Assessments of Social Capital at the Community Level

A key, but under-utilized, relevance of multilevel models for social capital and health research is that it enables researchers to develop "un-confounded" measures of social capital from survey data aggregated up to the group level (Subramanian, Lochner, & Kawachi, 2003a). A common approach to assessing community or neighborhood level social capital involves surveying residents about their perceptions and behaviors, e.g. the extent to which they trust their neighbors; participate or engage in civic groups; or undertake acts of reciprocity. These individual responses are then aggregated to measure the level of social capital within the community (see chapter 3 by Trudy Harpham).

While this approach is commonly used, it is potentially problematic for an analysis that seeks to evaluate neighborhoods in terms of their social capital, since the observed differences between neighborhoods on social capital could be confounded by the characteristics of residents that constitute neighborhoods. At the same time, since information is originally collected as individual responses, such information, arguably, offers greater analytical scope for the understanding of social capital both at the level of individuals and at the level of neighborhoods.

In instances when community social capital is based upon aggregating individual information, one could utilize a standard multilevel model to refine the neighborhood measures of social capital. Consider the classic two-level hierarchical model:

$$y_{ij} = \beta_0 + \beta x_{ij} + (u_{0j} + e_{0ij}) \tag{7}$$

where, y_{ij} is the response on a social capital question or questions for individual i in neighborhood j; x is a vector of continuous and categorical individual covariates (e.g. age, sex, socioeconomic status) for that individual; u_{0j} is the random displacement for neighborhood j, assumed to be normally distributed with a mean of zero and variance σ_{u0}^2; and e_{0ij} is the individual- or the level-1 residual, assumed to be identically, independently, and normally distributed with mean zero and a variance σ_{u0}^2. In model (1) the regression and variance parameters take on the following interpretations: β_0 (associated with a constant, x_{0ij}, which is a set of 1s, and therefore, not written) is the average level of social capital across all neighborhoods; *β is a vector of regression coefficients associated with the vector of individual covariates;* σ_{u0}^2 represents the between-neighborhood variation in individual social capital response, conditional on individual (compositional) covariates; and σ_{u0}^2 represents the between-individual within-neighborhood variation.

The underlying random structure (variance-covariance matrix, represented as Ω) of the model specified in model (1) is typically specified as: $Var[u_{0j}] \sim N(0, \sigma_{u0}^2)$; $Var[e_{0j}] \sim N(0, \sigma_{e0}^2)$; and $Cov[u_{0j}, e_{0ij}] = 0$. Model (1) is usually referred to as the "random-intercepts" or "variance components" model, since it allows us to partition variation according to the different levels, with the variance in y_{ij} being the sum of σ_{u0}^2 and σ_{e0}^2; this in turn also allows us to ascertain the degree of similarity between two randomly chosen individuals within a neighborhood, expressed as: $\rho = \dfrac{\sigma_{u0}^2}{\sigma_{u0}^2 + \sigma_{e0}^2}$ (Goldstein, 2003).

Note that model (1) estimates a variance based on the observed sample of neighborhoods. While this is important to establish the overall importance of neighborhoods as a unit or level, model (1) also allows us to estimate for each level-2 unit: $\hat{u}_{0j} = E(u_{0j} \mid Y, \hat{\beta}, \hat{\Omega})$. The quantity is $\hat{u}_{0j}$ referred to as "estimated" or "predicted" residuals, or using Bayesian terminology, as "posterior" residual estimates, and is calculated as $\hat{u}_{0j} = r_j \times \dfrac{\sigma_{u0}^2}{\sigma_{u0}^2 + \sigma_{e0}^2 / n_j}$, where σ_{u0}^2 and σ_{e0}^2 are as defined above, r_j is the mean of the individual-level raw residuals for neighborhood j, and n_j is the number of individuals within each neighborhood j. This formula for $\hat{u}_{0j}$ uses the level-1 and level-2 variances and the number of people observed in neighborhood j to scale the observed level-2 residual (r_j). As the level-1 variance declines or the sample size increases, the scale factor approaches 1, and thus estimated $\hat{u}_{0j}$ approaches r_j.

These neighborhood-level residuals are "random variables with a distribution whose parameter values tell us about the variation among the level-2 units"

(Goldstein, 2003). Another interpretation is that each $\hat{u}_{0j}$ estimates neighborhood j's departure from expected mean outcome. This interpretation is premised on the assumption that each neighborhood belongs to a population of neighborhoods, and the distribution of the population provides information about plausible values for neighborhood j (Goldstein, 2003).

Consequently, one can develop a model-based indicator of community social capital that is now adjusted for observed factors that are likely to influence individual perceptions of trust. This can be accomplished by adding $\hat{\beta} + \hat{u}_{0j}$ or equivalently $\hat{\beta}_{0j}$ which is the predicted average levels of trust in a community. The perspective developed above has implications for the ways in which we measure and specify contextual exposures such as "percent reporting mistrust" (Subramanian et al., 2003a). Typically, as mentioned earlier, these are usually based on raw proportions, i.e. aggregating individual responses to their neighborhood. In an analysis of the Community Survey data from the Project on Human Development in Chicago (PHDCN), Subramanian et al. (2003a) used the predicted residuals from survey items inquiring about trust in order to derive "cleaned" measures of neighborhood trust. This measure can then be used in the "second-stage" model that regress individual health outcomes on community social capital of the form specified in equation (4).

1.5. Social Capital as a Contextual Influence on Health: The Importance of Scale

As is evident from the foregoing discussion, social capital can influence health at several different levels of action: at the individual level, at the level of residential communities, schools, or work places, as well as at even broader levels of spatial aggregation (such as states, regions, and countries). In turn, the scale at which social capital is conceptualized and measured requires careful theorizing about the differences in mechanisms through which it is hypothesized to affect health outcomes.

When researchers conceptualize social capital as the resources that individual access through their networks, the relevant mechanisms involved in the production of health include: social influence, social engagement, and the exchange of social support. An extensive literature in health psychology and public health has elaborated on these pathways and mechanisms (Berkman & Glass, 2000; Cohen, Underwood, & Gottlieb, 2000). For example, being integrated within a social network brings individuals under the influence of others in the same network, which serves to regulate their health behaviors (an observation dating back to Durkheim, 1897). Needless to add, social influence can cut both ways. If others in a network disapprove of smoking and drunk driving, individuals who are part of that network will be more likely to refrain from those behaviors. If on the other hand, the individual belongs to a tightly-knit network of injection drug-users or a cult obsessed with mass suicide, we might expect social capital in such instances to be damaging to health. Social networks are also the conduit ("the wiring") through which various forms of social support (information, advice, cash loans, etc) are exchanged within relationships. In turn, social support is believed to promote wellbeing through its ability to buffer stress – either by positively affecting the individuals' appraisals of their ability to cope with a stressful situation, or by directly supplying the resources required to deal with the stressful perturbation (Cohen, Underwood, & Gottlieb, 2000; Kawachi & Berkman, 2001).[5]

There is some debate as to whether trust measured at the individual level constitutes a genuine indicator of social capital (see chapter 3 by Trudy Harpham for further discussion on this issue). Those who argue against using trust as an indicator of social capital point out that an individual's perception of trust can be either a precursor of social capital or a consequence of it, but not actually a part of social capital itself (Lin, 1999). We tend to agree with the view that *individual* trust (most commonly ascertained by questions such as "Do you agree that most people can be trusted?") is problematic as an indicator of individual social capital – though for a different reason than the one commonly offered. The reason why we would view individual trust as potentially problematic is because it overlaps with the assessment of hostility in health psychology. Hostility refers to a personality trait that many studies have shown to be a risk factor for cardiovascular disease (Kubzansky & Kawachi, 2000; Matthews, 1988). Although the assessment of the hostility complex involves several components (including anger and aggression), one of the key constructs is mistrust of others. Thus, our view is that the evidence linking individual mistrust to health outcomes may be confounded by hostile personality traits. On the other hand, when perceptions about trust are *aggregated* to the group level, we would argue that it is no longer a measure of personality but a measure of the *trustworthiness* of people in the group. Moreover we would argue that the trustworthiness of a group is: (a) a collective property possessed by the group; (b) a resource that facilitates collective action; and hence (c) a valid measure of social cohesion.[6]

Turning now to community social capital, a different set of pathways and mechanisms needs to be invoked to explain the relationships to health outcomes than the ones just described for the case of individual social capital. At the community level, social capital (or more precisely, social cohesion) is hypothesized to influence health through processes such as collective socialization, informal social control, and collective efficacy (Coutts & Kawachi, 2006; see also chapter 11 by Kathleen Cagney and Ming Wen). Collective socialization refers to the role of community adults – not just a child's own parents – in shaping child development, behaviors, and health outcomes. A related concept, informal social control, refers to the capacity of a group to regulate the behavior of its members according to

---

[5] We hasten to add that some forms of social support can also be negative, for example a critical and judgmental partner might exacerbate a potentially stressful situation).

[6] We use the term "valid" here to denote content validity, i.e. that trust properly belongs to the construct of social cohesion. Whether the perceptions expressed by individuals are reliable (dare we say "trustworthy") or not is another matter (see chapters 3 and 7 for further discussion).

collectively desired (as opposed to forced) goals. In other words, in contrast to externally enforced actions (such as a police crackdown), informal social control focuses on "the effectiveness of informal mechanisms by which residents themselves achieve public order" (Sampson, Raudenbush & Earls, 1997). An example of informal social control that is relevant to health outcomes is the community's ability to regulate "deviant" health behaviours among its youth, such as drug use and under-age smoking. Finally, collective efficacy, which is the neighborhood counterpart to the concept of individual efficacy, refers to the global willingness of residents to intervene on behalf of the common good (Sampson, Raudenbush, & Earls, 1997). In terms of measurement, collective efficacy is conceptualized as the combination of informal social control and neighborhood social cohesion. According to the theory of collective efficacy, the willingness of local residents to intervene for the common good depends crucially on the presence of mutual trust and solidarity among neighbors (Sampson, Raudenbush, & Earls, 1997). The pathways through which neighborhood collective efficacy may influence health outcomes include – *in addition* to informal control over deviant behaviors – the ability of residents to extract resources and to respond to threatened cuts in public services (such as the closure of health clinics), as well as their ability to engage in sustained collective action to manage neighborhood physical hazards (e.g. the location of toxic waste sites) (Browning & Cagney, 2002; Kawachi & Berkman, 2000).

At a still broader level of spatial aggregation, a number of empirical studies have examined the association between state-level (Kawachi, Kennedy, & Glass 1999; Kawachi, Kennedy, Lochner, & Prothrow-Stith, 1997) or country-level (Helliwell & Putnam, 2004; Lynch et al., 2001) indicators of social cohesion and population health outcomes. Once again, the mechanisms underlying the demonstrated links between social capital and health are thought to be different at these broader levels than at the community or individual levels. Research has found that: (a) there are marked variations in the levels of social cohesion across broad geographic areas, and (b) the variations in social cohesion are strongly correlated with the degree of income inequality across the same areas (Kawachi et al., 1997; Putnam, 2000). Proceeding from these observations, we have theorized that the erosion of social cohesion is a critical mechanism through which inequality in the distribution of income is damaging to population health (Kawachi et al., 1997; Kawachi & Kennedy, 2002). Across the US states, for example, state-level measures of income inequality are tightly (and negatively) correlated with indicators of social cohesion, such as the degree to which residents agree that "most people can be trusted" and "most people are helpful". In turn, states that are both unequal and low in social cohesion tend to be less generous with respect to the provision of public goods – which may help to explain their lower levels of health achievement (Kawachi & Kennedy, 2002). In societies with a more egalitarian distribution of economic resources than the United States – such as Sweden (Islam, Merlo, Kawachi, Lindstrom, Gerdtham, 2006a in press) or New Zealand (Blakely et al., 2006) – neither income inequality nor social cohesion has been found to be associated with population health outcomes. The income inequality hypothesis has generated considerable debate.[7] Nevertheless, recent evidence from experimental economics appears to be broadly consistent with the theory that economic inequality erodes social cohesion, and that lower levels of cohesion in turn results in reduced willingness to cooperate in the provision of public goods (see chapter 7 by Lisa Anderson & Jennifer Mellor for a description of these experiments).

1.6. Three Charges Against Social Capital

Social capital remains a contested concept in public health not just on account of the criticisms which have already been mentioned – such as the elusiveness in the way it is conceptualized and defined, or the tendency to hawk it as a panacea for public health whilst downplaying its negative aspects. Several additional charges have been leveled at "social capitalists" by critics who remain skeptical about the utility of "investing" in social capital as a public health improvement strategy (Pearce & Davey Smith, 2003). We highlight three of them in this section.

First, mapping the presence of social capital across diverse communities without an accompanying analysis of power differentials raises the risk of "blaming the community" for its problems (Muntaner, Lynch, & Davey Smith, 2001). It is tempting but wrong-headed to diagnose community pathology (high crime rates, poor health status) as the consequence of residents' unwillingness to cooperate with each other or to trust their neighbors. As we have argued in the previous section, social capital does not arise in a vacuum or magically rain down from the sky on a few selected (and lucky) communities; but rather, social capital is itself shaped by broader structural forces operating at the level of communities, such as historical patterns of residential mobility (e.g. the influx of immigrants, shifts in local labor markets), municipal investment in housing and local infrastructure, as well as policies that perpetuate residential segregation or the planned shrinkage of services and amenities. In short, it is much more challenging to develop durable network ties, to organize collective activities, to trust strangers in your community, etc, when the community is unstable, deprived, socially isolated and abandoned without hope or prospects for a better future. Accordingly, the goal of mapping social capital should never yield to simplistic prescriptions like exhorting community members to act nicer to each other. Building social capital must be thought of as a complement to broader structural interventions (e.g. improving access to local labor markets), not as a replacement for them (Szreter & Woolcok, 2004).

This brings us to the second major criticism leveled at social capital, which is that building social cohesion has been peddled by some as a "cheap" way to solve the problems of poverty and health inequalities, notably by Third Way politicians who cite it as a tool to justify the abrogation of the state's responsibilities to

---

[7] For recent surveys of the state of the evidence from dissenting corners of the debate, see Subramanian and Kawachi (2004), Lynch et al. (2004) and Wilkinson and Pickett (2006)

provide for the welfare of its citizens. After all, it would be far cheaper to suggest that the poor help each other than for the state to pump millions of dollars into anti-poverty programs. Alarm bells were raised in several quarters when the World Bank started to talk the language of social capital in their strategic documents during the 1990s (Fine, 2001). As we have tried to emphasize, a strategy to improve community outcomes by exhorting the poor to pull themselves up by their bootstraps is unlikely to succeed or be sustainable. A critique related to the charge that social capital has been hijacked by Third Way politicians is the complaint that the language of social capital has stripped politics and power relations out of the analysis of health inequalities (Muntaner, 2004; Navarro, 2002; Navarro, 2004;). There is cogency and moral force to this argument, at least in macro analyses of how social cohesion at the societal level shapes patterns of population health. Careful historical analyses – such as Szreter and Woolcock's (2004) discussion of the role played by linking social capital in shaping the sanitary reforms in 19th century Britain – show how politics and power relations can be brought back into the analysis of social capital and health.

The third and final criticism of social capital that we wish to highlight here pertains to the lack of clarity about the policies and interventions needed to build social capital. Assuming policy makers want to improve both the material infrastructure of deprived communities and to shore up their social capital, how do we advise them to go about achieving the latter? Social capitalist have been frequently (and perhaps unfairly) accused of advocating a return to traditional communitarian values; of wanting to turn the clock back to some idealized notion of "what a community ought to be like", in which neighbors cooperate to bring in the harvest or raise barns (or some other more contemporary equivalent). In reality, as everybody knows, there is no practical way to recreate past forms of network connections – nor would it be necessarily desirable to do so. While demonstrations of interventions to boost social cohesion remain sparse, there is growing consensus about a few principles.

First, no magic recipe exists for building social capital that we are aware of. Social capital often arises as a by-product of social relationships, and few of us consciously "invest" in our social ties with the explicit aim of getting something out of them later. This raises the question about whether social connections can be manufactured de novo, or whether we should be focusing on mobilizing or strengthening existing social ties. According to the Social Capital Building Toolkit, developed by the Saguaro Seminar of the Kennedy School of Government at Harvard University (Sander & Lowney, 2005), our best chances of building social capital at the community level is by making a series of "smart bets". An example of a smart bet would be using established principles of community organizing to encourage the formation of neighborhood-based associations. This raises another question. Before rushing off to organize one's neighbors into a block group, it is critical to recognize that it is not only the overall level of social capital that matters, but also the type of social capital. Thus for example, widely scattered weak ties are more effective at disseminating information, whereas strong and dense connections are more effective for collective action

(Chwe, 1999). As Sobel (2002, p. 151) cautions: "People apply the notion of social capital to both types of situation, Knowing what types of networks are best for generating social capital requires that one be specific about what the social capital is going to be used to do". Moreover, theory would suggest that it is not sufficient (or may be even harmful) to build bonding social capital among unemployed youth. It would be more helpful instead to build bridging capital between unemployed youth and employed adults to provide access to role models and mentoring (Sander & Lowney, 2005).

Any strategy to build social capital needs to pay close attention to the *distribution* of costs and benefits, including the possibility of unintended consequences. A gendered analysis of social capital would suggest that the mobilization and provision of support to others in the community tends to fall disproportionately on the shoulders of women. A health promotion strategy that supports one group in the community (e.g. men) at the expense of burdening another group (women) would only lead to a zero-sum outcome.

Lastly, in order to be sustainable, a social capital investment strategy requires more than the donated voluntary efforts of conscientious citizens. Investing in social capital requires real money and resources, and hence involvement of both the state and the private sector that are committed to such a strategy. Historically, the sustenance of social cohesion has depended on state support and stewardship, not just on voluntarism and the energy of communities (Szreter & Woolcock, 2004). Ultimately the most compelling economic rationale for governments to be involved in building social capital is that community cohesion – as a collective asset – produces externalities, i.e. collateral benefits to the rest of society that reach beyond the immediate members of networks. Because these externalities are intangible, the benefits may not become apparent except during a community crisis (such as in the aftermath of a hurricane or some other disaster). When left in the hands of private initiatives, economic theory suggests that communities will tend to under-invest in the production of such collective assets.

1.7. Structure of the Book

Our book is structured in two parts, with the first part (chapters 2 through 7) dealing with alternative approaches for measuring social capital, and the second part (chapters 8 through 13) dealing with the empirical evidence on social capital and health as well as broader applications of the concept for public health practice and interventions.

As we have alluded to already, researchers have adopted a variety of approaches for conceptualizing and measuring social capital. In chapter 2, Martin van der Gaag and Martin Webber describe the development of instruments to measure individual social capital, following the theoretical traditions of Bourdieu (1980), Burt (1992), Flap (1999), and Lin (2001). The authors describe three such instruments and their respective strengths and limitations: the name generator, the position generator, and the resource generator. In chapter 3, Trudy Harpham summarizes the most prevalent approach for measuring community social capital in current public health research, viz. social surveys. A variety of instruments has been developed for use in diverse cultural settings. The chapter provides a succinct introduction to the key issues involved in designing such surveys, evidence for the validity and reliability of existing instruments, and an assessment of the methodological shortcomings of existing surveys as well as suggested solutions.

Survey-based instruments are clearly aligned with the social cohesion school of social capital (in which individual responses are aggregated up to the community or other group level). By contrast, Cynthia Lakon, Dionne Godette, and John Hipp present a lucid account of the conceptualization and assessment of social capital from a network perspective (chapter 4). Responding to the charge that public health researchers have privileged the social cohesion account of social capital (Moore et al., 2005), these authors suggest alternative approaches based on the assessment of ego-centered networks and whole network analysis. Their suggestions hold promise for both re-directing empirical research towards a network-based definition of social capital and for delivering new insights into mechanisms and designing interventions to enhance health.

Richard Carpiano (chapter 5) clearly sympathizes with the view that empirical research on social capital needs to move beyond current conceptions that emphasize communitarianism and social cohesion. His essay attempts to bring social capital back to Bourdieu's original notion of social capital as resources embedded in durable network ties, and to integrate Bourdieu's theory within a broader framework for investigating the influence of neighborhood contexts on health.

Qualitative and ethnographic approaches enable researchers to focus on questions that survey-based approaches cannot reach, and allow us to increase understanding by adding conceptual and theoretical depth to knowledge. In chapter 6, Rob Whitley provides a review of studies that have used this approach, and discusses some of the unique insights generated by the qualitative approach. Like others in this book, Whitley cautions against "narrowly focused studies utilizing social capital as a proxy for the social world [that] may be missing important elements of the lived, communal experiences" of individuals.

The Measurement section concludes with a contribution from two economists, Lisa Anderson and Jennifer Mellor on experimental approaches to studying social capital (chapter 7). As the authors note, economists by training tend to be wary of perceptions and opinions (e.g. concerning the trustworthiness of others) obtained through self reports. Many have been equally skeptical of the use of social capital indicators derived from secondary sources of data (such as measures of civic engagement, political participation, or volunteering), which are apt to be only tangentially related to the key constructs of interest. Enter the experimental paradigm. Some economists such as Edward Glaeser have attempted to directly assess social capital by dropping stamped envelopes (addressed to the researchers) on random street corners and counting the proportion that are picked up by strangers and mailed back (Glaeser et al., 2000). The authors of chapter 7 describe an approach based on an experimental paradigm in which cooperation is directly observed through so-called trust games.

Part II of the book includes systematic reviews of empirical studies linking social capital to physical health outcomes (chapter 8), mental health outcomes (chapter 9), and health-related behaviors (chapter 10). The burgeoning literature on social capital and health almost guarantees that any systematic review will likely be outdated by the time it is published. Nevertheless, the important contribution of these chapters consists of the way in which the individual authors have attempted to draw out the emerging patterns of associations of social capital with specific health outcomes across different study designs (ecological, individual, multi-level), different cultural contexts, as well as different ways of measuring social capital.

The chapter by Daniel Kim, S.V. Subramanian and Ichiro Kawachi finds fairly consistent evidence of an association between social capital and physical health (chapter 8), although the evidence is strongest for self-rated health, and much more sparse for objective health outcomes, such as the incidence of cardiovascular disease. Also, as noted earlier, a relationship between social capital and physical health has been more consistently found in societies with high levels of economic inequality, whereas the links are much weaker or nonexistent in more egalitarian societies (a point also noted in a recent review by Islam et al., 2006b). The chapter by Astier Almedom and Douglas Glandon (chapter 9) reveals that the evidence linking social capital to mental health outcomes is more sparse (sixteen studies) compared to those focusing on physical health outcomes (over fifty studies). More importantly, Almedom and Glandon highlight several issues where our understanding of mechanisms remains incomplete, and they conclude with a plea for more inter-disciplinary investigations of social capital incorporating ideas and methods from qualitative research. In chapter 10, Martin Lindström summarizes the studies linking social capital to health behaviors including alcohol and drug use, smoking, physical activity, diet, and sexual behavior. If the relationship between social capital and health is truly causal, the effect is likely to be mediated by the way it influences health-related behaviors. Therefore the better we can understand the links to health behavior, the more insight we are likely to gain into the causal mechanisms linking social capital to health outcomes (both positive and negative).

In chapter 11, Kathleen Cagney and Ming Wen focus on the empirical evidence linking community social capital to health outcomes in the elderly. As these authors argue, the elderly deserve special attention as a group because their health is often closely tied to circumstances in the communities in which they "age in place". The chapter challenges researchers to refine their theories, measurements, and methods to better understand the ways in which social capital influences health outcomes in this demographic group.

The final two chapters of the book take us into the realm of policies and interventions. In chapter 12, Vish Viswanath explores the application of social capital to the field of health communications. His essay examines both how social capital can help to predict the success or failure of mass media campaigns (and potentially harnessed to improve the design and delivery of health messages), as well as how concepts in communication can shed light back on the different forms of capital (bonding and bridging). Finally, chapter 13 connects social capital to the highly topical subject of disaster preparedness and recovery. In the wake of the September 11 attacks, Hurricane Katrina and outbreaks of avian 'flu in Asia, public health preparedness in anticipation of disasters, pandemics and terrorist attacks has become a pressing concern for federal, state, and local agencies. The chapter by Howard Koh and Rebecca Cadigan provides a timely reminder of the salience of social capital for community disaster preparedness. As the authors argue, the long term value of activities carried out by agencies across the country to prepare for disaster consists in the way they build social capital. In turn, the social capital of communities turns out to be a critical ingredient of recovery following disasters (Kawachi & Subramanian, 2006).

The writer Jorge Luis Borges lamented the gradual debasement of philosophical ideas over time. According to Borges, once an idea is accepted by the public, a theory that originally took an entire book to develop later ends up being dispensed with in a short paragraph, then eventually consigned to a footnote (Borges, 1939/1998). Judging by the multiplicity and complexity of voices expressed in this book, we remain confident that social capital is in little danger of falling by the wayside, and that studying its relationship to health will remain an active field of scholarship for decades to come.

References

Aitkin, M., & Longford, N. T. (1986). Statistical modelling in school effectiveness studies. *Journal of Royal Statistical Society A, 149*, 1–43.

Berkman, L. F., & Glass, T. (2000). Social integration, social networks, social support, and health. In L. F. Berkman & I. Kawachi (Eds.), *Social Epidemiology* (pp. 137–173). New York: Oxford University Press.

Blakely, T. A., & Woodward, A. J. (2000). Ecological effects in multi-level studies. *Journal of Epidemiology and Community Health, 54*, 367–374.

Blakely, T., Atkinson, J., Ivory, V., Collings, S., Wilton. J., & Howden-Chapman, P. (2006). No association of neighbourhood volunteerism with mortality in New Zealand: a national multilevel cohort study. *International Journal of Epidemiology, 35*, 981–989.

Blakely, T., & Subramanian, S. V. (2006). Multilevel studies. In M. Oakes & J. Kaufman (Eds.), *Methods for Social Epidemiology* (pp. 316–340). San Francisco: Jossey Bass.

Borges, J. L. (1939). Pierre Menard, Author of the *Quixote*. In J. L. Borges, *Collected Fictions* (1998). New York: Penguin Books.

Bourdieu, P. (1980). Le capital social. Notes provisoires. *Actes de la Recherche en Sciences Sociales, 3*, 2–3.

Bourdieu, P. (1986). The forms of capital. In J. G. Richardson (Ed.), *The Handbook of Theory: Research for the Sociology of Education*. New York: Greenwood Press.

Browne, W. J., Subramanian, S.V., Jones, K., & Glod Stein, H. (2005). Variance partitioning in multilevel logistic models that exhibit overdispersion. *Journal of Royal Statistical Society A, 168*(3), 599–613.

Burt, R. S. (1992). *Structural holes: the social structure of competition*. Cambridge MA: Harvard University Press.

Browning, C. R., & Cagney, K. A. (2002). Collective efficacy and health: neighborhood social capital and self-rated physical functioning in an Urban Setting. *Journal of Health and Social Behavior, 43*, 383–399.

Caughy, M. O., O'Campo, P. J., & Muntaner, C. (2003). When being alone might be better: neighborhood poverty, social capital, and child mental health. *Social Science & Medicine, 57,* 227–237.

Chwe, M. S. (1999). Structure and strategy in collective action. *American Journal of Sociology, 105,* 128–156.

Cohen, S., Underwood, L. G., & Gottlieb, B. H. (2000). *Social support measurement and intervention. A guide for health and social scientists.* New York: Oxford University Press.

Coleman, J. S. (1990). *Foundations of social theory.* Cambridge, MA: Harvard University Press.

Coutts, A., & Kawachi, I. (2006). The urban social environment and its impact on health. In N. Freudenberg, S. Galea, & D. Vlahov (Eds.), *Cities and the health of the public* (pp. 49–60). Nashville: Vanderbilt University Press.

Durkheim, E. (1897, 1951). *Suicide: a study in sociology.* Glencoe, IL: Free Press.

Fielding, A. (2004). The role of the Hausman test and whether higher level effects should be treated as random or fixed. *Multilevel Modeling Newsletter, 16*(2), 3–9.

Fine, B. (2001). *Social capital versus social theory: Political economy and social science at the turn of the millennium.* London: Routledge.

Flap, H. D. (1999). Creation and returns of social capital: a new research program. *La Revue Tocqueville, XX,* 5–26.

Gittell, R., & Vidal, R. (1998). *Community organizing: Building social capital as a development strategy.* Thousand Oaks, CA: Sage Books.

Glaeser, E. L., Laibson, D. I., Scheinkman, J. A., & Soutter, C. L. (2000). Measuring trust. *Quarterly Journal of Economics, 115*(3): 811–846.

Goldstein, H. (2003). *Multilevel statistical models* (3rd ed.). London: Arnold.

Goldstein, H., Browne, W. J., & Rasbash, J. (2002). Partitioning variation in multilevel models. *Understanding Statistics, 1,* 223–232.

Helliwell, J. F., & Putnam, R. D. (2004). The social context of well-being. *Proceedings of the Royal Society B: Biological Sciences, 359,* 1435–1446.

Islam, M. K., Merlo, J., Kawachi, I., Lindstrom, M., & Gerdtham, U.-G. (2006a). Social capital and health: Does egalitarianism matter? A literature review. *International Journal of Equity in Health, 5*(1), 3.

Islam, M. K., Merlo, J., Kawachi, I., Lindstrom, M., Burstrom, K., & Gerdtham, U.-G. (2006b in press). Does it really matter where you live? A panel data multilevel analysis of Swedish municipality level social capital on individual health-related quality of life. *Health Economics, Policy and Law.*

Kawachi, I., Kennedy, B. P., Lochner, K., & Prothrow-Stith, D. (1997). Social capital, income inequality, and mortality. *American Journal of Public Health, 87,* 1491–1498.

Kawachi, I., Kennedy, B. P., & Glass, R. (1999). Social capital and self-rated health: A contextual analysis. *American Journal of Public Health, 89,* 1187–1193.

Kawachi, I., & Berkman, L. F. (2000). Social cohesion, social capital, and health. In L. F. Berkman, & I. Kawachi (Eds.), *Social Epidemiology* (pp. 174–190). New York: Oxford University Press.

Kawachi, I., & Berkman, L. F. (2001). Social ties and mental health. *Journal of Urban Health, 78*(3), 458–467.

Kawachi, I., & Kennedy, B. P. (2002). *The health of nations.* New York: The New Press.

Kawachi, I. (2006). Commentary: Social capital and health – making the connections one step at a time. *International Journal of Epidemiol, 35*(4), 989–993.

Kawachi, I., & Subramanian, S. V. (2006). Measuring and modeling the social and geographic context of trauma. *Journal of Traumatic Stress, 19*(2), 195–203.

King, G. (1997). *A solution to the ecological inference problem: Reconstructing individual behavior from aggregate data.* Princeton: Princeton University Press.

Kubzansky, L. D., & Kawachi, I. (2000). Affective states and health. In L. F. Berkman, & I. Kawachi (Eds.), *Social Epidemiology* (pp. 1213–1241). New York: Oxford University Press.

Lin, N. (1999). Building a network theory of social capital. *Connections, 22*(1), 28–51.

Lin, N. (2001). *Social capital. Theory and research.* New York, NY: Aldine de Gruyter.

Loury, G. (1992). Theeconomics of discrimination: getting to the core of the problem. *Harvard Journal of African American Public Policy I*, 91–110.

Lynch, J. W., Davey Smith, G., Hillemeier, M. M., Shwa, M., Raghunathan, T., & Kaplan, G. A. (2001). Income inequality, the psychosocial environment and health: comparisons of wealthy nations. *Lancet, 358*, 194–200.

Lynch, J.W., Davey Smith, G., Harper, S., Hillemeier, M., Ross, N., Kaplan, G.A., & Wolfson, M. (2004). Is income inequality a determinant of population health? Part 1. A systematic review. *The Milbank Quarterly, 82*(1): 5–99.

MacLeod, J. (1987). *Ain't no makin' it. Leveled aspirations in a low-income neighborhood.* Boulder, CO: Westview Press.

Matthews, K. A. (1988). Coronary heart disease and Type A behaviors: update on and alternative to the Booth-Kewley and Friedman (1987) quantitative review. *Psychological bulletin, 104*, 373–380.

Mitchell, C. U., LaGory, M. (2002). Social capital and mental distress in an impoverished community. *City & Community*, 1, 195–215.

Moon, G., Subramanian, S.V., Jones, K., Duncan, C., & Twigg, L. (2005). Area-based studies and the evaluation of multilevel influences on health outcomes. In A. Bowling & S. Ebrahim (Eds.), *Handbook of health research methods: Investigation, measurement and analysis* (pp. 266–292). Berkshire, England: Open University Press.

Moore, S., Shiell, A., Hawe, P., & Haines, V. A. (2005). The privileging of communitarian ideas: Citation practices and the translation of social capital into public health research. *American Journal of Public Health, 95*, 1330–1337.

Muntaner, C., Lynch, J., Davey Smith, G. D. (2001). Social capital, disorganized communities, and the third way: Understanding the retreat from structural inequalities in epidemiology and public health. *International Journal of Health Services, 31*(2), 213–237.

Muntaner, C. (2004). Commentary: Social capital, social class, and the slow progress of psychosocial epidemiology. *International Journal of Epidemiol, 33*, 674–680.

Navarro, V. (2002). A critique of social capital. *International Journal of Health Services, 32*(3), 423–443.

Navarro, V. (2004). Commentary: Is capital the solution or the problem? *Int J Epidemiol 33*, 672–674.

Pearce, N., & Davey Smith, G. (2003). Is social capital the key to inequalities in health? *American Journal of Public Health, 93*(1), 122–129.

Portes, A. (1998). Social capital: Its origins and application in modern sociology. *Annual Review of Sociology, 24*, 1–24.

Putnam, R. D. (1993). *Making democracy work: Civic traditions in modern Italy.* Princeton, NJ: Princeton University Press.

Putnam, R. D. (2000). *Bowling alone: The collapse and revival of American community.* New York: Simon and Schuster.

Raudenbush, S. (1989). "Centering" predictors in multilevel analysis: choices and consequences. *Multilevel Modelling Newsletter, 1*(2), 10–12.

Raudenbush, S., & Bryk, A. (2002). *Hierarchical linear models: Applications and data analysis methods.* Thousand Oaks: Sage Publications.

Sampson, R. J., Raudenbush, S. W., & Earls, F. (1997). Neighborhoods and violent crime: a multilevel study of collective efficacy. *Science, 277,* 918–924.

Sander, T. H., & Lowney, K. (2005). *Social Capital Building Toolkit,* version 1.1. Cambridge, MA: Harvard University J. F. Kennedy School of Government. Accessed at: www.ksg.harvard.edu/saguaro/pdfs/skbuildingtoolkitversion1.1.pdf.

Sobel, J. (2002). Can we trust social capital? *Journal Economic Li, XL,* 139–154.

Stack, C. B. (1974). *All our Kin: Strategies for survival in a black community.* New York: Harper & Row.

Subramanian, S. V., Kim, D., & Kawachi, I. (2002). Social trust and self-rated health in US communities: a multilevel analysis. *Journal of Urban Health, 79*(4 Suppl 1), S21–34.

Subramanian, S. V., Lochner, K. A., & Kawachi, I. (2003a). Neighborhood differences in social capital: a compositional artifact or a contextual construct? *Health Place, 9*(1), 33–44.

Subramanian, S. V., Jones, K., & Duncan, C. (2003b). Multilevel methods for public health research. In I. Kawachi & L. F. Berkman (Eds.), *Neighborhoods and health* (pp. 65–111). New York: Oxford University Press.

Subramanian, S. V. (2004). Multilevel methods, theory and analysis. In N. Anderson (Ed.), *Encyclopedia on health and behavior* (pp. 602–608). Thousand Oaks, CA: Sage Publications.

Subramanian, S. V., & Kawachi, I. (2004). Income inequality and health. What have we learned so far. *Epidemiologic Reviews, 26,* 78–91.

Subramanian, S. V., Glymour, M. M., & Kawachi, I. (2007 in press). Identifying causal ecologic effects on health: a methodologic assessment. In S. Galea (Ed.), *Macrosocial determinants of population health.* New York: Springer Media.

Szreter, S., & Woolcock, M. (2004). Health by association? Social capital, social theory, and the political economy of public health. *International Journal of Epidemiology, 33*(4), 650–667.

Varshney, A. (2002). *Ethnic conflict & civic life. Hindus and muslims in India.* New haven: Yale University Press.

Wilkinson, R. G., & Pickett, K. E., (2006). Income inequality and population health: a review and explanation of the evidence. *Society Science & Medicine, 62*(7), 1768–1784.

Ziersch, A. M., & Baum, F. E. (2004). Involvement in civil society groups: Is it good for your health? *Journal of Epidemiology Comm Health, 58,* 493–500.

Part I
Measurement of Social Capital

2
Measurement of Individual Social Capital
Questions, Instruments, and Measures

MARTIN VAN DER GAAG AND MARTIN WEBBER

The idea that social relationships can be conceptualized as potentially productive, "social" additions to personally owned resources has been welcomed as an attractive, explanatory mechanism in many areas of social and economic research. The assessment of resources embedded in social networks, potentially available to individuals or the larger community as a whole, has gradually become an established extension to conceptual models which may provide useful, additional explanations for many research questions with socio-demographic aspects. Although still enmeshed in debates about the meaning of "social capital", health researchers are also gradually realizing the explanatory potential of this concept to health outcomes. However, the translation of this idea into valid and reliable quantification has proven to be cumbersome, as the number of leads that can be followed in matters of operationalisation and measurement have proved labyrinthine; this has resulted in many incomparable measures and instruments (Flap, 1999, 2004).

Conceptualized in its individual form, social capital refers to all possible kinds of resources potentially owned by social network members, which may become available to a focal individual as a result of mutual investments in a shared past, of which the social relationships with these network members form evidence (Van der Gaag & Snijders, 2004). A definition of social capital at this individual level remains quite close to its original analogy with more traditional notions of financial and material "capital", which have been developed and accepted in the academic world for more than 200 years (see e.g. beginnings by Quesnay, 1766) – the idea that relationships can be invested in and form "capital" that may harvest returns in the future is, similar to human and cultural capital, directly derived from economy. Perhaps this is the reason that when defined at the individual level by leading scholars (Bourdieu, 1980; Burt, 1992; Flap, 1999, 2004; Lin, 2001), social capital shows much less variation in the number and nature of dimensions specified than collective level social capital, where large differences between various conceptualizations are prevalent (Coleman, 1988; Putnam, 1993).

For the development of systematic, comparable social capital measurement instruments, the perspective of individual level social capital offers the most simple and clearly defined units of measurement – a focus on the individual avoids the common interpretation problems in analyses that stem from the use of aggregated data, in which the problem of "modifiable area unit" may be encountered. The methodology of individual social capital research is essentially based on social network research, a well-established research area within which many insights for operationalization, and tools for data collection have been readily developed.

In this chapter, we aim to provide an overview of current methods and instruments for the measurement of individual social capital, and to the various methodological concerns that shape these methods. A first section introduces research questions and theoretical issues that shape the desired characteristics of social capital measurement. A second section discusses ways to construct social capital indicators from available data. A final and third section discusses the three main measurement instruments for individual social capital currently available: the name generator, the position generator, and the resource generator. As an illustration of advanced measurement in individual social capital research, we conclude the chapter with an example from a recent study using the resource generator instrument for a UK sample.

2.1. Questions That Shape Measurement

The use, design, and quality of social capital measurement can only be judged when its eventual applications are made explicit. Disregarding any specific, topical domains such as the job market, status attainment, personal well-being, health issues, etc., social capital research questions can be categorized into three main issues.

The first and most important of these is that individual social capital research considers an inequality question, based on the presumption that people equipped with "better" social capital will succeed better in attaining their goals (Flap, 2004; in the section "measures" we will further specify which characteristics of social capital could be considered "better" social capital). Generally, four explanatory mechanisms for this hypothesis are specified. Social network members and their resources are expected to be helpful in goal attainment because they 1) significantly add to an individual's collections of personal resources, such as his cultural, human, material, and political capital (e.g. the social network may provide more useful information about jobs than can be gathered by an individual on the market), 2) provide unique resources that cannot be produced or purchased to satisfaction individually (e.g. love, friendship, emotional support, and opportunities for reproduction are poorly available on the market), 3) may actively provide help without asking (e.g. by means of recommendations), and 4) form the identity of one's social network to the "outside world", which may work as an advertisement for an individual (Lin, 1999a, 2001; Van der Gaag, 2005:40).[1] Summarized, the

---

[1] Each of these mechanisms also provides unique forms of *social liability* – a term proposed by Leenders and Gabbay (1999) to identify negative experiences specifically caused by social network members. This chapter does not explicitly discuss such negative sides to social capital.

general issue regarding social capital is to investigate its *productivity*, and shed light on the question whether social networks are actually helpful in attaining individuals' goals.

Social capital is a complex, latent construct with several dimensions: in its individual form it refers to social relationships with alters[2] with different personal characteristics, various social resource collections, and, in some lines of social capital research, also patterns of relationships between network members (network structure). Therefore, a second, main research issue considers the question which configuration, which part, or which resource domain of social capital is productive in a certain context. Empirical findings have shown that to find a job, or attain higher social status through one's social network, social capital should be specific; it is necessary to know the right people with the right resources in order to climb the social ladder (Flap & Völker, 2001; Lin, 1999b). On the other hand, in order to find a house, or to enjoy company in general, rather unspecific social capital (as indicated by having a large social network) seems to be sufficient. Apparently, the resources responsible for such outcomes, which concern any member in the population, may successfully be passed on through any network member (Van der Gaag & Snijders, 2003; Van der Gaag, 2005:191–194). Summarized, not all kinds of relationships and resources represented by social capital are important at the same time, and specific configurations of these have distinct roles in its productivity in distinct contexts. These types of questions can therefore be labeled as investigations about social capital's *goal specificity* (Flap, 1999, 2002). As yet, knowledge about which social capital dimensions are responsible for any productivity is still fragmented.

If some configuration of social capital is productive for individuals in a certain context, this also implies decreased opportunities for those lacking it, and reproduction of inequality through the use of social capital (Flap, 1991, 2004; Lin, 2001:99–124). Therefore, a third main social capital research issue is the *identification of advantaged and deprived groups,* or the question how social capital is distributed over the general population (Flap, 1991, 2002, 2004). Eventually, studies addressing this issue may provide the translation of social capital research into future policy advice.

Making these research questions explicit is necessary because these directly shape social capital measurement at the level of operationalization and indicator construction. As will be discussed in the next section, so far many researchers have operationalized social capital into single, and rather unspecific indicators of "something useful about the social network". Social capital research in exploratory stages, aimed at uncovering *the existence* of a relationship between individual social capital and its productivity, may indeed harvest meaningful, if not very specific, results from using a single indicator. However, the desire to identify *which*

---

[2] In ego-centered social network research, the focal individual of a social network is denoted as "ego", wheras any, unspecified social network member is denoted as an "alter". For reasons of fluidity, we also use these terms throughout this chapter.

part or quality of social capital is responsible for any effect directly requires the development of multiple social capital indicators, each tuned towards specific sub dimensions; the same is true for almost all questions about the distribution of social capital over the population. Although some researchers have already emphasized the need to construct multiple measures for social capital at an early stage (e.g. Campbell, Marsden, & Hurlbert, 1986), most of them have not recognized the need to use multiple measures to measure social capital full yet.

2.2. Measure Construction

A latent, complex construct with several dimensions offers many opportunities for measurement – in the case of social capital perhaps even too many. Systematic research into its productivity and goal specificity has been slow in development and has seen the construction of many different, incomparable measures; often, these seem to have been developed based on available data rather than valid operationalization. The main cause for this is, however, that for many research domains more specific ideas about the productivity of social capital are difficult to establish firmly. Social capital investigators are often confronted with the fact that they do not really know which indicators could be essential to explain their studied outcomes: will an hypothesized effect stem from the presence of specific alters, types of relationships, social resources, the structure or size of the social network, all of these, or some of these aggregated into some useful combination? In the overview below, we discuss the potential value of several principles as a basis for social capital measures.

Social network structure Since individual social capital research gradually evolved from social networks research, it is not surprising that many authors have operationalized social capital from a structural point of view. Assessing the relative advantage of an individual's position in a social network, such social capital measures are calculated from data matrices about relationships in networks with clear boundaries, of which all members participate in research (see overview by Borgatti, Jones, & Everett, 1998). Many of these studies are investigations to which some form of entrepreneurship is the central topic, locating advantageous positions in environments characterized by competition. Therefore, most measures are based on the expected added value from sparse networks full of "structural holes" (Burt, 1992), containing few relationships between alters, and capitalizing on the idea of accessing diverse information at minimal costs. This preconception is not universally transferable to other research domains, such as personal health, in which social capital functioning within an environment conducive to trust and network closure can often seem more beneficial (Coleman, 1990). Single measures of network structure could serve as indicators in social capital productivity research, but these only refer to patterns of relationships, not explicitly to social resources, leaving explanations of any productivity effects rather implicit. However, the need for well-defined boundaries to local populations also reduces their usefulness, since research applications in the health domain usually require data samples of general population in such settings opportunities for the calculation of structural social capital measures are severely limited.[3]

Presence of specific alters Other social capital measures are based on data from ego-centered social network research, which results in traditionally structured data sets. Most of these depart from theoretical notions regarding one single dimension of social capital; often, this concerns the existence of specific relationships or (groups of) specific alters. For example, Granovetter's (1973) classic argument about the strength of weak ties refers to the theoretical advantage of weaker relationships in the attainment of instrumental goals; subsequently, the proportion of weak ties in a person's social network can be used as a social capital measure. In a health context, where the attainment of expressive goals is often more central, indicators of the presence of strong ties in the social network (e.g. the proportion of strong ties among all relationships) could be considered useful. Such measures do not directly refer to social resources however, and their inclusion in explanatory models only tells us something very general about social network effects. Instead of relationships, another perspective is the identification of specific classes of network members. Since neighbors, friends, family members, etc. give access to specific sets of social resources (Felling, Fiselier, & Van der Poel, 1991), measures indicating the presence of alters with specific *roles* can serve as indirect social capital indicators. However, for insight into the productivity and nature of these social resources, additional data will be needed. Checking for specific role-players in social networks is also marked by the problem that not all productive roles are easily labeled – while these may indeed be potentially helpful it is, for example, not very productive to ask respondents to list "intriguing, vague acquaintances" in their network. Other specific classes of network members are formed by socio-demographic denominations, such as alters of specific age, gender or ethnicity. The nature of any specific social resources attached to socio-demographic positions also remains very implicit, and their beneficial effects as social capital are also possibly very population-specific. Since the theoretical meaning of such indicators can therefore be very different between social capital studies, their ad hoc inclusion usually also adds to the incomparability of findings. Only one indicator of social capital directly referring to specific, productive persons in the network has found systematic use – this is discussed in the section about the "position generator" measurement instrument.

Newer ideas for social capital indicators have moved away from any specific presumptions about useful categories and configurations of persons and relationships, and aim to characterize an individual's social network as a whole on more general, morphological grounds.

Volume One of the first notions used to characterize an individual's social capital was formulated by Bourdieu (1980) in terms of volume, or the total amount of

---

[3] It is possible to calculate network structure indicators from ego-centered data by asking respondents whether, and how well their network members know each other (see section "name generator"). Such observations are unreliable, however.

social resources one has potential access to. Having remained largely intuitive, the idea is that having "more" social capital is productive as a result of all four mechanisms specified earlier, and adds to sustain the production of individual well-being. Following this argument, it would be logical to construct measures of social capital volume as cumulative indicators of "all resources" of "all members" of an individual social network. This meets with the problem that, apart from the fact that measurements of "all resources" of "all members" are susceptible to reliability and boundary problems, this would require the collection of extensive sets of data per individual (see section "name generator"). Therefore, measuring social capital volume to any detail has not become very popular in this form. The use of social network size as a social capital volume indicator, counting the number of different alters mentioned in an interview, can be seen as a more economical version, omitting resource measurements. This measure could be used as a single indicator to detect goal-*un*specific effects of social capital, where any productivity stems from the sheer number of people one knows (see section "questions"). However, an extended rationale that the more people one knows, the more resources they will generally represent, and the more helpful the network will be, is perhaps a bit limited. Using measures of social capital volume in explanatory analysis also has limitations in terms of content validity. Theoretically, not all social capital available in a social network can or will contribute to the attainment of goals: most goals are attained by the use of personally owned resources, [4] and there will be many duplications of resources between alters. For most social resources, it is not the question how much or how many of them are present in the social network in order to be helpful (which is implicit in cumulative counting), but whether at least one instance of them is present at all. Summarized, multiple alters giving access to the same resources can be unnecessary, inconvenient, or normatively restricted to give help (Van der Gaag & Snijders, 2004).[5] An inventory of all resources may therefore require the collection of much superfluous information.

---

[4] This argument gets even more important when we realise that because it creates an obligation to pay back services in the future, using social capital is also costly. For some goals, using social capital is also awkward for the seeker of help – it is quicker and more practical to clean one's dishes oneself. Having social capital of some quality is therefore not an immediate, automatic blessing. For the attainment of most goals individuals are self-sufficient, either through the direct use of personal resources, or by buying solutions (goods and services) on the market. Only a small proportion of potentially accessed resources is used; when asked about the resource generator instrument, a number of participants commented that they would probably not ask for a number of the resources they had access to (Webber & Huxley, submitted).

[5] Several alters providing similar resources could be seen as "insurance" for a certain kind of help, because across relationships the opportunities for alters to actually provide help will vary over time. However, a possible lack of an opportunity to exchange help will only block very specific social capital transactions – usually, helping is without hurry. Furthermore, in many social networks there is an established order among network members who has to help first; help is therefore less easily mobilised from other than "usual" alters. Therefore, having social network "extras" in theory shows diminishing returns.

Diversity A logical further specification of social capital volume is its diversity: an account whether elements of different kinds are represented in the social network by at least one instance. Several authors have proposed the idea that specific resources and relationships can be located and accessed more successfully when more differentiation in alters, resources and relationships is present in the network, hence resulting in better social capital (Burt, 1992; Erickson, 1996, 2003; Flap, 1991; Granovetter, 1973; Lin, 2001; see also Erickson, in Lin & Erickson, forthcoming). Social capital diversity measures can be constructed in a straightforward way for relationships (e.g. variation in relationship strength or role), alters with specific characteristics (e.g. variation in gender, age groups, ethnicity, etc.), but operationalizations most valid in terms of social capital are those establishing the more explicit resource diversity of a person's social network (e.g. variation in alters' education, occupational prestige, etc.). So far, diversity measures are general, single social capital indicators making the most of their parsimony, incorporating robust content validity, while being sufficiently transferable to diverse social capital contexts to enable comparisons between studies.

Social resources While being the most obvious indicators for the concept of social capital, measures referring to resources of social network members were neglected for a long time. Perhaps the problem *which* of all possible social resources should be indicated by social capital measures, and how these should result in indicators, was central to this omission. The history of the concept of "capital" shows that its operationalization has always been complex, even when usually referring to relatively straightforward financial and material resources only (Hennings, 1987). For social capital, this question is even more complex, since the idea of "social resources" may refer to any collection of resources owned by network members. In the traditional categorization of capital used in the social sciences, social capital therefore includes the financial (money), human (education and skills), cultural (symbolic knowledge), and political capital (power) of network members. Investigations of the productivity, and especially of the goal specificity of social capital, should therefore ideally be capable of indicating which of these classes of social resources help individuals to attain their goals; hence a good social capital measurement instrument should contain separate indicators for each of these collections – within any research domain.[6] However, since the number of *possible* social resources that can be distinguished seems almost infinite, it is difficult to point out exactly which resources should be included in indicators of social resources from each of these classes.

---

[6] A measurement instrument constructed this way will be capable of specifying the productivity of social capital as follows. If none of these indicators are significant predictors for a central outcome, there is apparently no effect of social capital. If one, or some of these indicators are significant predictors, social capital is productive and goal specific – productivity then results from knowing the *right* people. If all of these indicators prove significant predictors for an outcome with comparable magnitudes, there is a very unspecific effect of social capital – the effect may then result from knowing *enough* people.

There are two ways to deal with this problem. A first solution is the conversion of various "social resources" into a single currency – this is the basis of the "position generator" measurement model, where social resources are expressed as the job-specific prestige of network members' occupations (see section "position generator"). A second option is to use some form of concretely listed, potentially useful social resources. Starting from a theoretical classification, for each capital collection some useful examples can be the basis for questionnaire items. This is the basis for the "resource generator" measurement instrument, which is explained in a separate section below.

2.3. Instruments

The translation of theoretical presumptions about social capital measurement into questionnaire items meets with the problem that a general perspective on the wording of questions needs to be chosen. When we wish to understand the role of social capital in attaining outcomes at the personal level, it is important to distinguish between accessing and mobilizing social capital (Flap, 2004; Lin, 1999a) – after all, not all potentially accessed social capital is mobilized, and furthermore, asking respondents questions about whether they could access social resources versus whether they have used social resources potentially retrieves very different answers. Both ways of questioning bring along specific measurement problems.

When we ask questions about having *access* to certain social resources (such as the questions listed in Table 2.1), the quality of the data remains rather hypothetical. Answers to such questions may contain considerable unreliability, and in case of social capital, social desirability.[7] In addition, unused social capital is probably not as well memorized as used social capital – people who actively use their networks will more clearly remember the contents of their networks. Moreover, of many resources people do not know whether they are owned by personal network members, because they are context specific, not commonly encountered in social exchange, or knowledge about them is limited to intimate confidents. Furthermore, as discussed earlier (see section "volume") measurement of a collection of unused social capital points towards superfluous measurements, because most of the potentially accessed social capital will never be used.[8] In predictive analyses, this eventually reduces amounts of explained variance in productivity and goal specificity questions.

Other, but more serious problems are encountered when we would ask respondents questions about the *mobilization* of resources only. Questions about the use of help from network members operate from a retrospective time perspective by definition. This introduces the need for a pre-specified time frame (e.g. use in the

---

[7] Especially in an interview situation, respondents will want to avoid they are seen as "social losers", and are eager to indicate they have access to a diverse social network.

[8] See note 4.

TABLE 2.1. Empirically determined domain specific cumulative social capital measurement scales for UK sample, based on a resource generator with stem question "Do you personally know anyone with the skill or resource listed below that you are able to gain access to *within one week* if you needed it?" (N = 295; sample of south London and Doncaster electoral registers); popularity and scale fit of individual items and scale diagnostics.

Do you know anyone who.....? Domestic resources	% "yes"	$H_i{}^a$
A17 – knows a lot about DIY	84	0.40
B3 – help you to move or dispose of bulky items	81	0.43
B4 – help you with small jobs around the house	88	0.58
B14 – get you cheap goods or "bargains"	53	0.54
B15 – help you to find somewhere to live if you had to move home	65	0.56
B16 – lend you a large amount of money	46	0.59
B17 – look after your home or pets if you go away	86	0.51

n = 276, H^b = 0.52, ρ^c = 0.78

Expert advice	% "yes"	H_i
A7 – has a professional occupation	88	0.60
A12 – knows a lot about government regulations	43	0.58
A13 – has good contacts with the local newspaper, radio or t.v.	18	0.46
B1 – give you sound advice about money problems	70	0.49
B2 – give you sound advice on problems at work	70	0.58
B8 – give you careers advice	50	0.52
B9 – discuss politics with you	59	0.52
B10 – give you sound legal advice	55	0.49
B11 – give you a good reference for a job	85	0.61

n − 266, H = 0.54, ρ = 0.83

Personal skills	% "yes"	H_i
A1 – can repair a broken-down car	72	0.34
A3 – is a reliable tradesman	76	0.39
A6 – is good at gardening	83	0.45
A9 – works for the local council	43	0.32
A11 – can sometimes employ people	56	0.36
A15 – knows a lot about health and fitness	65	0.36

n = 279, H = 0.37, ρ = 0.69

Problem solving resources	% "yes"	H_i
A4 – can speak another language	60	0.45
A5 – knows how to fix problems with computers	77	0.39
A8 – is a local councillor	23	0.54
B5 – do your shopping if you are ill	90	0.34
B7 – lend you a small amount of money	90	0.41

n = 287, H = 0.42, ρ = 0.60

[a,b] Loevingers homogeneity index indicating individual item fit in scale (H_i) and scale homogeneity (H) (see text)

[c] Scale reliability index as calculated by software MSP5 for windows

last three or six months), and may result in unreliability of data in terms of specific memory effects. In addition, the action of using social capital is an outcome of a decision process that is influenced by personal wealth (e.g. more wealth could make social capital less useful), the individual need for help in general (e.g. being of old age or ill health increases the need for support), and one's personality, including an individual's propensity to ask for assistance. Therefore, information about the use of social capital is not only unreliable to some extent, but also confounded by many other important variables.

In comparison, the mobilization perspective seems more problematic than the access perspective (Van der Gaag & Snijders, 2004). Therefore, we advise investigators to use highly standardized versions of questionnaires using the access perspective. Perhaps ideally, social capital measurement instruments would include questions from both perspectives; however, time and resources will often prevent inclusion in questionnaires. The development of social capital questionnaire forms has largely followed three models, which can all be adapted to both the access and use perspective on social capital.

2.3.1. Name Generator

The oldest measurement tool for individual social capital stems from 1970s social network research. It comprises an extensive social network inventory performed with a combination of "name generator" and "name interpreter" questions. Originally designed for the estimation of social network size, and the identification of social network structure and contents, the method comprises two or three rounds of data collection. In the first "name generator" part, a systematic list of queries asks the respondent to mention names of persons he or she knows, which are recorded by an interviewer. A second, "name interpreter" part collects information about all alters listed in the first part, comprising the relationships with the focal individual and alter attributes, among which questions about any social resources embedded in these relationships. (A third, optional round is sometimes added to assess existing relationships between alters; for an example, see Flap, Völker, Snijders, & Van der Gaag, 2004).

This procedure was the main method of social capital data collection until the mid 1990s and still is the staple instrument for studies of social network structure. While various types of name generating questions have been tested (e.g. Van Sonderen, Ormel, Brilman, & Van Linden van den Heuvell, 1990), the "exchange" type name generator proposed by McCallister and Fischer (1978) was eventually most widely used; its most famous example is the single "core"-network identifying item "with whom do you talk about personal matters?", recurrent in annual rounds of the US General Social Survey (Burt, 1984; Marsden, 1987; for various early forms see Marsden, 1990).

For social capital research, the name generator / interpreter combination can provide very detailed social network and social capital information. It is the only social capital measurement instrument that identifies single alters and their various attributes, which enables the study of individual network structure, relationship-specific attributes and relationship multiplexity – research issues closely related to social capital. The wealth of possible information collected with this tool has also led to an abundance of differently calculated social capital measures (see section "measures").

The costs of data collection with name generators can be high. Dependent on the limits set to the allowed number of alters to be mentioned in response to each question, interviews can become lengthy and repetitive when large networks are encountered, and many interpretative (such as social capital) questions are added. Even though this specific part of the information is usually later deleted, some respondents also become suspicious when asked to identify their network members. Moreover, the central idea of making a complete resource inventory of individual social networks theoretically retrieves much superfluous data (see section "volume"). The flexibility of the design of name generator / interpreter sets has led to many different versions. Although several name generator questions have become relatively standardized, there is no general agreement on which questions to include for alter identification in social capital studies. Therefore, results of social capital studies using name generators are often difficult to compare.

2.3.2. Position Generator

A measurement method focusing more on the presence of social resources than relationships in networks is the "position generator" (Lin & Dumin, 1986; Lin, Fu, & Hsung, 2001) – an instrument deliberately designed to cover social capital in the "general" life of the modern Western individual, without considering specific areas of goal attainment, life domains, or subpopulations. A position generator typically asks about a systematic list of 10–30 different occupations whether the respondent "knows" anyone having this occupation; subsequently, it is checked whether people in these positions are known as family members, friends, and acquaintances. Social capital data from the position generator are based on the idea that the occupations of network members represent social resource collections that can be quantified with job prestige measures. Based on a model of an hierarchically modeled society, following Lin's theories of social resources and social capital (Lin, 1982, 2001), the most important underlying assumptions of this measurement model are that having access to persons with high-prestige occupations gives 1) access to large resource collections, and 2) such alters may exert important influence in their (second-order) social networks.

The position generator instrument has been consistently applied in research since its first publication, and has gradually become a popular measurement instrument in individual social capital research (for an overview of recent research see Lin & Erickson, forthcoming). The construction of social capital measures from position generator data has developed into largely standardized sets; three measures directly derived from Lin's social capital propositions (Lin, 2001:61–63) are most frequently used in research: *highest accessed prestige* is an indicator based on the hypothesis that accessing high prestige network members leads to the generation of higher returns (Lin, 2001:62). Two other position generator measures are indicators of beneficial diversity (see "measures"): *range in accessed prestige* is calculated as the difference in prestige between the highest and lowest occupation accessed, while *number of different positions accessed* is the total number of different occupations in which a respondent knows anyone.[9]

Because it takes much less interview time than sets of name generators and name interpreters, the position generator is more respondent-friendly. Moreover, since this measurement model is firmly rooted in theory, the logic and theoretical rigor behind its operationalization enables a systematic development of versions for every society in which occupations, occupational prestige or job-related socioeconomic indices have been catalogued. These characteristics make the instrument appealing for systematic comparisons of returns to social capital between populations. However, although its aim is to be "content free" (Lin, Fu, & Hsung, 2001), position generator data rather emphasize the identification of social capital productive for instrumental use: accessing social prestige is not relevant for every social capital question (e.g. receiving emotional support from a surgeon is not better than from a cleaner), and alters without any identifiable job prestige can still be very relevant and useful social capital (e.g. home-makers have no official occupation or job prestige, but are essential network members to many people) (Van der Gaag, Snijders, & Flap, forthcoming). Especially when applied in the domain of health studies, the validity of position generator data may therefore show some systematic shortcomings.

Using position generator data for research into the goal specificity of social capital is difficult. The amalgamation of social resources into social prestige measures prevents the design of multiple indicators that each refer to specific social resource collections. One way to construct more specific indicators is to establish separate indicators for the financial and cultural resources attached to each of the included occupations, which can subsequently be used as social capital sub-dimensions (see dimensional analyses in Flap & Völker, 2001; Webber, 2007). Another is to specify the positions for male and female network members separately (Erickson, 2004).[10]

Position generator data are liable to some problems regarding their validity and reliability. Ideally, respondents say "yes" to included positions because they actually know someone in a specified occupation. However, respondents can also do so when this occupation only somewhat resembles the occupation of someone they know,

---

[9] Some of these measures show little variation in scores, especially when few items (<15) are included in the instrument. Less often used position generator measures without this disadvantage are the *average accessed prestige* (introduced by Campbell, Marsden, & Hurlbert, 1986), calculated as the mean of the prestige of all occupations in which the respondent knows anyone, and *total accessed prestige*, a social capital volume measure, calculated as the cumulative prestige of all accessed occupations (Boxman, Flap, & Weesie, 1992:47–48; Hsung & Hwang, 1992).

[10] A third method to construct more specific measures from position generator data is the performance of latent trait analyses on the sets of items (Van der Gaag, 2005:ch.6; Van der Gaag, Snijders, & Flap, 2006). This method is further explained in section "resource generator".

while both could be rated at various levels of job prestige (e.g. "community worker", "civil servant", and "member of armed forces") (Webber, 2007). "False positive" answers can be given when people interacted with only professionally are mistaken for personal network members (e.g. teachers, doctors, members of clergy, sales people, and directors of firms should not be included as positions). Some occupations may sound too salient to confess not to know anyone having it (e.g. artists or managers) while this is not the case. Some studies have shown that people are only vaguely aware of the actual professions of their network members (Laumann, 1969). Lower educated respondents sometimes do not fully understand the question asking to imagine occupations and "fill" them with people they actually know. In a recent UK validation study, participants were however found to unambiguously refer to persons they actually knew in specified occupations, which showed good to excellent test-retest reliability (Webber, 2007).[11]

2.3.3. Resource Generator

The "resource generator" (Snijders, 1999; Van der Gaag & Snijders, 2005) offers a new development in measuring social capital by using a "checklist": in an interview situation, access is checked against a list of useful and concrete social resources, for which exchange is considered acceptable (see Table 2.1). This method combines the economy of the position generator with the content validity of the name generator / interpreter method, because of its vivid measurement of social resources. In particular, when potential respondents are involved in the construction of the instrument, a valid list of relevant resources can be readily obtained and the questions can be phrased clearly to obtain a reliable response (Webber and Huxley, Submitted).

Some methodological issues need further study. While its data are concrete and its administration is quick, resource generator items have validity problems similar to the position generator – of many social resources it is unknown how much people actually know about their social network members. Furthermore, the inclusion of actual resource items in instruments is difficult to achieve with any theoretical rigor. The examples of social capital included in the instrument need to be potentially productive, exchangeable, acceptable to ask for, and memorable for the respondent. Since most of these characteristics are culturally dependent, developed versions of resource generator instruments are strongly bound to a specific population. Another problem proves to be that the popularity of the items is rather high: respondents very easily give an affirmative answer to questions whether they could access resources in their social networks; this also indicates susceptibility for socially desirable answers (Van der Gaag & Snijders, 2005).

---

[11] Occupations can also prove to be unsuitable for inclusion in a position generator because they are not very well known in the general population, such as "academic researcher", "laboratory technician", and "fishmonger" (Webber, 2007).

The construction of single social capital indicators from resource generator data can proceed in a theory-guided fashion (a single volume/diversity indicator can be constructed from its data as the sum score of access to all different items, whereas multiple indicators could be constructed for all sub domains included in its items), but the data are also suited for an empirical construction of measures (Van der Gaag & Snijders, 2005). This method comprises the construction of population-specific sets of multiple, domain-specific social capital measures by dimensional analysis of data. The idea behind this is that by checking the associations between all included items the latent structure of social capital is identified for a specific population, in which groups of strongly correlated items point towards the existence of separately accessed social capital domains. Since social capital data are typically of an ordinal nature, factor-analytic models such as e.g. Principal Components Analyses (designed for use with normally distributed data of at least 5 categories) are generally not suitable to accomplish such dimensional reductions. Instead, models from Item Response Theory are more appropriate (see e.g. Van der Linden & Hambleton, 1997).

The Resource Generator-UK (RG-UK) (Webber & Huxley, Submitted) provides a good example of such an analysis. The content validity of the items and questions for this instrument was established through a qualitative process of focus groups and an expert panel. This resulted in a pool of 35 usable social resources items which were used to explore the social capital domain structure of this population. Explorative analyses were performed using Mokken scaling (Mokken, 1997), a non-parametric item response theory method that aims to find robust and one-dimensional scales within sets of items. It begins by taking pairs of items with the strongest associations and continues by gradually including other well-fitting items until a scale has been formed that does not improve any further when other items are added.

Cumulative scale analyses was performed using MSP5 for Windows (Molenaar & Sijtsma, 2000). This uses Loevinger's H-coefficients (Loevinger, 1947) to express the fit of specific items within a scale and for the homogeneity of the scale as a whole. Uncorrelated items produce values of $H = 0$, whereas perfectly homogenous scales produce values of $H = 1$. Conventionally, scales with $H \geq 0.3$ are useful, $H \geq 0.4$ are medium strong and $H \geq 0.5$ are strong scales. The Mokken scaling method allows for each item to appear in only one scale. The procedure eliminates items that do not fit within any scale if their item homogeneity (H_i) falls below a set value, conventionally $H_i = 0.3$ (Mokken, 1997). Further, a reliability coefficient (ρ) is calculated for each scale. Values above 0.6 are conventionally taken as indications of sufficient reliability (Molenaar & Sijtsma, 2000).

Data for scaling and item reduction in the RG-UK was obtained from a postal pilot survey of individuals on the electoral register in south London and Doncaster in south Yorkshire (N = 295). The 27 items together form a homogeneous scale ($H = 0.37$) with high reliability ($\rho = 0.89$). The RG-UK scale and its subscales have good test-retest reliability (full validity and sample details are reported elsewhere) (Webber & Huxley, Submitted). Using explorative Mokken scaling, four consistent internal domains were found within the instrument, each referring to a distinct dimension of an individual's social capital (Table 2.1). Firstly, the domestic resources scale refers to resources that may be required to assist daily living and improve one's living conditions. These are quite common resources with four of the seven being accessible to over 80% of this sample. Secondly, the expert advice scale contains skills that are important for the employment market or are associated with the domain of the professions. Empirically, this is the strongest scale ($H = 0.54$, $\rho = 0.83$). Thirdly, the personal skills scale draws together a range of attributes that are important for "getting the job done". It includes tradesmen, mechanics and gardeners, though a less obvious fit in this scale is someone who can employ others. Finally, a seemingly disparate group of items came together to form the problem solving resources scale. These could all be useful in difficult situations that could become very frustrating for individuals if they were not resolved.

Within-scale item correlations were positive and significant (Table 2.2). Table 2.2 groups the items within their scales in order of popularity, starting with the rarest resource in each scale. This shows that if one has access to someone who could lend a large amount of money (B16), one is more likely to have access to other resources within the domestic scale such as someone who could get cheap goods (B14) or could help one find somewhere to live if one had to move home (B15), for example. Similarly, if one knows someone with good contacts with the local media (A13) one is also likely to know someone knowledgeable about government regulations. The same is true for the other two scales. Moreover, since the scales have a cumulative character, individuals who have access to rare social resources are likely to also have access to more common social resources included in the same scale. Most of the items are correlated with items from other scales, though none is correlated with every other item. This is further evidence of the separate sub-domains of social capital that can be accessed through informal networks.

A further pilot tested for an association between these scales and common mental disorders such as depression and anxiety. Using postal questionnaires sent to a random sample of 1000 people on the electoral registers in the same two areas as mentioned above, 335 respondents completed the RG-UK and the twelve item General Health Questionnaire (GHQ) (Goldberg & Williams, 1988), a well validated self-completed instrument that assesses the likely presence of a common mental disorder (further details reported elsewhere) (Webber & Huxley, Submitted). Further study of the distribution of social capital sub-domains across the population illustrate that increasing age result in diminishing access to expert advice. Occupational status is an important variable across all sub-domains except domestic resources. Additionally ethnicity and likely presence of a common mental disorder also appear to be important variables (Webber & Huxley, in press: Table3).

On the GHQ, 27.3% (n = 91) of the sample scored three or above, the threshold value for a probable common mental disorder. Table 2.3 indicates that looking after the home or being unemployed increase the odds of having a common mental disorder, whereas having a low status occupation appears to be a protective

TABLE 2.2. Inter-Item correlations of empirically determined resource generator scales (N = 295; sample of south London and Doncaster electoral registers).

Item	Scale 1: Domestic resources							Scale 2: Expert advice									Scale 3: Personal skills					Scale 4: Problem solving resources					
	B16	B14	B15	B3	A17	B17	B4	A13	A12	B8	B10	B9	B1	B2	B11	A7	A9	A11	A15	A1	A3	A6	A8	A4	A5	B5	B7
Scale 1																											
B16	1																										
B14	0.37	1																									
B15	0.44	0.39	1																								
B3	0.28	0.27	0.36	1																							
A17	0.24	0.20	0.23	0.23	1																						
B17	0.34	0.30	0.35	0.29	0.28	1																					
B4	0.26	0.33	0.29	0.31	0.45	0.42	1																				
Scale 2																											
A13	ns	ns	ns	ns	ns	0.12	0.25	1																			
A12	0.32	0.22	0.28	0.17	0.22	0.21	0.17	0.25	1																		
B8	0.28	0.23	0.32	0.23	0.22	0.16	0.21	0.17	0.32	1																	
B10	0.27	0.26	0.26	0.24	0.21	0.13	0.16	0.21	0.42	0.31	1																
B9	0.29	0.21	0.33	0.17	ns	0.16	0.17	0.16	0.37	0.45	0.44	1															
B1	0.32	0.23	0.33	0.24	0.26	0.17	0.12	0.16	0.40	0.36	0.35	0.32	1														
B2	0.34	0.34	0.34	0.33	0.29	0.23	0.29	0.16	0.27	0.36	0.33	0.33	0.50	1													
B11	0.24	0.22	0.22	0.22	0.19	0.21	0.17	0.12	0.40	0.27	0.31	0.31	0.36	0.21	1												
A7	0.24	ns	0.28	ns	0.15	0.15	0.12	0.12	0.27	0.22	0.28	0.28	0.26	0.26	0.42	1											
Scale 3																											
A9	0.16	0.17	ns	0.13	0.18	0.17	0.13	0.17	0.32	0.13	0.19	0.18	0.17	0.18	0.21	0.16	1										
A11	0.26	0.26	0.24	0.26	0.25	0.29	0.17	0.14	0.25	0.26	0.28	0.16	0.32	0.20	0.32	0.27	0.21	1									
A15	0.19	0.18	0.22	0.28	0.29	0.17	0.15	0.21	0.40	0.18	0.27	0.29	0.22	0.23	0.31	0.34	0.33	0.22	1								
A1	0.17	0.21	0.20	0.22	0.29	0.29	0.15	ns	0.19	0.17	0.19	0.17	0.14	0.17	0.17	0.13	0.15	0.23	0.22	1							
A3	0.21	0.19	0.23	0.31	0.34	0.16	0.15	0.17	0.14	ns	0.26	0.18	0.28	0.32	0.23	0.27	0.18	0.27	0.37	0.45	1						
A6	0.21	0.19	0.28	0.21	0.24	0.16	0.17	0.21	0.13	ns	0.15	0.18	0.18	0.19	0.24	0.27	0.21	0.23	0.23	0.23	0.31	1					
Scale 4																											
A8	0.19	0.16	0.21	ns	0.18	0.19	ns	0.21	0.33	0.14	0.19	0.23	0.23	0.14	0.16	0.19	0.44	0.18	0.15	0.15	0.21	0.13	1				
A4	0.12	ns	0.18	ns	0.12	ns	ns	0.13	0.32	0.22	0.22	0.28	0.26	0.22	0.17	ns	0.23	0.16	0.17	0.21	0.17	0.24	0.24	1			
A5	0.12	ns	0.18	0.15	0.22	0.12	ns	ns	0.24	0.17	0.19	0.16	0.27	0.28	0.23	0.21	0.25	0.23	0.19	0.31	0.34	0.21	0.16	0.29	1		
B5	0.12	0.22	0.22	0.26	0.29	0.43	0.41	ns	0.19	0.23	0.14	ns	0.21	0.14	0.17	0.15	0.15	ns	ns	ns	0.16	0.18	0.18	0.16	0.19	1	
B7	0.25	0.28	0.26	0.12	0.26	0.26	0.20	ns	0.14	0.27	0.15	0.22	0.24	0.27	0.24	0.15	ns	ns	0.15	0.12	0.15	0.12	0.13	0.13	0.19	0.34	1

Pearson correlations: **p < 0.01**, p < 0.05

TABLE 2.3. Logistic regression models with predictive factors for common mental disorder[a] including none, one general resource generator social capital sum score measure, and four domain specific social capital resource generator measures (N = 335, sample of south London and Doncaster electoral registers).

Model	Variable	Odds ratio (95% CI)	p
No social capital variables	Looking after the home[1]	6.11 (1.83–20.45)	0.003
$R^2 = 14.2\%$, $\chi^2(22) = 51.05$, p = 0.0004	Unemployed[1]	5.28 (1.04–26.80)	0.044
	SOC 7–9[1]	0.18 (0.04–0.86)	0.032
RG-UK total score	Looking after the home[1]	4.58 (1.30–16.09)	0.018
$R^2 = 17.3\%$, $\chi^2(23) = 51.80$, p = 0.0005	Age	0.96 (0.92–0.99)	0.012
	RG-UK total	0.93 (0.87–0.99)	0.029
	SOC 7–9[1]	0.18 (0.04–0.91)	0.038
RG-UK sub-scales	Looking after the home[1]	5.54 (1.51–20.38)	0.010
$R^2 = 18.7\%$, $\chi^2(26) = 55.73$, p = 0.0006	Age	0.96 (0.93–0.99)	0.017
	SOC 7–9[1]	0.19 (0.04–0.95)	0.043

[1]Contrast group = SOC groups 1–3 (Office for National Statistics, 2000)

[a] Common mental disorder measured with twelve item General Health Questionnaire (GHQ) (Goldberg and Williams, 1988), GHQ; dichotomisation scoring under 3/3+

Only variables significant at p<0.05 tabulated

factor in this sample. When access to social resources is included in the model, it becomes apparent that the volume or diversity of accessible social capital is a protective factor for mental health. However, when the total scale score is replaced by the four sub-domain scores, this effect disappears. This suggests that in this context social capital has an unspecific effect, and that having access to a diversity of social resources across all domains, resulting from having an extensive social network, is important for the prevention of mental disorder;.

As this data is cross-sectional it is not possible to determine the direction of any causal relationships between these variables. However, there are a number of possible explanations. An absolutely low level of resources may act as a vulnerability factor in the development of common mental disorder. Also, the loss of previously accessible and valued resources may increase vulnerability or act as a trigger for an episode. It is also possible that access to resources may diminish as common mental disorders persist, possibly as a result of diminished social interaction and exchange through social withdrawal.

Further work is underway in which the RG-UK is being used in a cohort study of people with depression in London. Studies of this nature will further our understanding of how access to social capital affects recovery or influences the chronicity of illness. The hypothesis being tested is that those with access to a larger number of resources will have a faster rate of recovery over a six month period. Early results from this study suggest that people access resources within their networks after the acute phase of illness has passed. These resources may assist recovery in a number of ways. In addition to the various forms of advice, help and support that can be obtained from informal social networks, people with chronic illnesses may improve their employment or promotion prospects by having more resourceful networks which, in turn, may assist recovery, for example (Webber, 2005). It will be instructive to learn how the different domains of social capital contribute to recovery.

2.4. Conclusion

Recent methodological research has shown that measures calculated from different social capital measurement instruments indicate very different aspects of social capital, and that separate measures from separate instruments also have different predictive value for different outcomes of social capital. Therefore, the selection of measurement instruments should be careful, and according to specific research interest, for which a general research strategy has been proposed (Van der Gaag, 2005:181–205; Van der Gaag & Snijders, 2003). Researchers are therefore advised to use two social capital measurement instruments in questionnaires whenever possible: one instrument aiming to measure the presence of specific social resources, which may identify social capital sub domains and illustrate the usefulness of particular resources (such as the resource generator), and one instrument that is more structurally comparable to other studies (preferably the position generator).

Social capital measurement instruments to be used in health studies ideally need extensive pre-testing to ensure their validity and reliability in the population being investigated. When effects of the presence of network structure or particular alters and/or relationships are not specifically investigated, studies including name generators are not recommended for reasons of efficiency. Resource generators work best if they are sufficiently large to contain a number of sub-domains of social capital so that specific groups of resources can be identified as influencing the outcome being studied. If specific resources are identified as useful in a particular population for preventing illness or enhancing recovery from it, more specific interventions can be designed to maximize the availability of, or access to, them.

References

Borgatti, S. P., Jones, C., & Everett, M. G. (1998). Network measures of social capital. *Connections, 21*, 27–36.

Bourdieu, P. (1980). Le capital social. Notes provisoires. *Actes de la Recherche en Sciences Sociales, 3*, 2–3.

Boxman, E., Flap, H. D., & Weesie, H. M. (1992). Informeel zoeken op de arbeidsmarkt. [Informal search on the labour market.] In S. Jansen & G. L. H. Van den Wittenboer, (Eds.), *Sociale Netwerken En Hun Invloed* (pp. 39–56). Meppel: Boom.

Burt, R. S. (1984). Network items and the general social survey. *Social Networks, 6*, 293–339.

Burt, R. S. (1992). *Structural holes: the social structure of competition.* Cambridge MA: Harvard University Press.

Campbell, K. E., Marsden, P. V., & Hurlbert, J. S. (1986). Social resources and socio-economic status. *Social Networks, 8,* 97–117.

Coleman, J. (1988). Social capital in the creation of human capital. *American Journal of Sociology, 94,* S95–S120.

Coleman, J. (1990). *Foundations of social theory.* Cambridge/London: Belknap Press of Harvard University Press.

Erickson, B. H. (1996). Culture, class, and connections. *American Journal of Sociology, 102,* 217–251.

Erickson, B. H. (2003). Social networks: the value of variety. *Contexts, 2,* 25–31.

Erickson, B. H. (2004). The distribution of gendered social capital in Canada. In H. Flap & B. Völker (Eds.), *Creation and returns of Social Capital* (pp. 27–50). London: Routledge.

Felling, A., Fiselier, A., & Van der Poel, M. (1991). *Primaire relaties en sociale steun.* [Primary relations and social support.] Nijmegen: ITS.

Flap, H. D. (1991). Social capital in the production of inequality. A review. *Comparative Sociology of Family, Health, and Education, 20,* 6179–6202.

Flap, H. D. (1999). Creation and returns of social capital: a new research program. *La Revue Tocqueville, XX,* 5–26.

Flap, H. D. (2002). No man is an island. In E. Lazega & O. Favereau (Eds.), *Conventions and structures* (pp. 29–59). Oxford: Oxford University Press.

Flap, H. D. (2004). Creation and returns of social capital. In H. Flap & B. Völker (Eds.), *Creation and returns of social capital* (pp. 3–24). London:Routledge.

Flap, H. D., & Völker, B. (2001). Goal specific social capital and job satisfaction: effects of different types of networks on instrumental and social aspects of work. *Social Networks, 23,* 297–320.

Flap, H. D., Völker, B., Snijders, T. A. B., & Van der Gaag, M. P. J. (2004). Measurement instruments for social capital of individuals. Document including SSND questionnaire social capital items http://www.xs4all.nl/~gaag/work.

Goldberg, D., & Williams, P. (1988). *A user's guide to the general health questionnaire.* Windsor: NFER-Nelson.

Granovetter, M. (1973). The strength of weak ties. *American Journal of Sociology, 78,* 1360–1380.

Hennings, K. H. (1987). Capital as a factor of production. In J. Eatwell, P. Newman, M. Ilgate (Eds.), *The new palgrave. A dictionary of economics, Vol.1* (pp. 327–333). London etc.: MacMillan.

Hsung, R., & Hwang, Y. (1992). *Job mobility in Taiwan: job search methods and contacts status.* Paper presented at the XII International Sunbelt conference on Social networks, February 13–17, San Diego, California, USA.

Laumann, E. O. (1969). The social structure of religious and ethnoreligious groups in a metropolitan community. *American Sociological Review, 34,* 182–197.

Leenders, R. Th. A. J., & Gabbay, S.M. (Eds.). (1999). *Corporate social capital and liability.* Boston: Kluwer Academic.

Lin, N. (1982). Social resources and instrumental action. In P. V. Marsden & N. Lin (Eds.). *Social structure and network analysis* (pp. 131–145). Beverly Hills: CA, Sage.

Lin, N. (1999a). Building a network theory of social capital. *Connections, 22,* 28–51.

Lin, N. (1999b). Social networks and status attainment. *Annual Review of Sociology, 25,* 467–487.

Lin, N. (2001). *Social capital: a theory of social structure and action.* Cambridge: Cambridge University Press.

Lin, N., & Dumin, M. (1986). Access to occupations through social ties. *Social Networks, 8,* 365–385.

Lin, N., & Erickson, B. (forthcoming). *Social capital: advances in research.* New York: Oxford University Press.

Lin, N., Fu, Y., & Hsung, R. (2001). The Position Generator: measurement techniques for social capital. In N. Lin, K. Cook, R. S. Burt (Eds.). *Social capital: theory and research* (pp. 57–84). New York: Aldine De Gruyter.

Loevinger, J. (1947). A systematic approach to the construction and evaluation of tests of ability. *Psychological Monographs,* 61.

Marsden, P. V. (1987). Core discussion networks of Americans. *American Sociological Review, 52,* 122–131.

Marsden, P. V. (1990). Network data and measurement. *American Review of Sociology, 16,* 435–463.

McCallister, L., & Fischer, C. (1978). A procedure for surveying personal networks. *Sociological Methods and Research, 7,* 131–148.

Mokken, R. J. (1997). Nonparametric models for dichotomous responses. In W. J. Van Der Linden, & R. K. Hambleton (Eds.), *Handbook of modern item response theory* (pp. 351–368). New York: Springer.

Molenaar, I. W., & Sijtsma, K. (2000). *User's manual. MSP5 for Windows.* A Program for Mokken scale analysis for polytomous items, Groningen: iecProGAMMA.

Office for National Statistics. (2000). *Standard occupational classification 2000.* London: The Stationary Office.

Putnam, R. (1993). *Making democracy work: Civic traditions in modern Italy.* Princeton: NJ: Princeton University Press.

Quesnay, F. (1766). Observations sur l'intérêt de l'argent. [Observations on financial interest]. *Journal d'Agriculture, du Commerce et des Finances,* 151–171.

Snijders, T. A. B. (1999). Prologue to the measurement of social capital. *La Revue Tocqueville, 20,* 27–44.

Van der Gaag, M. P. J. (2005). *Measurement of individual social capital.* Groningen: Ph.D dissertation.

Van der Gaag, M. P. J., & Snijders, T. A. B. (2003). *A comparison of measures for individual social capital.* Paper presented at the conference "Creation and returns of Social Capital"; october 30–31, Amsterdam, The Netherlands.

Van der Gaag, M. P. J., & Snijders, T. A. B. (2004). Proposals for the measurement of individual social capital. In H. D. Flap & B. Völker (Eds.), *Creation and returns of social capital* (pp. 199–217). London: Routledge.

Van der Gaag, M. P. J., & Snijders, T. A. B. (2005). The Resource Generator: measurement of individual social capital with concrete items. *Social Networks, 27,* 1–29.

Van der Gaag, M. P. J., Snijders, T. A. B., & Flap, H. D. (forth coming) Position Generator measures and their relationship to other social capital measures. In N. Lin, B. Erickson (Eds.), *Social capital: advances in research.* Oxford: Oxford University Press.

Van der Linden, W. J., & Hambleton, R. K. (1997). *Handbook of modern item response theory.* New York: Springer.

Van Sonderen, E., Ormel, J., Brilman, E., & Van Linden van den Heuvell, Ch. (1990). A comparison of the exchange, affective, and role-relation approach. In C. P. M. Knipscheer & T. C. Antonucci (Eds.), *Social network research: Methodological questions and substantive issues* (pp. 101–120). Lisse: Swets & Zeitlinger.

Webber, M. (2005). Social capital and mental health. In J. Tew (Ed.), *Social perspectives in mental health. Developing social models to understand and work with mental distress* (pp. 90–111). London: Jessica Kingsley Publishers.

Webber, M., & Huxley, P. (2006). *Measuring access to occupational prestige: The validity and reliability of the Position Generator-UK.* Kings College London: Institute of Psychiatry.

Webber, M. (2007) "Access to social capital and improvement in depressive symptoms", unpublished PhD thesis, Institute of Psychiatry, King's College London.

Webber, M., & Huxley, P. (in press) Measuring access to social capital: The validity and reliability of the Resource Generator-UK and its association with common mental disorder in the UK general population. *Social Science and Medicine.*

3
The Measurement of Community Social Capital Through Surveys

TRUDY HARPHAM

This chapter is about quantitative surveys of social capital within general community-based health surveys. It assumes that the investigation of social capital is only part of a larger survey that includes, at the least, additional questions on health-related outcomes, attitudes or behaviour. It therefore focuses on key issues that should be addressed when designing social capital measures but acknowledges that such measures need to be limited in order to be kept in proportion to the overall survey. It aims for a minimalist but theoretically strong approach.

Various instruments are referred to including the World Bank's Social Capital Assessment Tool (SOCAT, Grootaert & Van Bastelaer, 2002) and the Adapted Social Capital Assessment Tool (ASCAT, Harpham, Grant, & Thomas, 2002).

3.1. The Components of Social Capital

3.1.1. Cognitive Versus Structural

In health research, there is growing recognition of the need to separate structural from cognitive social capital because the two components have different relationships with health outcomes. For example, generally speaking, high levels of cognitive social capital are associated with good mental health but high structural social capital is sometimes associated with poor mental health (for examples of studies and exploration of the hypotheses as to the reasons for these associations see De Silva et al., 2006).

Structural social capital refers to what people *do* (associational links, networks) which could be objectively verified (by observation or records). Cognitive social capital refers to what people *feel* (values and perceptions) and is thus subjective. Within structural social capital it is important to separate formal networks (recognized groups related to school, sports, religion, politics or hobbies) from informal networks (friends, family, neighbours, work colleagues). Again, this is because the two forms may have different patterns of associations with health (e.g., Ziersch & Baum, 2004).

51

3.1.2. Bridging Versus Bonding

Bonding social capital is the strong ties with people in the same community that enable you to 'get by'. Bridging social capital is the formal and informal links with other communities that enable people to 'get ahead'. Bridging implies links between individuals in different structural positions of power and can refer to links up *and* down. It thus can incorporate the subset of linking social capital that usually refers only to links with external sources of power such as local government and other controlling forces. Linking social capital is the concept that brings governance (the relations between civil society and the state) into studies of social capital.

3.1.3. Things that are not Social Capital

This chapter takes the view that in most health research, social capital is hypothesized as being a resource (a determinant) of health. While it is acknowledged that health status can determine social capital (and indeed, as most research is cross-sectional we cannot distinguish the causal route), most interest is in social capital as a potential mechanism for improving health. One of the main problems in social capital research has been the tendency to measure lots of things that are not social capital and to lump them under the heading of social capital. While such factors may be on the causal route between social capital and health, it is important not to dilute the definition of social capital.

There now seems to be more rigorous thinking about empirically distinguishing between social capital and its outcomes. If the general conceptual framework for social capital and health has a 'mean and lean' concept of social capital on the left hand side and health outcome(s) on the right then there is room for intermediate outcomes (or proximate determinants to use another form of language) in the middle. And it is in this middle ground that things become fuzzy. Topics which are sometimes regarded as social capital but that can be more correctly and usefully regarded as intermediate variables between social capital and health include:

– Sense of belonging
– Enjoyment of area
– Desirability to move/stay
– Neighbourhood quality/desirability (noise, graffiti, litter, greenery, facilities)
– Security/crime

Collective action is another concept that is difficult to place in any conceptual framework of social capital and health. It covers political action such as demonstrating or campaigning and is thus very culture-specific. In writing about the SOCAT, Grootaert and Van Bastelaer (2002) acknowledge that 'unlike most of the indicators of structural and cognitive social capital, collective action is an output measure. Its usefulness stems from the fact that in the vast majority of settings, collective action is possible only if a significant amount of social capital is available' (p. 55). The SOCAT measures the extent, type and assessment of the willingness towards collective action. In a space- and time-limited questionnaire a more general and useful question might be the one used in the UK General Household Survey's social capital component: 'By working together, people in my neighbourhood/community can influence decisions that affect the neighbourhood/community' (answered in a Likert scale).

3.1.4. Reference Area

One of the most difficult problems in social capital research is defining 'community' in a standardized, meaningful way to respondents. Most studies use a geographical area of reference, even though it might be vaguely stated, for example, 'around here'. However, there is a growing interest in the social capital of non-spatial communities, for example work, school, religious and family groups. The definition of these latter sorts of communities poses fewer problems because questions can be phrased about 'people you work with/go to school with', 'people from the same church/mosque/temple' and 'family members'.

When using a spatial community the main decision is whether to use an officially recognised area, such as an electoral ward or postcode area, or to qualitatively explore respondents' constructions of community and then to use the most meaningful definition in the quantitative survey. Here, the practice of geographers in the 1970s might be usefully resurrected: the use of mental maps where people are asked to draw a map of their 'community' with salient points marked on it. Although the resulting areas will inevitably be different, commonality may enable a more meaningful area to be referred to than some official designation. The SOCAT includes a group mapping exercise to define community.

The problem of defining community will vary by context. For example, community is a word almost never used by elderly respondents in the UK (Blaxter & Poland, 2002). However, in Vietnam where the 'commune' is a resilient and highly meaningful geographical construct, no such problems are encountered (Tuan et al., 2005).

Whatever the reference area, it is important to consider whether questions refer to the community in general or the respondent's perception alone. For example: 'do people around here tend to trust each other?' or 'do you tend to trust people around here?'. Surveys often have an unhelpful mix of both types of questions (see comments on the Health Survey of England (HSE) below).

3.1.5. Reference Period

The challenge of logical consistency in the reference (or recall) period between social capital measures and health measures is often ignored. When it comes to cognitive structural capital it only makes sense to ask about current feelings. However, when asking about behaviour, in order to tap into structural social capital, a standardized reference period should always be provided (e.g., "in the last month have you joined in the activities of any of the following groups?"). Arguably, this should match up with the reference period used for the health outcome measure (e.g. in the last month have you experienced any of the following problems?) However, the exposure variable may take time to have an impact on the health indicator of interest, so different reference periods might be used according to the hypotheses being tested. This issue needs consideration and explicit decisions about the reference periods selected.

3.1.6. Individual Versus Ecological Social Capital

This chapter takes the view that both individual (compositional) social capital (following Bourdieu) and ecological (contextual) social capital (following Putnam) should be measured. Again, the argument for this is that the two forms of social capital have been found to have different associations with health. Although Van Deth (2003) argues that distinguishing between the two conceptualizations of social capital (individual versus ecological) is important 'because it implies the selection of quite different research strategies' (p. 84) this chapter will argue that aggregating individual responses is still the best way to obtain an ecologic measure. However, it accepts that questions still remain about whether aggregate survey data about, say, individual trust really measure the amount of trust available as a collective good for all citizens.

Once the reference area is defined, analysis of ecological social capital is only possible if a large enough sample of communities is included in the research design. This begs the question of 'what is large enough?' and a return to the sampling principles of the 1980s coverage surveys of the Expanded Programme of Immunization (EPI) in developing countries might be useful (Bennet, Woods, Liyanage, & Smith, 1991). These advocated a 30-cluster (community) approach and although the sample will depend on the research questions, this approach is a good starting point.

The search for valid, directly observable, collective, ecologic indicators continues (Harpham et al., 2002). Various ecological, community-level indicators have been proposed such as: paid newspaper circulation, congregation size, union membership, number of voluntary organizations, volunteering rates, number of blood donations, voter turnout, donations to charities, crime rates and the famous 'letter drop' whereby a stamped, addressed letter is dropped in the street and the number of people who pick it up and post it is regarded as an indicator of social capital. Most of these are very culturally specific and thus limit comparability. Moreover, they do not represent a collective measure of social relations in a community. So, we still rely on aggregating individual responses to represent the level of social capital in a community. Community social capital is typically measured on an ordinal scale, or as dichotomous, Categorized as high or low levels of different sorts of social capital(see below). The main methodological weakness of this approach is that any differences in social capital between communities can be confounded by the characteristics of the individuals living in those communities. This emphasizes the need to measure a thorough range of potential confounding factors (see below).

3.2. Networks

The need to identify the structure of social relations is a core part of any measure of social capital. The most rigorous method is classic network analysis, but as this chapter is assuming constrained resources such demanding analysis is not considered further here. (See chapter 4 for further discussion of network analysis.) As a more minimalist approach, this chapter advocates the measurement of the *extent*, the *nature* (informal/formal), and the *intensity* of the links.

The types of formal local organizations to be included in the measurement of social capital must be qualitatively explored before the design of any quantitative instrument. A question arises as to whether to include both formal and informal groups. As the relationship with health outcomes may differ it is usually advisable to include both, and as the analysis of social support (see below) usually maps back onto network links, it is advisable to cover both informal and formal sources when measuring networks *and* support.

Although the nature of networks analysed will vary according to context, the following will be appropriate in most studies:

Informal
Family in the household
Family outside the household
Friends
Co-workers

Formal
Groups related to:
Politics
Education
Employment (including trade union)
Faith
Sports/music/dance/drama/other hobbies
Well-being (individual or neighbourhood)
Finance/credit
Age/gender/ethnic-specific (e.g. women, youth, parent)

For example the HSE asks about participation in 14 types of associations ranging from political to music and dance groups. The ASCAT combines the question about networks with the question about support from the network as follows:
SAY: *Now I am going to ask some questions about your community, the place that you live which is called (name of place).*

1) In the last 12 months have you been an active member of any of the following types of groups in *name of place*?

Read list in the table 3.1 and record whether a member under 'group code', record the positive answers and then ask about support.

TABLE 3.1. ASCAT questions on social networks and support.

Group code	Group type	Member? 1 = yes 2 = no	In the last 12 months, did you receive from the group any emotional help, economic help or assistance in helping you know or do things?		
			Emotional	Economic	Know/ do things
01	Community organization (i.e., executive council, residents group)				
02	Food distribution groups (i.e., glass of milk program, communal kitchen, mother's club)				
03	Political group				
04	Religious/parish group				
05	Sports/social group				
06	Committees for health, water, or electricity				
07	School groups (e.g., parent/teacher association)				
08	Vigilante groups (e.g., the Ronda)				
09	Other (specify)				

NB: The groups listed will be specific to each country (this is for Peru).

The extent of networks can be measured by the number of groups in which a person is active, and the intensity can be measured by the frequency of involvement (a minimum approach might be to ask if involvement has occurred in the last six months).

3.2.1. Civic participation/Citizenship

These are non-group-based relations such as signing a petition, contacting a local politician/councillor, or attending a protest/council meeting. They can be subsumed in a general question such as 'In the last (recall period) have you done something for your neighbourhood as a whole?'

3.2.2. Social Support

Here we are discussing *perceived* social support so it is regarded as part of cognitive social capital. As social support has long been recognized as a buffer against stressors that can cause ill health, we know more about how to measure it in surveys. At the minimum, it is worth separating out instrumental (help to do things), emotional

TABLE 3.2. ASCAT questions on support from non-groups.

		Support code 1 = yes 2 = no
01	Family	
02	Neighbours	
03	Friends who are not neighbours	
04	Community leaders	
05	Religious leader	
06	Politicians	
07	Government officials/civil service	
08	Charitable organisations/NGO	
09	Other: specify	

NB Bridging social capital questions could be added to these – i.e., asking about membership of groups outside the community and support received from individuals/organisations from outside the community.

(help to feel things), and informational (help to know things) support as all these can be hypothesized to have different associations with health outcomes.

The Health Survey for England (HSE) presents seven statements: 'there are people I know – amongst my family or friends – who: do things to make me happy; make me feel loved; can be relied upon no matter what happens; would see that I'm taken care of if I needed to be; accept me just as I am; make me feel an important part of their lives; give me support and encouragement'. Note that there is no reference area defined here. In the 2002 HSE this problem was partly addressed by asking people whether 'this area is a place where neighbours look after each other'.

The ASCAT asks about support from non-groups in the following way:
SAY: *Now I am going to ask some questions about individuals who have given you support in the last 12 months*

1) In the last 12 months, have you received any help or support from any of the following, this can be emotional help, economic help or assistance in helping you know or do things?

Read list in the table 3.2 and record whether any support was received under support code.

3.2.3. Trust

Arguably, trust can be seen as a pre-disposing factor for social capital rather than being a part of social capital itself. This relates to the argument that cognitive elements predispose people to certain actions or behaviours. However, the position of this chapter is that it is part of social capital and this is certainly the position of nearly all studies of social capital and health.

One of the main problems with questions about trust in social capital research is the fact that a reference area (see above) is omitted. Asking about general trust may reflect certain perceptions of the world that have no relation to life within a defined community. For example, the HSE and the European Social Survey (ESS) measure trust with the question 'generally speaking, would you say that most people can be trusted or you cannot be too careful in dealing with people?' The ESS additionally asks 'do you think that most people would try to take advantage of you if they got the chance, or would they try to be fair?' and 'would you say that most of the time people try to be helpful or that they are mostly looking out for themselves?' Most of these questions are drawn from the famous World Values Survey. These measures of generalized trust or trust in strangers (sometimes referred to as thin trust) are gradually being abandoned in favour of questions that refer to familiar/personal trust (thick trust).For example, the SOCAT asks 'do you think that in this community people generally trust one another in matters of lending and borrowing?' The A-SCAT asks 'In general, can people in this community be trusted, or only some people, or people can't be trusted?'

Sometimes trust has been measured by asking about behaviours that require trust (e.g., looking after a child). As these are outcomes of trust they are best avoided.

It is important to separate out social trust (in individuals) from institutional/ civic or political trust. And in most cultural contexts it is probably important to measure both at the community level. The most common way to measure institutional trust is to simply list the relevant local institutions and then ask to what extent they are trusted.

3.2.4. Reciprocity

Reciprocity is the willingness to help others with the expectation that the favour would be returned when needed. Unlike trust it implies a two-way relationship. It can be measured by asking about norms or behaviours. The ASCAT asks about a norm: 'In general, people around here are willing to help each other out' (followed by a Likert scale). Questions which focus on the behavioural outcomes of reciprocity could include: 'In the past six months, how often have you helped neighbours?'

3.2.5. Informal Social Control

Informal social control (ISC) is a community's collective capacity to act in their best interests, fuelled by shared norms, which produce community sanctions. ISC, together with social cohesion, formed the scale of collective efficacy in the well-known Sampson, Raudenbush, & Earls (1997) Chicago study. Questions tend to revolve around perceptions of the likelihood of people in the community acting if something bad was being done (children showing disrespect to an adult, someone spraying graffiti, children playing truant, fighting, the threat of a closure of a community facility etc). ISC overlaps with collective action and thus suffers the same problems of arguably being an outcome of social capital (see above).

3.3. What to Control For?

Because the main 'exposure' is community, length of residence should be recorded. A minimum list of other obvious potential confounding factors includes:

Gender
Ethnicity
Socio economic status
Age
Home ownership
Education
Employment

3.4. Validity and Reliability

Unfortunately Van Deth's (2003) plea that *'assessing the validity of each measure of social capital in different settings (both cross-cultural and longitudinal) should be standard practice among empirical researchers in this area'* has not been heeded. In a review of 28 studies of social capital and mental health, De Silva (2006) found that only four included any validity testing. In a broader review of social capital and health studies, eleven studies did conduct some validation of their social capital tool, nine using psychometric validation such as factor analysis to assess internal validity. All of these studies found the tools they validated were able to distinguish between the different theoretical constructs of social capital, and therefore to have acceptable discriminant validity. However, in a field where no gold standard measure is available to assess concurrent validity, a broader approach to validation is necessary (De Silva et al., 2006). Psychometric validation does not contain any analysis from the respondents' viewpoint, a perspective that is vital in order to understand how respondents interpret the questions and therefore what the tool is actually measuring. Two of the eleven studies did use such cognitive validation techniques.

De Silva et al. (2006) assessed different aspects of construct validity using psychometric techniques including factor analysis and an assessment of face and content validity of a shortened version of ASCAT in Peru and Vietnam. This was followed by an in-depth cognitive assessment of the respondents' viewpoint through qualitative interviews. As a minimum validation strategy, any study of social capital and health should include cognitive validation of social capital measures as it is relatively low-cost and time-limited (in Peru and Vietnam about 20 qualitative interviews were undertaken in each country). This will be most useful when done as part of a pilot/pre-test activity so that results can be incorporated into the main survey. In addition, most health surveys need to assess reliability (repeatability) so a repeat survey of a small sample of respondents is advisable.

3.5. Measuring the Social Capital of Children

There is little experience of measuring the social capital of children. Issues around the measurement of social capital of children include: separation of intra- and inter-household social capital and the meaning of 'community' for children.

Most studies have measured social capital outside the family, though Coleman (1988) does make the distinction between social capital within and outside the family: social capital within the family is 'the relations between children and parents (and, when families included other members, relationships with them as well)' (p. 110). Coleman operationalizes family social capital into five components with measures linked to each: family structure, quality of parent-child relations, adult's interest in the child, parents' monitoring of child activities and extended family exchange and support. Winter (2000) and Ferguson (2006) provide reviews of family/child social capital research. Morrow (1999) has shown how both Putnam's and Coleman's work have taken a top-down view of the effect of parents on children with the focus being on parents' ability to invest in their children's well-being or future. 'A more active conceptualisation of children, drawing on the sociology of childhood . . .would explore how children themselves actively generate, draw on, or negotiate their own social capital, or indeed make links for their parents, or even provide active support for parents' (Morrow, 1999, p. 751). She goes on to suggest that many of the studies that measure social capital seem to assume that individual children are only influenced by family structure and school. They do not measure the broader social context, such as friends, social networks, and out-of-school activities like paid work and children's activities in their communities. In other words they play down children's agency and overemphasise the influence of parents on children's lives. Morrow suggests that social capital currently is poorly specified as it relates to children and that any future empirical measure of the social capital of children should include tapping into sense of belonging and integration into local communities and sense of self-efficacy. Morrow (2000) also points out that 'young people's 'communities' more often constitute a 'virtual' community of friends based around school, town centre and street, friends' and relatives' houses, and sometime two homes, rather than a tightly bound easily-identifiable geographical location' (p. 150).

3.6. Conclusion

De Silva's review of 28 studies of social capital and mental health (2006) found the following methodological weaknesses (Table 3.3):

TABLE 3.3. Weaknesses of measures of social capital.

Included measures that do not reflect common definitions of social capital	10
Secondary analysis of survey questions not originally designed to measure social capital	6
Did not measure both aspects of social capital (cognitive and structural)	12
Combined different aspects of social capital into one score	10
Provided no information on validity of social capital measure	24

This chapter has addressed these and other methodological weaknesses and has recommended practical solutions. Although Van Deth (2003) suggests that each component of social capital must have multiple item measurement and that sophisticated data reduction techniques should then be used, this assumes that the researcher has the capacity and resources to do this. This chapter has taken a more pragmatic position and has tried to identify trends, items and issues that will be useful to researchers who have only limited scope for social capital methodological research. It is possible to achieve a desirable balance between theoretical relevance and feasibility. It is important that all health researchers who are measuring social capital take on board the latest methodological lessons from the burgeoning literature on social capital.

References

Bennet, S., Woods, T., Liyanage, W., & Smith, D. (1991). A simplified general method for cluster sample surveys of health in developing countries. *World Health Statistical Quarterly, 44*, 98–106.

Blaxter, M., & Poland, F. (2002). Moving beyond the survey in exploring social capital. In C. Swann & A. Morgan, *Social capital for health: Insights from qualitative research.* London:Health Development Agency.

Coleman, J. S. (1988). Social capital in the creation of human capital. *American Journal of Sociology, 94*, S95–S120.

De Silva, M. (2006). A systematic review of the methods used in studies of social capital and mental health. In K. McKenzie & T. Harpham (Eds.), *Social capital and mental health.* London:Jessica Kingsley.

De Silva, M., Harpham, T., Tuan, T., Bartolini, R., Penny, M. & Huttly, S. (2006). Psychometric and cognitive validation of a social capital measurement tool in Peru and Vietnam. *Social Science and Medicine, 62*(4), 941–953.

Ferguson, K. (2006). Social capital and children's wellbeing: a critical synthesis of the international social capital literature. *International Journal of Social Welfare, 15*, 2–18.

Grootaert, C., & Van Bastelaer, T. (2002). *Understanding and measuring social capital.* Washington DC:World Bank.

Harpham, T., Grant, E., & Thomas, E. (2002). Measuring social capital within health surveys: Some key issues. *Health Policy and Planning, 17*(1), 106–111.

Morrow, V. (1999). Conceptualising social capital in relation to the well being of children and young people: a critical review. *Sociological Review, 47*(4), 744–765.

Morrow, V. (2000). 'Dirty looks' and 'trampy places' in young people's accounts of community and neighbourhood: implications for health inequalities. *Critical Public Health, 10*(2), 141–152.

Sampson, R., Raudenbush, S., & Earls, F. (1997). Neighbourhood and violent crime: a multilevel study of collective efficacy. *Science, 277*(5328), 918–927.

Tuan, T., Harpham, T., Huong, N. T., De Silva, M., Huong, V., Long, T., et al. (2005). Validity of a social capital measurement tool in Vietnam. *Asian Journal of Social Science, 33*(2), 208–222.

Van Deth, J. W. (2003). Measuring social capital: orthodoxies and continuing controversies. *International Journal of Social Research Methodology, 6*(1), 79–92.

Winter, I. (2000). Towards a theorized understanding of family life and social capital. *Australian Institute of Family Studies Working Paper* number 21. (www.aifs.org.au/institute/pubs/wp21).

Ziersch, A., & Baum, F. (2004). Involvement in civil society groups: Is it good for your health? *Journal of Epidemiology and Community Health, 58,* 493–500.

4
Network-Based Approaches for Measuring Social Capital

Cynthia M. Lakon, Dionne C. Godette, and John R. Hipp

A variety of disciplines, ranging from sociology to public health, have struggled with the conceptualization and measurement of social capital. Differences in the approach used to measure social capital may contribute to variations in the observed relationships between social capital and individual and population health across studies. As well, the heavy reliance on communitarian measures of social capital in public health may truncate the field's understanding of the relationship between social capital and health (Moore, Shiell, Hawe, & Haines, 2005).

While much of the public health literature has relied upon the communitarian view of social capital, researchers (e.g., Borgatti, Jones, & Everett, 1998; Lin, 2001; Moore et al., 2005) are now calling for the study of social capital as a relational construct. From this point of view, social capital is an inherent property of social relationships, the resources they hold, and the social networks they make up. Hence, social network concepts and methodology provide a useful mechanism for measuring social capital.

Despite the burgeoning literature on social capital that spans numerous disciplines, few studies utilize network measures of this construct. Prior studies within the fields of sociology and communications have explored structural, functional, and positional network based measures of social capital. The goal of this chapter is to define key terminology relating to social networks and to discuss how social network constructs may be used to measure social capital in public health research. The chapter provides a general overview of basic network measures of social capital, including structural, positional, and functional measures of network ties, with respect to both egocentric and whole networks. The chapter closes with a glossary of relevant social network terms (see Appendix 1), and a brief orientation to egocentric networks and sociometric networks (see Appendix 2)—readers unfamiliar with social network methodology and nomenclature may wish to consult these appendices before reading the main text.

4.1. Social Network Measures

Social capital has been conceptualized and measured using both egocentric amd sociomatric network measures. Egocentric networks are defined from the vantage point of a focal individual or "ego," for some role relationship (e.g., friends or coworkers). Egocentric networks do not include all relationship ties known to the focal individual. Instead, egocentric network measures are based on those who fulfill certain role relationships for a respondent, for instance, his or her five best friends. Examples of egocentric measures are the size and density of a network. Sociometric networks are based on information on all the respondents in a social system with defined boundaries (e.g., a school). Sociometric measures allow the measurement of social capital both as an individual level construct and as a group level construct. This chapter will provide a general overview of egocentric and sociometric measures of social capital. The network measures covered in this chapter draw largely from those discussed in Borgatti et al. (1998).

Published studies primarily focus on three domains of network characteristics as measures of social capital 1) *functional* measures, which reflect the content of network ties (e.g., supportive qualities of network ties); 2) *structural* measures, which describe how people in a network are connected to one another; and 3) *positional* measures, which reflect actors' positions in a network. Functional measures focus on the content of network ties. For example, they may assess whether specific ties provide network resources such as types of social support that include: information, tangible aid, emotional support, or other network resources. While there has been some acknowledgement that such resources are generated and embedded in network structures (Lin, 2001), functional measures specifically focus on the content provided by individual ties. Structural measures move beyond individual ties and focus on the linkages between actors in either an individual's network (egocentric measures) or in the larger overall network (sociometric measures). For example, structural measures can be used to test whether the density of ties promotes or inhibits the flow of resources, information, and influence through a network. Positional network measures are specific to sociometric network studies, and can be used to test whether certain network positions confer power and other resources via influence and advantage to network actors. In this view, specific actors have the power to influence how resources flow and are distributed within a network, and differentially affect access to resources and opportunities.

4.1.1. Egocentric Measures of Social Capital

Egocentric networks are measured at the level of the individual, and they require the respondent to provide information on those they name in their network. These measures generally focus on either the specific ties—their *function*—or on the relations among those ties—their *structure*.

4.1.1.1. Egocentric Functional Measures of Social Capital

When studying the function of ties, researchers often focus on the resources, the information, or the influence that a particular tie provides. Theoretical guidance is required to determine which resources are important for the outcome being studied. In work conducted by Van der Gaag and Snijders (2005), an approach is described in which such resources are defined by the researcher in advance of collecting data.

The content provided by network ties is particularly important in relation to health and health behavior. Several studies suggest relationships between social ties and health outcomes (Blazer, 1982; Cassel, 1976; Cobb, 1976; Coyne & Lazarus, 1980; Gottlieb, 1981; House, Landis, & Umberson, 1988; House, Robbins, & Metzner, 1982; Schoenbach, Kaplan, Fredman, & Kleinbaum, 1986). Studies suggest that the quality and number of network ties are negatively related to mortality risk (Berkman & Syme, 1979; House et al., 1982; Schoenbach et al., 1986; Seeman, Kaplan, Knudsen, Cohen, & Guralnik, 1987). These relationships generally hold (Berkman, 1986) across age, gender, and health status (Berkman & Syme, 1979; Schoenbach et al., 1986; Seeman et al., 1987). Likewise, content of ties is important for fostering positive or negative behaviors. Evidence from at least one study indicates that among adolescent and young adult injection drug users, social influences, namely emotional support conferred by ties to sexual partners, was positively correlated with risky needle use behaviors (Lakon, Ennett, & Norton, 2006).

A key network resource generated from ties is *social support*. Social support is defined as " . . . the functional content of relationships, such as the degree to which the relationships involve flow of affect or emotional concern, instrumental or tangible aid, information, and the like" (House & Kahn, 1985). Emotional support is based on closeness, connection, and belongingness (Schaefer, Coyne, & Lazarus, 1981). Instrumental support includes the provision of physical aid and services in mundane and emergency situations (Schaefer et al., 1981). Informational support includes the provision of informational resources.

Social support may be a key social process that is a source of social capital embedded in network ties. Wellman and Frank (2001) describe the potential for social capital embedded in supportive ties in our "personal communities," which are comprised of ties to friends, family, and important significant others in our lives. Such network capital may take on the form of emotional, instrumental, and informational support, providing people with both material and emotional aid, and a sense of connection and belongingness. Thus, studies measuring the presence of social support in a respondent's network often ask whether any ties in their network provide a particular type of support.

An alternative approach to measuring the resources provided by particular ties is to simply focus on the *tie strength*. Tie strength is a " . . . (probably linear) combination of the amount of time, the emotional intensity, the intimacy (mutual confiding), and the reciprocal services which characterize the tie" (Granovetter, 1973, p. 1361). In a study of best friend ties, closeness was the strongest indicator of tie strength (Marsden & Campbell, 1984).

Tie strength can generate social capital through a number of mechanisms. Strong ties may be more likely than weak ties to generate social support (Wellman, 1979). The strength of ties may also influence the amount of social regulation that can be exerted through a network, with stronger ties associated with increased regulatory influences (Flache & Macy, 1996). Within a community sample, tie strength was positively associated with the provision of emotional support, companionship, and minor services (Wellman & Wortley, 1990).

However, there are possible negative effects of strong, supportive ties. Some supportive ties can require very high relational investments, and over time, the ego may feel depleted and undermined if the relationship is too much work and not mutually beneficial. In addition, strong ties may not be consistently supportive—only providing support under certain circumstances (Wellman & Wortley, 1990). Weak ties have some inherent advantages as they may be more likely than strong ties to link people across social groups (Granovetter, 1973). These linkages result in access to new information and resources, and may be more effective than strong ties in conducting information through a network (Granovetter, 1973). While very close ties can increase access to emotional and instrumental support, they may simultaneously decrease access to information from outside resources (Hall & Wellman, 1985).

Numerous measures of tie strength exist. Marsden and Campbell (1984) suggested that tie strength measures the closeness of ties, where close friends are strong ties and more distant friends are weaker ties. For example, a question assessing tie strength might ask respondents to rate how close they are to each person in their networks. Other measures of tie strength include frequency of contact, the duration of the contact, whether the tie is emotionally supportive, and whether it is *multiplex* (Marsden & Campbell, 1984).

Multiplexity requires measuring network ties on more than one dimension, such as the role relationships (e.g., spouse, friend, and coworker) in which social network members know each other (Fischer, Jackson, Steuve, Gerson, Jones & Baldassare 1977). A multiplex tie is one that is based on knowing a person in two or more relationship contexts. Thus, multiplexity reflects overlap between an individual's social networks. In contrast, uniplex ties are defined by a single role relationship. Multiplexity can be measured as the proportion of people named in a respondent's network (e.g., friendship network) that are also named in one or more of a respondents' other networks, where the denominator of this proportion is the number of alters named in the respondent's friendship network.

Multiplex ties may facilitate the generation of social capital in a network. Such ties may increase resources in a network, as multiplex ties are more likely than uniplex ties to provide support (Kapferer, 1969). Also, multiplexity may increase the regulatory aspects of a tie (Krohn, 1986). Hence, if a multiplex tie provides support and other resources in one relationship context, it may also be more likely to provide the resources in other contexts. This may be due to social control and the need to maintain social standing across relationship contexts.

Network heterogeneity measures the diversity of alters' backgrounds with respect to various attributes. The choice of the attributes to study must be guided by theory, and can include such standard demographic measures as gender, age, or race.

For example, the ethnic heterogeneity (EH) in a network k is usually calculated based on a Herfindahl index (Gibbs & Martin, 1962) based on particular characteristics. When calculating the racial/ethnic heterogeneity of a network based on four racial/ethnic groups, it takes the following form:

$$EH_k = 1 - \sum_{1}^{j=J} G_j^2$$

where G represents the proportion of the network of ethnic group j out of J ethnic groups. Subtracting from 1 makes this a measure of heterogeneity.

Studies have suggested that network heterogeneity may be an important source of social capital since alters with a diversity of attributes likely provide a broad diversity of resources to the ego that are beneficial (Burt, 1983). Thus, this assumes that diversification of network resources may enhance social capital.

Compositional quality is the number of alters who possess characteristics that are of interest to ego (e.g., generosity, power) (Borgatti et al., 1998). While network heterogeneity focuses on the diversity within a network, network compositional quality focuses on the presence of specific characteristics of theoretical importance. This measure is particularly important in studies of social support, with considerable evidence that network composition provides social support (Hirsch, 1980; Walker, McBride, & Vachon, 1977). A common approach to measurement is to have the respondent report how many people in their network provide them with some type of support. For example, a question assessing the amount of emotional support garnered from an ego's friendship network might take on the following form for respondents who had been asked to name their five best friends:

Of the people you named in your friendship network, whom do you talk to when you need to discuss a personal problem?

Emotional support, conferred by the alters, may be measured as a proportion of the number that provide support (i.e., the number of people who provided support divided by the total number in the friendship network) or as an absolute number of people providing support. The choice of whether to use an absolute number versus a proportion depends on the research question one seeks to answer.

4.1.1.2. Egocentric Structural Measures of Social Capital

Structural network characteristics move beyond a focus on individual ties and view the linkages between network members (Israel, 1982). This includes such measures as size and density. *Network size* is the number of alters that an ego is directly connected to. The relationship between network size and social capital is straightforward: the larger one's network is, the greater the likelihood that any one person has diverse resources that the ego might need (Borgatti et al., 1998). For example, if there are many alters in one's egocentric friendship network, then the likelihood of gaining more support from any one of those alters is higher than if the network were smaller. Indeed, studies have found a positive relationship between network size and measures of social capital (Burt, 2000), and between network size and the number of alters who may provide social support (Wellman & Frank, 2001). Studies also indicate that larger networks may generate more instrumental and emotional support resources (Bott, 1957; Kapferer, 1969) than smaller networks (Seeman & Berkman, 1988).

Despite this empirical evidence, the relationship between network size and social capital may be vulnerable to omitted variable biases and spuriousness. For instance, it may be important to take into account 1) who the ties are to, since some individuals may be better able to provide resources than others (Lin, 1990); 2) the strength of the ties, 3) whether the ties are characterized as amicable (e.g., friendship bonds); and 4) whether the bonds enhance or detract from the ego's personal resources and social standing, as some ties may enhance one's resources while other ties can deplete or even exploit them. For example, Wellman and Frank (2001) found that the likelihood of receiving mundane support in everyday life situations as well as emergency support from alters was greater among egos who reported being close to a small number of alters. Wellman and Frank (2001) concluded that having closer ties can sometimes balance having a small number of network ties.

Egocentric **network density** moves beyond a simple count of the number of members in the network to take into account the extent to which alters know one another. Thus, a respondent is providing information on the relationships between the alters in their network. Density is measured by dividing the number of pairs of alters who know one another by the total number of connections that could exist among them. If n is the number of alters named in an ego network, then the equation for density for undirected ties is:

$$Density = \Sigma(alters\ who\ know\ one\ another)/(n(n-1))/2)$$

The denominator is the number of possible ties between network members with undirected linkages.[1]

The relationship between network density and social capital is likely nuanced. The evidence for whether denser social networks provide more network resources such as social support is mixed: on the one hand, some studies have found a positive relationship between dense networks and social support (Walker, McBride, & Vachon, 1977), specifically more emotional and instrumental support (Israel, 1982). On the other hand, other studies suggest that dense networks are not necessarily supportive and health enhancing (Hall & Wellman, 1985). Similarly, the role of dense networks in spreading influence

---

[1] Generally in egocentric measures the report on ties between alters is "undirected." That is, the respondent is simply asked whether alter "A" is friends with alter "B". In some instances, the researcher may ask for "directed" ties: that is, does "A" know "B", and does "B" know "A". Because the latter requires a considerable degree of information on the part of the respondent to report accurately, such an approach is more common in sociometric studies (in which both person "A" and person "B" can both directly report whether they know each other). In such an instance, density is measured as: *Density = Σ(alters that know one another) /n(n-1)* where all terms are as defined above.

and information has important implications for measuring social capital. For instance, densely connected networks are likely important for influencing the behavior of the ego respondent. In densely connected networks, social sanctioning may be particularly effective when the alters all know one another. However, densely connected networks are likely inimical for the diffusion of information and other resources from the outside into the network. For instance, if most or all of the alters know one another, then it's unlikely that any network member will introduce new information, violate existing network sanctions, or introduce new resources and ideas into a network, all of which may limit the generation of new social capital resources. In support, a study found a negative association between density and social capital, wherein the latter was measured by performance of managers in an organization (Burt, 2000).

4.1.2. Sociometric Measures

Sociometric network measures are indicators of whole networks. Such network measures require relational data, which unlike egocentric network data is measured from the vantage point of all individuals that comprise the network under study. Therefore this type of data is relational and describes a system of all actors in the network. An important initial step for sociometric studies is determining the *boundary* of the network. This may be facilitated by studying an organization with a natural boundary, such as a school, as it may be clear who does and who does not attend the school. Thus, researchers using data sets such as Add Health (e.g., Bearman, Moody, & Stovel, 2004) can study how information and influence diffuse through the network in a school and impact health behavior outcomes. Other studies have examined how network social influence diffuses through school-based networks in relation to cigarette smoking behaviors among youth (e.g., Valente, Hoffman, Ritt-Olson, Lichtman, & Johnson, 2003; Valente, Unger, & Johnson, 2005; Lakon & Valente, 2005). For other research questions—such as studying the injection drug user population in a city—determining the boundary of networks of injection drug users is not always straight-forward, as injectors are often transient, making network boundaries hard to define and sociometric studies extremely difficult to undertake.

In sociometric studies, relational data are presented in matrices and represent the ties between members of the network. Both the rows and the columns of the matrix represent the persons in the network. For instance, a 10 person network is represented by a 10x10 matrix: the first row and the first column represent the first person, the second row and the second column represent the second person, and the rest follows suit for the others in the network. Thus, in the case of directed ties, the row indicates which other network members an actor sends resources to (or whatever the links in the network represent). If person 1 sends resources to person 2, then the cell in row 1, column 2 will be given a value of 1. If they do not send resources to this person, then this cell will have a value of 0. The same example can be applied to a matrix displaying whether people in a network know one another: if person 1 knows person 2, then the cell in row 1 column 2 will be given a value of 1. These conventions can be generalized to *valued* networks, in which each cell may represent the strength of the relationship (i.e., the frequency of sending support, a measure of the tie strength, etc.). Alternatively, a matrix can be constructed in which the rows represent individuals, and the columns represent the groups they affiliate with—these are referred to as affiliation network matrices. For more information on both types of matrices, see Wasserman and Faust (1994). Once this matrix is constructed, various network measures can be constructed utilizing matrix algebra.

Sociometric measures can be categorized as two types: 1) *positional measures* focus on the position of persons within the network, and 2) *structural measures* focus on the structure of the entire network. The latter move beyond the focus on the position for a particular individual to focus on structural effects for all members of the network.

4.1.2.1. Sociometric Positional Measures of Social Capital

Positional measures reflect the location of actors in a network, and generally focus on either the *centrality* of the actor, or the *bridging* location of the actor in the network. There are numerous measures of centrality, such as degree, betweenness, eigenvector, and closeness centrality (Wasserman & Faust, 1994).

Degree centrality is a measure of how directly connected one is to most others in a network. If an actor is connected to most others in a network directly, then that actor is in an advantageous position to transmit and receive influence. There are two types of degree centrality. One is *in-degree*, which is the number of actors that report knowing a particular actor. The other is *out-degree*, which is the number of actors a particular actor reports knowing. The higher the degree centrality of an actor, the more directly connected the actor is in a network. Therefore, the more readily the actor is able to access network resources, the more social capital the actor has.

Betweenness centrality is a measure of the extent to which an actor lies between other actors on the shortest paths linking them. An actor high in betweenness centrality (C_B) may, through direct and indirect linkages, influence proximal actors, through both direct and indirect pathways (Friedkin, 1991). Consider the probability that a communication between actors takes a particular pathway. If we assume that a communication is likely to pass through the shortest route between actors, and that a *geodesic* is the shortest path linking two actors, then g_{jk} is the number of *geodesics* linking actor j and actor k. If all geodesics between the actors are a possible route for the communication, the probability any one of them is chosen is $1/g_{jk}$. Secondly, the probability that actor "i" takes part in the communication between actor j and k is $g_{jk}(n_i)$, which is the number of geodesics linking the two actors that contain actor "i" (Wasserman & Faust, 1994). The equation for the betweenness index for actor n_i, from actor j to actor k for nondirectional ties (Freeman, 1979) is:

$$C_B(n_i) = \sum_{j<k} g_{jk}(n_i) / g_{jk}$$

This index is a measure of the extent to which an actor lies between other actors in a network.

Betweenness centrality may be positively related to social capital. Actors high in betweenness centrality are in the position to connect actors who would not otherwise be connected, hence generating new opportunities for information, influence, and resources (Borgatti et al., 1998).

Closeness centrality measures how far away an actor is to other actors in a network. An actor with low closeness centrality can quickly transmit influence through a direct or a short path to others. Closeness centrality (C_c) is measured (Sabidussi, 1996), where $d(n_i, n_j)$ is the number of lines in the shortest path linking actors i and j, and the total distance "i" from all of the other actors, summing from j = 1 to g, where g is the geodesic distance between all pairs of nodes is:

$$\sum_{j=1}^{g} d(n_i, n_j)$$

And the equation for closeness centrality is:

$$C_c(n_i) = [\sum_{j=1}^{g} d(n_i, n_j)]^{-1}$$

Closeness centrality is inversely related to social capital. The lower the distance to others in a network, the more likely that an actor can access resources from proximal others, which increases the likelihood of gaining more social capital (Borgatti et al., 1998).

Eigenvector centrality is a measure of how connected an actor is to those who are well connected to others in a network. Those occupying positions high on betweenness or eigenvector centrality may be in an advantageous position to and receive and transmit influence other actors through their connections to highly connected othersin more distant parts of a network. This measure assumes an actor's centrality is a function of how connected their contacts are to others. The equation can be expressed as:

$$(I - \beta \# Z)^{-1} * Z * W$$

where I is an identity matrix, Z is an N x N adjacency matrix showing all ties between residents, W is an N x 1 vector of 1's, # represents element-wise multiplication, and β is a value chosen to represent the power of the centrality score (Bonacich 1987; Moody, 2000). Because those high in eigenvector centrality are linked to well-connected actors, the former can tap into the rich informational and other resources that belong to those who are well connected in a network.

Besides focusing on the centrality of an individual within the entire network, another approach focuses on which individuals provide *bridges* between various subsections of the overall network. In general, bridges are links that connect disparate, unconnected groups of actors in a network. The seminal work of Granovetter (1973) on the strength of weak ties focuses on how weak ties link otherwise disconnected social groups. Assuming that weak ties bridged a network actor to groups outside his/her local social network (e.g., friends and family), Granovetter suggested that weak ties would provide access to resources outside the local sub-network, such as job contacts. Burt (1992) built on this insight in developing his theory of structural holes: the notion that disconnected groups in a network could benefit by a bridging tie linking them. Bridges can facilitate access to information outside of one's network and expose a network actor to new information and influence. Hence, bridges can generate social capital in a network because they link actors to disparate regions of a network. These bridges provide linkages to new and possibly diverse network resources that are not likely to be found in the actor's local networks.

Various indicators are used to measure bridging. For instance, Valente (2006) proposed a measure of bridging by " . . . systematically deleting existing links and adding non-existent links and summing the resultant changes in the network's average path length." Path lengths in networks are calculated by tracing a path from each member of the network to every other member, and counting the number of nodes that must be traversed to reach the destination. Thus, if Nancy and Ted are directly tied, the path length is one. However, if Ted and Fred both know Nancy, but do not know each other, then the path length between Ted and Fred is two (since the shortest path between them must go through Nancy). The intuition underlying Valente's measure is that if an important bridge person exists in a network, the shortest way to trace paths between nodes in the network will be to go through this person. Thus, eliminating the links to and from this person in the network will greatly increase the length of many paths to others in the network, and hence increase the average path length.

While measures of bridging are positional measures since they posit that certain network positions can confer social and other advantages, they are also structural since the intuition underlying structural holes is that social opportunities may be more likely to arise in diffusely connected network ties than densely connected ties. Thus, there are implications for other individuals in the network besides the bridge person: if a sub-network is not closed, that is, if all of the actors in the network do not know one another, then the network is more likely to span "structural holes" in the network. These "holes" or weak ties are conduits to subgroups outside the local network that may have diverse resources. While the individual providing the link outside of the local sub-network likely obtains advantages by garnering new and diverse resources, the other members of the sub-network also gain since this information is able to permeate their sub- network.

4.1.2.2. Sociometric Structural Measures of Social Capital

Sociometric structural measures can capture both individual social capital and aggregate level social capital. At the individual level, Burt(1992) suggests that **network constraint** relates to social capital. Network *constraint* measures how much alters constrain the ego. Constraint is calculated by summing the degree to which each of the alerts is connected to others in the personal network. Constraint is the extent to which " . . . all of ego's relational investments directly or indirectly involve a single alter" (Borgatti et al., 1998, pg. 6). A highly constrained network is one that contains fewer structural holes, and most actors are directly connected to one another or connected via a central actor. Conceptually similar to density, constraint uses more of the information available in the personal network than does density (T.W. Valente, personal communication, April 2006). A more constrained actor has less potential for engaging in actions that would lead to the generation of social capital resources. Hence, highly constrained network actors have fewer opportunities for diversifying their resources. Therefore, network constraint has been negatively related to social capital (Burt, 1992). To measure network constraint for an individual (Burt, 2000):

$$Cij = (p_{ij} + \Sigma_q p_{iq} p_{qj})^2$$

Where q is not equal to i or j, $p_{ij} = Z_{ij} / \Sigma_q Z_{iq}$ (the proportion of i's network time and energy invested in contact j), and Z_{ij} is the strength of the relationship between contact i and j. Summing these constraints for all network members yields the overall network constraint C.

Moving beyond the individual level, measures of aggregate social captial (i.e., at the full network level), capture the social accured by all members of a network. For example, density can be measured as a network level indicator of how well-connected actors are to one another. It is measured as the number of connected actors divided by the total possible connections that could exist between them (Scott, 2000):

$$L/(n(n-1)) \text{ (for directed ties)}$$
$$L/(n(n-1)/2) \text{ (for undirected ties)}$$

Where L = the number of lines (i.e., relationship ties between network members) in a graph and n = the number of nodes

The relationship between network level density and social capital is ambiguous (Borgatti et al., 1998). Depending on the nature of the relationships that characterize densely connected ties, network level density may be either positively or negatively related to social capital. For example, densely connected friendship ties may promote social capital, as the friendships themselves can be worthwhile and beneficial to actors. If, however, relationships are characterized by strain and conflict, densely connected ties may decrease social capital resources by inhibiting resource flow and slowing or blocking access to desired resources.

Centralization is a measure of the variability of the individual centrality values of the actors in a network. In an extreme instance, one actor is particularly central relative to other network members. Note that while *centrality* views the location of a single actor, *centralization* characterizes the entire network.

The centralization index for nondirectional relations is measured as (Wasserman & Faust, 1994):

$$C_A = \sum_{i=1}^{g} [C_A(n^*) - C_A(n_i)] / \text{Max} \sum_{i=1}^{g} [C_A(n^*) - C_A(n_i)]$$

where $C_A(n^*)$ = the largest value of the particular index that occurs across the g actors in the network, and $C_A(n_i)$ = is the actor centrality index. Intuitively, this measure is capturing the degree to which the network contains many central actors.

The effect of centralization on the social capital of the group is ambiguous. On the one hand, in a highly centralized network, one or very few actors are bridges between all others (all ties go through this person). While the centrality of this person certainly places them in a very strategic position, there is the risk that relying on this single person for the flow of information is less desirable than a more diffuse network with ties between many of the actors (but longer average path lengths as a result). On the other hand, one could argue that in highly centralized networks actors are more likely to be privy to informational flows, influence, and other resources because the distances between actors are smaller and actors can occupy positions that facilitate the flow of information. This would suggest that greater network centralization is related to more social capital.

Measures of social *cohesion* can also be used to measure the social captial of subgroups within the larger network. Numerous measures of cohesion have been proposed. For instance, Markovsky and Lawler (1994) proposed that the "reachability" of all actors in the group is an important characteristic of cohesive groups. That is, their measure estimates the degree to which a path can be traced from any group member to any other group member. Another approach uses the number of ties as a measure of cohesion. Moody and White (2003), however, point out that a limitation of such a measure is that while the elimination of a single tie would have little effect on the number of ties within the group, it could quite dramatically change the connectivity of a group. Thus, in a group in which one or two persons are the crucial links for disparate parts of the network, eliminating one link could greatly reduce the overall connectivity. Therefore, Moody and White (2003) proposed a measure in which "a group's cohesion is equal to the minimum number of actors who, if removed from the group, would disconnect the group."

Finally, the literature on *bridging* and *bonding* social capital suggests looking not only at the cohesion of groups within the larger network, but also how the groups are connected. This ties in with the previous discussion on the presence of bridging individuals within a network. In this literature, a full network consisting of several densely connected groups with minimal ties between the groups would be characteristic of *bonding social capital*. In such a structure, there would be considerable flow of information and support among members of a particular group, but little flow of support and information *between* groups. On the other hand, a full network in which groups existed (though perhaps slightly less dense), along with scattered bridging ties between the groups would be characteristic of *bridging social capital*. Such a structure would enable information and resource flow between the groups.

While the nascent work using bridging and bonding social capital has generally only used proxy measures of these constructs, one strategy would be to combine both the clustering coefficient of a network along with the average path length in the network. Such an approach underlies the burgeoning small world literature (Watts, 1999). Thus, the clustering coefficient captures the degree to which "clustered" groups exist in the network, while the average path length gives an indication of the presence of bridge persons in the network. The clustering coefficient can be measured in two ways: 1) as the average local density (i.e., first measuring the density of ties for the individual network of each actor in the larger network, and then computing the mean of these values); 2) the transitivity ratio (the proportion of closed triads).[2] Calculating the average path length was described above in the section on bridge persons.[3]

Although studying the overall network and highly connected subgroups within it is a challenging task, there is likely a high potential payoff from such a strategy for studies of health outcomes in which information flow within a community is important for understanding community level indicators of health, for example the transmission of a disease through a community or other population. One example of a study that used network structural indicators to examine community crime rates was Beyerlein and Hipp (2005), which used religious traditions as a proxy for a bridging and bonding network structure in studying crime rates in communities. This study found that while communities with more bridging social capital as measured by their proxy have less crime, those with more bonding social capital actually had higher rates of crime. A network explanation was given, positing that crime-inhibiting activities of such communities are weaker because of this disconnected network structure. Nonetheless, studies that could actually measure a community network structure rather than simply using proxies would potentially provide key insights for health-related outcomes.

Somewhat related to the notion of bridging and bonding is the concept of *homophily:* the extent to which people interacting in a network maintain close network ties to people who are similar based on various characteristics. Based on the notion that "birds of a feather flock together," this construct measures the propensity of individuals to select others similar on a particular construct when controlling for other network effects. To the extent that individuals only choose others similar to themselves, this can induce a bonding form of social capital for the overall network structure. Thus, some have suggested that homophily is negatively related to social capital (Borgatti, et al., 1998). Besides the possible impact for all the members of the network, having close ties to people like oneself can be limiting in that similar people may share the same ideas, values, and offer no new information into a social group.

---

[2] A triad is composed of three persons. Transitivity is the notion that if Fred likes Nancy, and Nancy likes Ted, then we expect it is more likely that Fred and Ted will like each other. If Fred and Ted were indeed friends, this would be considered a closed triad, whereas if they were not, it would be considered an open triad.

[3] An issue when measuring the average path length is what strategy to take when networks are not fully connected: in such an instance, some path lengths would have a value of infinity (since no number of links would traverse the network from one person to at least one other person in the network). One suggestion is to simply use a particularly large value (such as the maximum value of path lengths in the networks being studied). If the networks were of large enough size, the actual choice of value used would likely have little impact on the average path length value in the network. For smaller networks, this choice may not be so benign.

4.2. Conclusion

In sum, we have sought to present both egocentric and sociometric network measures of social capital in an accessible way for scholars across multiple disciplines. Although this chapter is by no means an exhaustive list of network measures of social capital, we believe that the measures presented here are important for furthering our understanding of social capital, across numerous fields and disciplines. Understanding social capital through a network lens involves continuing to explore associations and the theoretical reasons for how and why network measures are robust and valid indicators of social capital. We hope this chapter helps to advance future work in public health towards that end.

Appendix 1

Glossary

There are many terms that are used to understand concepts related to social capital and social networks; however, in this chapter, the focus is on terms that are most central to providing the reader with an understanding of social network concepts. This is not a comprehensive glossary of social network terms.[4]

Actor	People, organizations, communities, nation-states that make up a network.
Alter	The people who have relationships ties to an ego or focal actor in a network.
Centrality	The degree of prominence of actors in a social network.
Betweenness Centrality	The degree to which an actor lies on the shortest paths connecting others in the network.
Closeness Centrality	The degree to which an actor is close to other actors in the network.
Eigenvector Centrality	The degree to which an actor is connected to well connected others in a network.
Centralization	The variability in actor's centrality values for all actors in a sociometric network.
Closure	Occurs when all actors in a network know one another.
Cohesion	While many have defined this concept, one general definition is the solidarity existing among people who know one another.

---

[4] For a comprehensive list of terms and explanations, please refer to Wasserman and Faust (1994) Social Network Analysis: Methods and Applications or Hanneman and Riddle (2005) Social Network Methods.

Density	The extent to which all members of a network are linked to each other or the network is interconnected by direct or undirected ties.
Directed Ties	Ties that are directional, e.g., a tie going from actor A to actor B in a network, (i.e actor A reports knowing actor B)
Ego	The focal actor in an egocentric social network, the network is defined from the vantage point of this person.
Egocentric Network	A network defined from the vantage point of a single individual (focal person or ego) for some role relationship (eg., friendship)
Heterogeneity	The extent to which network members have diverse attributes.
Multiplexity	A tie characterized by more than one role relationship.
Node	A graphic representing an actor in a network diagram or sociogram.
Relation	The relationship between any pair of network across.
Social Capital	Refers to the resources available to actors through their social networks (features of social relationships) and accessed or mobilized in purposive actions.
Social Network	A finite set or sets of actors and their relations.
Social Tie	It establishes a linkage between a pair of actors.
Sociogram	A picture in which any social units are represented as points in two dimensional space, and relationships among pairs are represented by lines linking the points.
Sociometric Network	Actors in a social system with a defined boundary and the relations that exist among them. This type or a network is reffered to as a sociometic network, whole network, of full network.
Structural hole	A region in a social network where there are non-redundant sources of information due to weak ties spanning across otherwise unconnected groups.
Tie Strength	A combination of the amount of time, emotional intensity, intimacy and reciprocal services characterizing a tie, hence, the quantity of resources characterizing a relation.
Undirected Ties	Ties between two actors with no directionality, i.e., the tie from actor A to actor B is valued the same way if A reports knowing B and if B reports knowing A.

Appendix 2

4.2.1. Egocentric Networks

Egocentric networks are comprised of people identified by a focal person, and are usually defined for some specific role relationship (e.g., friendship) (Wellman, 1999). These networks do not include all of the social ties of the focal individual. They are defined from the point of view of a focal individual, person "f" (see Figure 4.1) for some role relationship (e.g., friendship), wherein

FIGURE 4.1. Egocentric network.

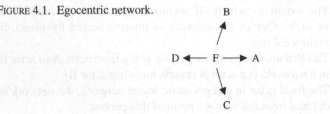

person A, B, C, and D are friends or "alters" whereas person F is referred to as the "ego" individual. Note that the three arrows are unidirectional to denote asymmetry in the tie from F to all others in the network. All three arrows are facing away from person F because it is person F that reports knowing each of the others in the network, while none of the others are asked whether they know the ego or any other alters.

4.2.2. Sociometric Networks

In contrast to egocentric networks, whole or sociometric networks include the universe of ties in a social system. For example, a whole network could be all of the social ties that exist between people in a high school class. The picture of all ties is referred to as a sociogram. The network picture below represents a hypothetical sociometric network of fourteen classmates and the friendship ties existing among them. The circles represent network actors while the lines connecting them represent social interactions between actors.

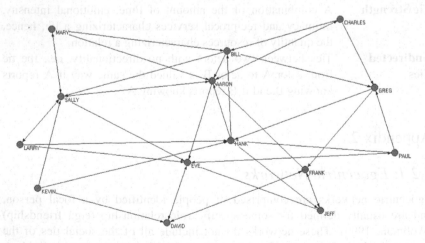

FIGURE 4.2. A hypothetical network of fourteen classmates and their friendship ties.

References

Bearman, S., Moody, J., & Stovel, K. (2004). Chains of Affection: The Structure of Adolescent Romantic and Sexual Networks. *American Journal of Sociology, 110*, 44–91.

Berkman, L. F., & Syme, S. L. (1979). Social networks, host resistance, and mortality: A nine-year follow-up study of Alameda County residents. *American Journal of Epidemiology, 109*, 186–204.

Berkman, L. F. (1986). Social networks, support, and health: Taking the next step forward. *American Journal of Epidemiology, 123*(4), 559–562.

Beyerlein, K., & Hipp, J. R. (2005). Social capital, too much of a good thing? American religious traditions and community crime. *Social Forces, 84*, 995–1013.

Blazer, D. G. (1982). Social support and mortality in an elderly community population. *American Journal of Epidemiology, 115*, 684–694.

Bonacich, P. (1987). Power and centrality: A family of measures. *American Journal of Sociology, 92*, 1170–1182.

Borgatti, S., Jones, C., & Everett, M. (1998). Network measures of social capital. *Connections, 21*(2), 36–46.

Bott, E. (1957). *Family and social network: Roles, norms, and external relationships inordinary urban families*. London: Tavistock.

Burt, R. S. (1983). "Range". In R. S. Burt & M. J. Minor (Eds.), *Applied network analysis* (pp. 176–194). Beverly Hills: Sage Publications.

Burt, R. S. (1992). *Structural holes*. Cambridge: Cambridge University Press.

Burt, R. S. (2000). The network structure of social capital. In R. I. Sutton & B. Staw (Eds.), *Research in organizational behavior, Vol. 22*. Greenwhich, Connecticut: JAI Press.

Cassel, J. (1976). The contribution of the social environment to host resistance. *American Journal of Epidemiology, 104*(2), 107–123.

Cobb, S. (1976). Social support as a moderator of life stress. *Psychosomatic Medicine, 38*(5), 300–314.

Coyne, J. C., & Lazarus, R. S. (1980). Cognitive style, stress perception, and coping. In I. L. Kutash & L. B. Schlesinger (Eds.), *Pressure point: Perspectives on stress and anxiety*. San Francisco, CA: Jossey-Bass.

Fischer, C. S., Jackson, R. M., Steuve, C. A., Gerson, K., Jones, L. M., & Baldassare, M. (1977). *Networks and places: Social relations in the urban setting*. New York: The Free Press.

Flache A., & Macy, M. W. (1996). The weakness of strong ties: Collective action failure in a highly cohesive group. *Journal of Mathematical Sociology, 21*(1–2), 3–28.

Freeman, L. C. (1979). Centrality in social networks: 1. Conceptual clarification. *Social Networks, 1*, 215–239.

Friedkin, N. E. (1991). Theoretical foundations for centrality measures. *American Journal of Sociology, 96*, 1478–1504.

Gibbs, J. P., & Martin, W. T. (1962). Urbanization, technology, and the division of labor: International patterns. *American Sociological Review, 27*, 667–677.

Gottlieb, B. H. (Ed.). (1981). *Social networks and social support*. Beverly Hills, California: Sage Publications, Inc.

Granovetter, M. S. (1973). The strength of weak ties. *American Journal of Sociology, 78*, 1360–1380.

Hall, A., & Wellman, B. (1985). Social networks and social support. In S. Cohen & S. L. Syme (Eds.), *Social support and health* (pp. 23–39). Orlando: Academic Press.

80   Lakon et al.

Hanneman, R.A., & Riddle, M. (2005). Introduction to social network methods. Riverside, CA: University of Califorina, Riverside.

Hirsch, B. J. (1980). Natural support systems and coping with major life changes. *American Journal of Community Psychology, 1980* (8), 159–172.

House J. S., & Kahn R. L. (1985). Measures and concepts of social support. In S. Cohen & S. L. Syme (Eds.), *Social support and health* (pp. 83–105). Orlando, FL: Academic Press, Inc.

House J. S., Landis K. R., & Umberson D. (1988). Social relationships and health. *Science, 241*, 540–545.

House, J. S., Robbins C., & Metzner, H. L. (1982). The association of social relationships and activities with mortality: Prospective evidence from the Tecumseh community health study. *American Journal of Epidemiology, 116*(1), 123–141.

Israel, B. A. (1982). Social networks and health status: Linking theory, research, and practice. *Patient Counseling and Health Education, 4*(2), 65–79.

Kapferer, B. (1969). Norms and the manipulation of relationships in a work context. In J. C. Mitchell (Ed.), *Social networks in urban situations: Analyses of personal relationships in Central African towns* (pp. 181–240). Manchester, England: Manchester University Press.

Krohn, M. D. (1986). The web of conformity: A network approach to the explanation of delinquent behavior. *Social Problems, 33*(6), S81–S93.

Lakon, C.M., Valente T.W. (2005). Relationships between individual and global level network characteristics and frequency of cigarette smoking among high school aged youth Paper presented at the American Public Health Association Philadephia, Pennsylvania.

Lakon, C. M., Ennett, S. T., & Norton, E., (2006) Mechanisms through which drug, sex partner, and friendship network characteristics relate to risky needle use among high risk youth and young adults. *Social Science & Medicine, 63*, 2489-2499.

Lin, N. (1990). "Social resources and social mobility: A structural theory of status attainment." In R. L. Breiger (Ed.), *Social mobility and social structure* (pp. 247–271). Cambridge: Cambridge University Press.

Lin, N. (2001). Social capital: Theory and research. In N. Lin, K. Cook, & R. S. Burt (Eds.), New York: Walter de Gruyter, Inc.

Marsden, P. V., & Campbell, K. E. (1984). Measuring tie strength. *Social Forces, 63*(2), 482–501.

Markovsky, B., & Lawler, E. J. (1994). A new theory of group solidarity. *Advances in Group Processes,* 11, 113–137.

Moody, J. (2000). *Span: SAS programs for analyzing networks: User's manual.* Columbus, OH: unpublished manuscript.

Moody, J., & White, D. R. (2003). "Social cohesion and embeddedness: A hierarchical conception of social groups." *American Sociological Review, 68*, 103–127.

Moore, S., Shiell, A., Hawe, P., & Haines, V. A. (2005). The privileging of communitarian ideas: Citation practices and the translation of social capital into public health research. *American Journal of Public Health, 95*(8), 1330–1337.

Sabidussi, G. (1966). The centrality index of a graph. *Psychomatrika, 31*, 581–603.

Schaefer, C., Coyne, J. C., & Lazarus, R. S. (1981). The health-related functions of social support. *Journal of Behavioral Medicine, 4*, 381–406.

Schoenbach, V. J., Kaplan, B. H., Fredman, L., & Kleinbaum, D. G. (1986). Social ties and mortality in Evans County, Georgia. *American Journal of Epidemiology, 123*(4), 577–591.

Scott, J. (2000). *Social network analysis, second analysis.* London: SAGE Publications.

Seeman, T. E., & Berkman, L. F. (1988). Structural characteristics of social networks and their relationship with social support in the elderly: Who provides support. *Social Science & Medicine, 26*(7), 737–749.

Seeman, T. E., Kaplan, G. A., Knudsen, L., Cohen, R., & Guralnik, J. (1987). Social network ties and mortality among the elderly in the Alameda county study. *American Journal of Epidemiology, 126*(4), 714–724.

Valente, T. W. (2006). *Bridges and potential bridges: Changing links to find critical paths and nodes in a network.* Paper presented at the International Sunbelt Social Networks Conference XXVI, Vancouver, Canada.

Valente, T. W., Hoffman, B., Ritt-Olson, A., Lichtman, K., & Johnson. C. A. (2003). Effects of a social-network method for group assignment strategies on peer-led tobacco prevention programs in schools. *Adolescent Health, 93*(11).

Valente, T. W., Unger, J., & Johnson, C. A. (2005). Do popular students smoke? The association between popularity and smoking among middle school students. *Journal of Adolescent Health, 37*(4), 323–329.

Van der Gaag, M., & Snijders, T. (2005). The resource generator: social capital quantification with concrete items. *Social Networks, 27,* 1–29.

Walker, K., MacBride, A., & Vachon, M. (1977). Social support networks and the crisis of bereavement. *Social Science & Medicine, 11,* 35–41.

Wasserman, S., & Faust, K. (1994). *Social network analysis: methods and applications.* Cambridge, UK: Cambridge University Press.

Watts, D. J. (1999). Networks, dynamics, and the small-world phenomenon. *American Journal of Sociology, 105,* 493–527.

Wellman, B., & Frank, K. (2001). Network capital in a multilevel world: Getting support from personal communities. In N. Lin, K. Cook, & R. S. Burt (Eds.), *Social capital theory and research* 223–274. New York: Walter de Gruyter, Inc.

Wellman B., & Wortley, S. (1990). Different strokes from different folks: Community ties and social support. *American Journal of Sociology, 96*(3), 558–588.

Wellman, B. (1979). The community question: The intimate networks of East Yorkers. *American Journal of Sociology, 84*(5), 1201–1231.

Wellman, B. (1999). *Networks in the global village.* Boulder, Colorado: Westview Press.

5
Actual or Potential Neighborhood Resources for Health
What Can Bourdieu Offer for Understanding Mechanisms Linking Social Capital to Health?

RICHARD M. CARPIANO

This chapter focuses on the importance of considering network-based resources and access to such resources in studying social capital and health for neighborhood or local community contexts. Specifically, it draws upon the work of French sociologist Pierre Bourdieu, whose conceptualization of social capital, as part of a more elaborate "practice theory" of the distribution of power in society (e.g., Bourdieu & Wacquant, 1992), has only recently received attention by health researchers for the study of social capital and, more broadly, socioeconomic determinants of individual and population health. Prior and on-going theoretical and empirical research are used to support the need to conceptualize neighborhood social capital as *resources* inhered within networks consisting of neighborhood residents—as well as potentially other neighborhoods and institutions—that may be used by residents for individual or mutual action. Discussion focuses on the issues concerning the incorporation of this Bourdieusian or resource-related theoretical perspective into future research on social capital and health.

5.1. Why Is a Bourdieusian Perspective Necessary?

To date, health research on social capital has almost exclusively relied upon political scientist Robert Putnam's (e.g., 1993, 1995, 2000) social capital theory (Moore, Shiell, Hawe, & Haines, 2005). However, this approach has received a variety of criticisms across several disciplines, including sociology (Lin, 2001; Portes, 1998), community development (DeFillipis, 2001), and social epidemiology (Muntaner & Lynch, 2002). In particular, the theory's heavy emphasis on interpersonal trust and norms of reciprocity downplays the importance of (1) the actual or potential resources that inhere within social networks and that may be used for personal or collective action (Carpiano & Kelly, 2005; Robert & Carpiano, 2005; Wakefield & Poland, 2005), and (2) power dynamics and how people access—or may be denied access to—these network-based resources (Morrow, 1999; Wakefield & Poland, 2005).

Bourdieu's (1986) social capital theory directly addresses these issues of resources and access. In thinking about how social class and other forms of inequality are socially reproduced (Bourdieu, 1986; Field, 2003), Bourdieu defined social capital as "the aggregate of actual or potential resources linked to possession of a durable network . . ." (1986, p. 248). These resources can be drawn upon by individual group members for pursuing individual or collective aims, either in the absence of, or in conjunction with, their own economic and cultural capital (e.g., education). In short, social capital constitutes *the resources that one possesses via being connected to others.* Conceptualizing social capital in this manner moves beyond concepts of trust and norms of reciprocity and necessitates consideration of more tangible network-based resources that people use for action. It considers that people differ vastly with regard to their social network composition and, thus, have unequal access to network-based resources, whether psychosocial, material, cultural, symbolic, or political in nature. Also, it recognizes the potential negative aspects (or "downsides") of social capital—particularly the exclusion of specific individuals from obtaining resources tied to a network (e.g., see Wacquant, 1998).

Bourdieu's approach is particularly useful when considering how neighborhoods and local areas impact residents' health and well-being. Extensive non-health research in community sociology has shown that the amount and quality of network-based resources are integrally linked to the socioeconomic conditions of the places in which people live (e.g., Small, 2004; Wacquant & Wilson, 1989). However, few health studies on social capital have, to date, used Bourdieu's conceptualization (Fassin, 2003), despite praise for its refinement (Portes, 1998) and increasing calls for its use in studying health inequalities due to its linkage to socioeconomic conditions (Baum, 2000; Carpiano, 2006; Carpiano & Kelly, 2005; Morrow, 1999; Muntaner & Lynch, 2002; Robert & Carpiano, 2005). Bourdieu's work on social capital has been overlooked by many health and non-health researchers, perhaps because some of his most elaborate work on the concept was published in French and, when translated, appeared in a sociology of education edited volume (Portes, 1998). Social capital researchers have been more likely to acknowledge Bourdieu's work versus actually incorporating it. Nevertheless, Bourdieu's theories of social action (e.g., *habitus* and *field*) have received significant attention in other areas of health research (e.g., nursing) and have now begun to see application in research on social determinants of health (e.g., see Cockerham, 2005; Frohlich, Corin, & Potvin, 2001; Veenstra, 2006).

5.2. A Bourdieu-Based Theory of Neighborhood Resources for Health

In prior work (Carpiano, 2004, 2006), I explicitly drew upon Bourdieu in conceptualizing a theoretical model of neighborhood social capital (see Figure 5.1) that considers social capital as conceptually distinct from its causes: "structural antecedents" (such as local area socioeconomic conditions) and social cohesion (which I contend, from a sociological perspective, more adequately captures

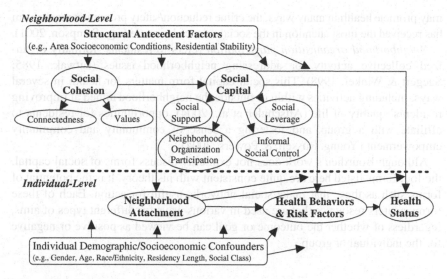

FIGURE 5.1. Conceptual model of neighborhood social capital processes on individual health outcomes.

aspects of Putnam's conceptualization of social capital). Extensive details about this model have been discussed previously, hence, my intention here is to focus on its consideration of the two most critical elements that are consistent with a Bourdieusian conceptualization of social capital: network-based resources and residents' differential access to such resources for use in pursuing a variety of ends.

5.3. Resources: Social Capital and its Four Forms

In an effort to better formulate resources, the model includes four "forms" of social capital: social support, social leverage, informal social control, and neighborhood organization participation. These forms have been extensively identified in prior community and urban sociology research as important for achieving a variety of outcomes.

Social support refers to a form of social capital that residents can draw upon to cope with daily problems (Briggs, 1998; Dominguez & Watkins, 2003) and is a critical determinant of health operating via numerous pathways (Thoits, 1995). *Social leverage* (Briggs, 1998; Dominguez & Watkins, 2003) is social capital that assists residents in accessing information pertaining to employment, child care, and other opportunities that afford individuals the possibility to minimize or avoid socioeconomic hardships that can negatively impact health and well-being (e.g., Cattell, 2001). *Informal social control* concerns residents' ability to collectively maintain social order (Sampson, 2001). It can affect health via the monitoring or surveillance of the local area and, thus, generate actual and perceived neighborhood safety (e.g., Altschuler, Somkin, & Adler, 2004). Although informal social control may promote health in many ways, the crime reduction/safety promotion mechanism has received the most attention in the social science literature (e.g., Sampson, 2001).

Neighborhood organization participation refers to residents' formally organized collective activity for addressing neighborhood issues (Litwak, 1985; Saegert & Winkel, 1998). This social capital form matters for health in several ways, including activities within or outside the neighborhood aimed at improving residents' quality of life (Altschuler et al., 2004), opportunities for residents to affiliate with a group, and fostering a sense of community and community empowerment (Young, Russell, & Powers, 2004).

Although Bourdieu's work does not explicitly discuss forms of social capital, the four forms listed here are quite consistent with his theory. It is the potential of forms such as these that make social networks useful for action. Each of these forms confers resources that are used in various ways for different types of aims, regardless of whether the outcome or goal can be viewed as positive or negative for the individual or group.

5.4. Residents' Access to Resources

A resource-based perspective also forces recognition of people's differential access or connection to forms of social capital. This issue necessitates considering individual residents' *neighborhood attachment* or degree to which a resident is integrated into a network (or even multiple networks) within the neighborhood. Such consideration can improve understandings about social capital by facilitating insights about power acquisition via neighborhood social networks (Morrow, 1999).

5.5. Empirical Research

While theoretical specificity is crucial for furthering research on social capital and health, for a theory to be useful for population health, it must be empirically testable (Carpiano & Daley, in press a, in press b). Although a resource-based approach to examining social capital is only beginning to emerge in health research, a handful of quantitative and qualitative health studies have considered aspects of this approach—with promising findings. Aspects of the theoretical ideas discussed above have been tested using two subsamples of the Los Angeles Family and Neighborhood Survey (L.A.FANS), a multi-level sample of families within 65 neighborhoods that represents one of the best publicly available US datasets for these issues.

5.6. Study 1: General Adult Sample

Carpiano's examination of social capital forms and health among adults (2004; 2007) produced findings consistent with prior theory, but, in some ways, contrary to public health ideas regarding the importance of social capital for health.

Carpiano (2004) found that higher neighborhood-level social support was positively associated with daily smoking and binge drinking (respective odds ratios of 1.59 and 1.79)—net of neighborhood socioeconomic disadvantage, residential stability, social cohesion (a composite measure capturing the level of trust and shared values in the neighborhood), the other social capital forms, and numerous individual-level demographic and socioeconomic confounders. In contrast, higher levels of social leverage and informal social control were associated with decreases in the odds of daily smoking and binge drinking (33% and 127% decreases in the odds, respectively).

While these findings are quite consistent with Bourdieu's theory—that social capital can produce both negative and positive consequences, they are intriguing for health research, which has tended to implicitly assume that social capital is only *health-beneficial*. Although smoking and drinking are often conceptualized as individual behaviors, they are commonly performed among groups. Consequently, the provision of social support social capital may offer opportunities for engaging in unhealthy as well as healthy behaviors. Not all social support may be beneficial.

Carpiano also examined whether access to resources (neighborhood attachment) moderated the relationship between social capital forms and health outcomes. For adults with a moderate level of neighborhood attachment (versus no/low neighborhood attachment), informal social control was associated with a health *advantage*, whereas neighborhood organization participation was associated with a health *disadvantage*.

The health benefits associated with informal social control for people with moderate neighborhood attachment are consistent with Durkheim's research on suicide (1951), which suggested that both low and high levels of attachment were detrimental for well-being. In some neighborhoods, highly attached residents may not be better off in terms of health because they might encounter: (1) more frequent obligations being imposed upon them to reciprocate favors (and provide resources to others) and/or (2) downward leveling norms or constraints put on their individual choices and behaviors due to strong neighborhood social mores. Both explanations are consistent with Portes' (1998) discussion of potential negative consequences of social capital.

The health disadvantage associated with neighborhood organization participation for those with moderate (versus no/low) attachment is also consistent with another issue raised by Portes (1998): social capital "free-riding." Residents with no/low attachment may benefit from formally organized groups concerned with the neighborhood (such as community associations or block clubs), but may not contribute their own time and resources towards these groups. Also, residents who are more attached to their neighborhood may receive more health risks from the demands of being involved in the neighborhood community, or their activities may be restricted to the neighborhood itself, which may be unsafe, unhealthy, or unable to provide sufficient resources to meet one's needs.

5.7. Study 2: Female Primary Caregivers

Arguing that neighborhood social capital may be more important for specific types of residents, Carpiano and Lee (2006) conducted analyses with a subsample of female primary caregivers. They similarly found that social capital forms were both positively and negatively associated with health.

While Carpiano and Lee's positive and negative results are also consistent with Bourdieu's theory, their findings obtained via testing interactions between social capital forms and neighborhood attachment suggest that, at least for this specific group, not all social capital forms may require extensive levels of network membership to access. Indeed, while some forms of neighborhood social capital may be restricted in use to particular residents, other forms may confer benefits that all may access simply via living in a particular neighborhood. However, in either situation, these benefits may be used in health promoting or health damaging ways.

5.8. Study 3: Ethnographic Research on Neighborhood Social Capital

The prior two studies examined social relationships in which certain types of resources inhere and are exchanged. However, due to the data upon which they rely, they are limited in their ability to fully examine what specific *types* of resources are exchanged and how they are beneficial or harmful for health. Therefore, identifying the types of resources that inhere within these forms of social capital and their relative utility for residential quality of life, health and well-being constitutes an important "next step" in elaborating a resource-based theory of neighborhood social capital for health.

With this issue in mind, I am presently conducting an ethnographic project in two predominantly African American, yet socioeconomically contrasted Milwaukee neighborhoods (Carpiano, 2005). One goal of this project is to identify resources that are most salient to residents across different types of neighborhoods. Although this study is on-going, the preliminary findings (based on interviews with residents and community organization service providers and observations at community meeting forums) suggest the importance of not only material, psychosocial, and political resources for achieving a variety of ends, but also informational resources (e.g., about local programs and services as well as drug houses and other dangers) and monitoring resources (e.g., possession of a number of neighbors who regularly surveil the local area for criminal or other potentially threatening activity). Integrally linked to discussions of these resources is the importance of considering how neighborhood social networks should be conceptualized as being constituted not only of residents, but also community-based organizations (CBOs) and other institutions inside the neighborhood (e.g., churches, schools, community health centers) and beyond the neighborhood (e.g., police, sanitation, and other city agencies, as well as private businesses). Consequently, the stock of social capital in a neighborhood is heavily dependent on the funding situations of these organizations and institutions (e.g., see Wacquant, 1998). These findings support the idea that social cohesion and trust in a community may not be enough to help a community or its residents achieve its aims, but that the resources found among residents and through their links to organizations and institutions likely matter as well.

5.9. Considerations for Future Research

Interest in applying a Bourdieusian perspective to the study of social capital and health is only beginning to emerge. Therefore, future research using this approach will require both qualitative and quantitative approaches.

As cogently noted by Frohlich and colleagues (2006), when one considers the type of data available in existing datasets, it becomes clear why a Putnam-based approach has been overwhelmingly favored compared to a Bourdieu perspective in what have, to date, been predominantly *inductive* investigations of social capital and health. The theoretical perspective chosen for any *deductive* study has implications for the types of measures and datasets one selects (Carpiano & Daley, 2007a; 2007b; Frohlich et al., 2007). However, to date, few public use datasets on neighborhood conditions in the US and elsewhere offer the variables necessary to test approaches informed by a Bourdieusian perspective (see Frohlich et al., 2006 for a further discussion of these epistemological issues).

Therefore, we need qualitative research to help us better understand: (1) the *processes* underlying neighborhood conditions and their implications for social capital available to network members (social capital both within and external to the neighborhood), and (2) the actions and goals in which social capital is put to use. Careful research on these questions will also be informative for creatively thinking about measures that may be used in quantitative, deductive studies. In fact, the formulation of the Bourdieu-based theoretical model I detailed above owes much to careful reading of qualitative research. Arguably, qualitative research has offered the social capital and health literature some of its greatest insights. Some examples include Klinenberg's (2003) study of the Chicago heat-wave, Erikson's (1976) examination of community ties torn apart following a flood disaster, and Cattell's (2001) comparative study of two English communities. Yet, quantitative research (particularly epidemiological research) has not kept pace and incorporated these insights.

While a resource-based approach can further our understanding of how social capital might matter in both good and bad ways for health, future work applying this approach will require datasets with resource-based social capital measures that capture more than just of the concept of social cohesion.

Some examples of potential measures include the extent—and capacity—to which residents:

1. do favors for one another, including provide child care, car rides, home maintenance/repairs, emotional support, money loans;
2. share information about jobs, social service and job training programs, health, medical care, child care; and
3. watch each other's property and personal safety, watch for/report criminal/delinquent activities,and monitor children; as well as
4. the extent, quality, and activities/initiatives of neighborhood informal and formal organizations, such as a block clubs, community boards, and community-based organizations with community organizing or social service aims. This includes organization activities/initiatives conducted alone or in conjunction with organizations and agencies located inside and outside the neighborhood.

Additionally, more extensive measures are needed to assess respondents' neighborhood attachment or placement within social networks both inside and outside of the neighborhood (e.g., proportion of a respondent's friends/family inside/outside of the neighborhood, extent to which one recognizes or interacts with neighbors, community leaders, and informal and formal community organizations).

Of course, numerous possibilities exist regarding the resources future studies should consider and the indicators used to measure them. Regardless of the resources considered, solid theoretical explication must underpin any analyses. Studies that simply regress health outcomes on a laundry list of neighborhood resource measures offer little for furthering our understanding of the mechanisms in which social capital operates for health (see Carpiano & Daley, 2007a; 2007b).

5.10. Conclusion

Pierre Bourdieu's social capital theory offers incredibly useful insight for understanding how social connections (whether in neighborhoods or in contexts that are more spatially-diffuse, such as personal networks) matter for health and well-being. However, health research on social capital to date has been heavily driven by the theoretical perspective of Robert Putnam, which, with its emphasis on features of social cohesion, has a number of limitations. While social cohesion may certainly be important for community health, overlooking the resources necessary to achieve a desired aim, as well as individuals' relative access to such resources, ignores two key factors in conceptualizing how social capital matters for understanding not only health disparities, but how quality of life and overall health can be maintained or improved within local communities.

For research on social capital and health to progress, it is essential for researchers and policy-makers to apply a wider range of theoretical perspectives on social capital. These include not only Bourdieu, but also James Coleman

(1988), Alejandro Portes (1998), Ronald Burt (2001), Nan Lin (2001), and other social scientists whom have devoted considerable theoretic and empirical attention to social capital and offer much for understanding health.

References

Altschuler, A., Somkin, C. P., & Adler, N. E. (2004). Local services and amenities, neighborhood social capital, and health. *Social Science & Medicine, 59*, 1219–1229.

Baum, F. (2000). Social capital, economic capital, and power: Further issues for a public health agenda. *Journal of Epidemiology and Community Health, 54*, 409–410.

Bourdieu, P. (1986). The forms of capital. In J. G. Richardson (Ed.), *Handbook of theory and research for the sociology of education* (pp. 241–258). New York: Greenwood.

Bourdieu, P., & Wacquant, L. J. D. (1992). *An invitation to reflexive sociology*. Chicago: University of Chicago Press.

Briggs, X. (1998). Brown kids in white suburbs: Housing mobility and the many faces of social capital. *Housing Policy Debate, 9*, 177–221.

Burt, R. S. (2001). Structural holes versus network closure as social capital. In N. Lin, K. Cook, & R. S. Burt (Eds.), *Social capital: Theory and research*. New Brunswick, NJ: Transaction Publishers.

Carpiano, R. M. (2004). *The forms of social capital: A sociomedical science investigation of neighborhood social capital as a health determinant using a Bourdieu framework*. Unpublished Doctoral Dissertation, Columbia University, New York.

Carpiano, R. M. (2005). *Come take a walk with me: Using action research to build theory and inform practice on community social capital, health and well-being*. Presented at the University of Wisconsin Department of Population Health Sciences Seminar Series, Madison, WI

Carpiano, R. M. (2006). Towards a neighborhood resource-based theory of social capital for health: Can Bourdieu and sociology help? *Social Science & Medicine, 62*(1), 165–175.

Carpiano, R.M & Daley, D. M. (2007a). A guide and glossary on post-positivist theory building for population health. *Journal of Epidemiology & Community Health, 60* (7), 564–570.

Carpiano, R. M., & Daley, D. M. (2007b). Theory building on the high seas of population health: Love Boat, Mutiny on the Bounty, or Poseidon Adventure? *Journal of Epidemilogoy & Community Health, 60*(7):574–577

Carpiano, R. M., & Kelly, B. C. (2005). What would Durkheim do? A comment on Kushner and Sterk's "The limits of social capital: Durkheim, suicide, and social cohesion." *American Journal of Public Health, 95*(12), 2120–2121.

Carpiano, R. M., & Lee, J. (2006). *Actual or Potential Neighborhood Resources and Access: Testing Ideas of Bourdieu's Social Capital Theory for the Health of Female Caregivers*. Paper presented at the Society for the Study of Social Problems annual meeting, Montreal, Quebec, Canada.

Caripiano, R. M. (2007). Neighbrhood social captial and adult health: An empirical test of a Bourdieu-based model. *Health & Place, 13*(3), 639-655.

Cattell, V. (2001). Poor people, poor places, and poor health: The mediating role of social networks and social capital. *Social Science & Medicine, 52*, 1501–1516.

Cockerham, W. C. (2005). Health lifestyle theory and the convergence of structure and agency. *Journal of Health & Social Behavior, 46*(1), 51–67.

Coleman, J. S. (1988). Social capital in the creation of human capital. *American Journal of Sociology,* 94, S95–121.

DeFillipis, J. (2001). The myth of social capital in community development. *Housing Policy Debate, 12,* 781–806.

Dominguez, S., & Watkins, C. (2003). Creating networks for survival and mobility: Social capital among African-American and Latin-American low income mothers. *Social Problems, 50,* 111–135.

Durkheim, E. (1951). *Suicide.* New York: Free Press.

Erikson, K. T. (1976). *Everything in its path: Destruction of community in the Buffalo Creek flood.* New York: Simon & Schuster.

Fassin, D. (2003). Le capital social, de la sociologie à l'épidémiologie: Analyse critique d'une migration transdisciplinaire. (full text in English at www.e2med.com/resp). *Revue Epidemiologie Sante Publique, 51,* 403–413.

Field, J. (2003). Social Capital. NewYork: Routledge.

Frohlich, K. L., Corin, E., & Potvin, L. (2001). A theoretical proposal for the relationship between context and disease." *Sociology of Health & Illness 23*(6), 776–797.

Frohlich, K. L., Dunn, J. R., McLaren, L., Shiell, A., Potvin, L., Hawe, P., et al. (2006). Understanding place and health: A heuristic for using administrative data. Health & Place, doi:10.1016/j.healthplace.2006.01.007.

Frohlich, K. L., Dunn, J. R., McLaren, L., Shiell, A., Potivn, L., Hawe. P., Dassa, C., & Thurston, W. E. (2007). Understanding place and health: A heuristic for using administrative data. *Health & Place, 13*(2), 299–309.

Klinenberg, E. (2003). *Heatwave: A social autopsy of disaster in Chicago.* Chicago: University of Chicago Press.

Lin, N. (2001). Building a network theory of social capital. In N. Lin, K. Cook, & R. S. Burt (Eds.), *Social capital: Theory and research.* New Brunswick, NJ: Transaction Publishers.

Litwak, E. (1985). *Helping the elderly: The complementary roles of informal networks and formal systems.* New York: Guilford Press.

Lochner, K. A., Kawachi, I., Brennan, R. T., & Buka, S. L. (2003). Social capital and neighborhood mortality rates in Chicago. *Social Science & Medicine 56,* 1797–1805.

Moore, S., Shiell, A., Hawe, P., & Haines, V. A. (2005). The privileging of communitarian ideas: citation practices and the translation of social capital into public health research. *American Journal of Public Health, 95,* 1330–1337.

Morrow, V. (1999). Conceptualising social capital in relation to the well-being of children and young people: A critical review. *Sociological Review, 47,* 744–765.

Muntaner, C., & Lynch, J. (2002). Social capital, class, gender and race conflict and population health: An essay review of *Bowling Alone*'s implications for social epidemiology. *International Journal of Epidemiology, 31,* 261–267.

Portes, A. (1998). Social capital: Its origins and applications in modern sociology. *Annual Review of Sociology 24,* 1–24.

Putnam, R. D. (1993). The prosperous community: Social capital and public life. *American Prospect, 13,* 35–42.

Putnam, R. D. (1995). Bowling alone: America's declining social capital. *Journal of Democracy, 6,* 65–78.

Putnam, R. D. (2000). *Bowling alone: The collapse and revival of American community.* New York: Simon and Schuster.

Robert, S. A., & Carpiano, R. M. (2005). *Our four cents: Future priority directions of research on neighborhoods, social capital, health, and aging.* Invited Position Paper for National Institute of Aging.

Saegert, S., & Winkel, G. (1998). Social capital and the revitalization of New York City's distressed inner-city housing. *Housing Policy Debate, 9*, 17–60.

Sampson, R. J. (2001). Crime and public safety: Insights from community-level perspectives on social capital. In S. Saegert, J. P. Thompson, & M. R. Warren (Eds.), *Social capital and poor communities* (pp. 89–114). New York: Russell Sage Foundation.

Small, M. L. (2004). *Villa Victoria: The transformation of social capital in a Boston barrio*. Chicago: University of Chicago Press.

Thoits, P. (1995). Stress, coping, and social support processes: Where are we? What next? *Journal of Health & Social Behavior*, Special Issue, 53–79.

Veenstra, G. (2007). Social space, social class and Bourdieu: health inequalities in British Columbia, Canada, *Health & Place 13*(1), 14–31.

Wacquant, L. J. D., & Wilson, W. J. (1989). The cost of racial and class exclusion in the inner city. *Annals of the American Academy of Political and Social Science, 501*, 8–250.

Wacquant, L. J. D. (1998). Negative social capital: State breakdown and social destitution in America's urban core. *Netherlands Journal of Housing and the Built Environment, 13*(1), 25–40.

Wakefield, S. E. L., & Poland, B. (2005). Family, friend, or foe? Critical reflections on the relevance and role of social capital in health promotion and community development. *Social Science & Medicine, 60*, 2819–2832.

Young, A. F., Russell, A., & Powers, J. R. (2004). The sense of belonging to a neighbourhood: Can it be measured and is it related to health and well being in older women? *Social Science & Medicine, 59*, 2627–2637.

6
Social Capital and Public Health
Qualitative and Ethnographic Approaches

ROB WHITLEY

Qualitative research is a broad umbrella term encompassing several specific methods and paradigms that rely on the collection, analysis and interpretation of non-statistical data. This is gathered principally through researcher-participant interaction and observation in real life settings[1] (Whitley & Crawford, 2005). Qualitative research generally aims for depth rather than breadth in description and analysis, with researchers becoming closely acquainted with one particular community or study setting. The main methods utilized in qualitative research (either in conjunction or isolation) are interviews, focus groups and (participant) observation. These methods are particularly useful in accessing the lived day-to-day experience of the relevant population, allowing investigators to intimately explore and understand phenomena from a "native" point of view. Social scientists have long relied on qualitative research to investigate the social world resulting in an extant body of respected methodological guidelines (e.g. Denzin & Lincoln, 2000; Glaser & Strauss, 1967; Miles & Huberman, 1994; Spradley, 1980). These are frequently consulted to steer design and analysis of rigorous qualitative research. There are many well-known studies utilizing qualitative research that have had a significant bearing on public health. One of the best known is that conducted by Goffman (1961) in asylums for the mentally-ill. Through regular interaction with staff and patients in situ, Goffman was able to describe and analyze the lived day-to-day experience of people within the institution, allowing him to formulate critical theory regarding the wisdom and benefit of widespread institutionalization in psychiatry.

One of the principal strengths of qualitative research, especially when applied to areas of emerging interest such as social capital, is that it allows for a full and complete empirical exploration of inchoate concepts and incipient ideas. Unlike most questionnaire research, qualitative investigation relies on open rather than closed questioning. In a reversal of traditional epistemological assumptions, study participants are considered the experts with researchers positioning themselves as

---

[1] Qualitative research is the term of preference in public health, though social scientists in other disciplines-most notably anthropology- often use the term "ethnography" to refer to the same concept. In honor of the public health tradition, the present paper utilizes the term "qualitative", respectfully noting that this is generally fungible with the term "ethnography".

enlightened lay-people. Pre-existing frameworks and definitions are not usually imposed in qualitative research; instead, these emerge from the data, rooted in the experience of ordinary people on the ground, rather than in the musings of cloistered academics in ivory towers. Resulting data can thus be conceptualized as a co-production of researcher and participants; the researcher compares and contrasts experiences of people on the ground with extant theory and literature on the topic under observation. Qualitative research thus has great potential to illuminate some of the ongoing debates regarding the definition, utility, applicability and impact of social capital in relation to public health.

6.1. Social Capital: Methodological and Conceptual Ambiguities

There are numerous acknowledged methodological and conceptual ambiguities with regards to social capital per se, and especially so as applied to public health. Papers are being increasingly devoted to this topic (Baum, 2000; Davey-Smith & Lynch, 2004; Muntaner, 2004; Navarro, 2004) indicating an indubitable exigency in clarifying well-founded concerns. In order to embed this review in current debates, I briefly outline some of the most pressing areas of ambiguity regarding inquiry into social capital and health (listed in Table 6.1 for ease of reference). These points are revisited throughout to ascertain how far qualitative studies are contributing to current controversies.

6.1.1. Varying Definitions

French sociologist Pierre Bourdieu and American political scientist Robert Putnam are generally considered to be the two most pre-eminent theorists of social capital. They take varying views regarding its definition. Bourdieu (1986) conceptualized social capital as an individual-level variable that was an aggregate of an individual's actual or potential ability to accumulate and access scarce social advantages and resources. He posited that individual biography (e.g. education) and networks (e.g. friends in high places) combined to give holders "a 'credential' which entitles them to credit, in the various senses of the word" (p249). In contrast,

TABLE 6.1. Methodological and conceptual ambiguities.

Methodological and conceptual ambiguities
• Varying definitions of the concept; Bourdieu's individual focus Vs Putnam's communitarian focus
• Lack of consensual agreement regarding appropriate unit of analysis/ level of affect; individual (micro), neighborhood (meso) or nation-state (macro)?
• Most studies have compared geographical areas. Differentials in social capital by other important socio-demographic variables (e.g. gender, ethnicity) are unexplored.
• Is there a downside to social capital?

Putnam's approach conceptualizes social capital as "features of social organizations, such as networks, norms, and trust that facilitate action and co-operation for mutual benefit" (1993: p35). Putnam's "communitarian" approach has some overlap and some discrepancy with Bourdieu's "network" approach. Both see benefit in group membership and activity. Bourdieu sees benefit as arising principally through the scope and influence of an individual's social network, which in itself is considered an outcome of individual biography. In contrast, Putnam's definition places more emphasis on horizontal civic and associational participation. Putnam further speculates that the benefit of social capital can diffuse throughout a locality by a form of social miasma, even to those contributing little to its creation and maintenance. By contrast, Bourdieu argued that benefit from social capital accrued strictly to individuals and their families. Qualitative research may be able to help unravel and unpack these two competing approaches to social capital research. Researchers can explore and elucidate the relative influence of individual networks, access to resources, collective norms and individual/ ecological trust on diverse aspects of health and well-being. Through its bottom-up epistemological orientation, qualitative research can explore social processes and mechanisms that are health-enhancing (or health damaging) without being beholden to a particular paradigm of social capital.

6.1.2. Units of Analyses and Scales of Effect

A corollary of the definitional haze regarding social capital is the choice of appropriate unit of analysis when studying social capital and health. Fukuyama (1995) suggested entire societies have levels of social capital. Putnam's early work focused on entire regions of Italy, but latterly he has focused on towns and neighborhoods. Kunitz (2004) makes a distinction between social capital in primary groups (intimate relationships) and secondary groups (voluntary associations). Bourdieu regarded social capital as primarily a property of individuals. The question of appropriate unit of analysis and scale of affect regarding social capital and health remains a bone of contention. Many studies of social capital have progressed without explicitly justifying their choice of unit of analysis. Thus theory, as well as data, is comparatively absent regarding the scale at which social capital operates. Again, open-ended qualitative investigation of people's everyday lives and behaviors could help determine the role of individual and spatial factors on health and illness.

6.1.3. Differentials in Social Capital

Bourdieu's theory implies differentials in levels of social capital between individuals of different socio-economic backgrounds whereas Putnam's theory implies differentials between geographical locations. Qualitative research could again explore these two viewpoints by examining variations in social capital by socio-economic status, neighborhood of residence and other relevant demographic variables such as gender and ethnicity. An approach focusing on theoretically at-risk groups would follow a proud tradition in qualitative research that gives voice to the silenced and disadvantaged, such as low-income women or vulnerable ethnic minorities (Benoit, Carroll, & Chaudhry, 2003; Fadiman, 1997; Graham, 1993). Unfortunately, most quantitative research has been sweeping in its approach, focusing as it has on very large samples recruited from divergent geographical contexts. These studies generally control for variables such as age, ethnicity and gender, rather than engaging in a discreet, theory-driven analysis of vulnerable sub-groups. Again, qualitative research is well-placed to enlighten thought in this area.

6.1.4. The Downside of Social Capital

Numerous commentators have argued that social capital has a frequently ignored downside. Portes (1998: p15) identified four negative consequences of social capital "exclusion of outsiders, excess claims on group members, restrictions on individual freedom and downward leveling norms". It is not difficult to imagine how these consequences could affect aspects of human health. Minorities could be excluded from plush new health services in ritzy white neighborhoods. Tight-knit families or communities low in financial capital may have excess claims on sick individuals to contribute to communal well-being, e.g. by caring for infant children whilst mothers go out to work. Individuals may feel restricted from participating in health promoting activities such as exercise, because of other demanding communal expectancies. Downward leveling norms could act to prevent individuals rising from deviant sub-cultures which foster health damaging activity such as substance abuse or unprotected sexual activity. These "fuzzy margins" of social capital have virtually never been explored in the quantitative literature on social capital and health. Reliant as the hypothesized mechanisms are on the exploration of local sub-cultures and the elucidation of hitherto un-chartered phenomena; qualitative research could considerably illuminate negativities associated with social capital.

6.1.5. Qualitative Studies of Social Capital and Health

As argued, qualitative research is well-suited to contribute to the resolution of the methodological and conceptual ambiguities previously outlined. It is thus somewhat surprising that the vast majority of recent research on social capital and health has relied on quantitative research, despite the fact that qualitative methods have long been used to elicit important aspects of the social world. In fact, one of the seminal works cited most frequently by social capital aficionados was at root a study relying on extended participant observation- De Tocqueville's (1961) "Democracy in America". This book chronicles the author's conclusions regarding contemporary American society based on a one-year journey around the continent in 1831-32. De Tocqueville noted, amongst other less-endearing characteristics (such as the insidious impact of slavery), that America was "a nation of joiners" and that this had a positive impact on various individual and supra-individual level variables. Despite the popularity of this book amongst proponents of social capital theory, little concomitant qualitative research has been conducted along-side the rapid rise of quantitative studies in recent years. Very few peer-reviewed papers have been published explicitly examining social capital and health through a qualitative lens. In a review published in 2001, Mackinko and Starfield noted the existence of only 10 empirical studies exploring the relationship between social capital and health, all of a quantitative nature. However Halpern (2004) noted that articles on social capital rose exponentially from the year 2000 onwards, giving cause for some optimism that new qualitative studies of social capital and health may begin to permeate the literature.

In light of these observations, I decided to set up systematic search criteria in order to elicit peer-reviewed papers focusing on social capital and health in the twenty-first century which would consequently be assembled and critically assessed in this chapter. Given the pre-identified paucity of studies pre-2000, I limited my search from January 2000 to March 2006 (the time of writing of this chapter). To ensure that papers were germane to health and of academic-quality (peer-reviewed), I used the search engine *med-line* to garner appropriate papers. Narrow search terminology was deliberately employed to ensure papers tangential to the main thrust of this review did not emerge. Titles, key words and abstracts were searched (with appropriate Boolean operators) for the terms "social capital", "qualitative" and "ethnographic". The aim was to extract papers that used social capital as a significant anchor of the underlying research. Acknowledging that some relevant studies may have escaped my attention, I took systematic efforts to ensure minimal leakage. The reference lists of papers gathered through the electronic search were manually searched for relevant studies hitherto concealed. Similarly I consulted recent peer-reviewed over-views of social capital and health (Almedom, 2005; Kunitz, 2004; Whitley & McKenzie, 2005) looking for relevant qualitative studies. Finally, I manually searched reference lists of the August 2004 special issue of the International Journal of Epidemiology devoted to the topic of social capital and health. These steps give confidence that all relevant studies have been harvested.

6.1.6. The Studies

Eleven studies emerged from the search, with appropriate details being given in Table 6.2 (see Table 6.2). As can be seen from the table, all bar one of the studies took place in high-income countries, six of the studies took place in England, two in Australia, one in Canada, one in the United States, and one in Peru/ Vietnam. Only one of the studies was conducted in rural locations (Peru/ Vietnam) with the rest being conducted in urban or semi-urban locations. Unlike many existing quantitative studies, none of the papers relied on secondary analysis, all data being purposely collected to examine the relationship of social capital to some aspect of health. Participants in most of the studies were recruited from the general population, though two papers focused on Afro-Caribbeans and another two focused on women. The two papers on Afro-Caribbeans were derived from the

Table 6.2. Qualitative studies of social capital and health; key characteristics.

First author	Year	Setting	Population	Sample size	Methods	Research question	Definition of/ orientation to social capital	Outcomes	Key findings
Boneham	2006	Northern English Town	Women aged 55–82	19	Interviews and focus group	"accounts of ill-health in the context of ageing were analyzed to explore the intricate ways in which social capital was created, maintained and linked to health"	Not specifically defined, Putnam invoked and quoted in the introduction	"Women's accounts of their health experiences"	Women use their networks to sustain a pro-active role in their own and other's health care.
De Silva	2006	Peru and Vietnam	Caregivers (almost all women) of young children	44	Interviews	Nested within a quantitative study evaluating the construct validity of the Social Capital Assessment Tool "qualitative cognitive interviews were conducted to explore what each question is actually measuring"	Based on Putnam "social capital is a way of describing social relationships within societies or groups of people"	"The respondent is asked a question from the SAS-CAT tool and then their thought processes behind their answers are probed"	Some items on the SCAT needed modification in light of qualitative interviews. The interviews revealed variable definitions of community, "active participation", group membership and "generalized trust" that needed further elucidation
Ziersch	2005	Adelaide suburbs	Residents	40	In-depth interviews	"explore the relationship between a number of elements of	"we draw on Bourdieu's conceptualization of social capital"	"We focus on residents' perceptions of their neighborhood	"thematic analysis linked physical neighborhood environment, perceptions of

Author	Year	Location	Sample	N	Method	Aim	Social capital conceptualization	Focus	Findings
								and the relationship with their health"	safety, civic activities and availability of services to health outcomes"
Whitley	2005	Inner-London	Residents and key-informants	32	Focus groups, interviews and ethnography	to explore how far deficits in social capital may be linked to high rates of neighborhood Common Mental Disorder (CMD)	Putnam's formulation of social capital as consisting principally of networks, trust, civic identity and reciprocity	Residents' satisfaction with components of social capital (as defined by Putnam) in the neighborhood	Residents expressed satisfaction with amenities, services, local trust and reciprocity. Lack of social capital is an inadequate explanation for high levels of CMD
Campbell	2004	South England Town	African-Caribbean mental health service users and other local community "stakeholders" from, or working with African-Caribbeans	30	Interviews and focus groups	We examine obstacles to participation by African-Caribbean lay people in local initiatives to improve mental health"	Bourdieu's conceptualization of social capital as "social relationships which may be drawn upon to advance a social group's interest"; also Putnam's distinction between "bridging" and "bonding" social capital.	To call attention to obstacles to participation in partnerships	Participation is colored by historical, economic and socio-cultural factors. These may act as obstacles to greater participation.

neighborhood life and neighborhood-based social capital, and health"

(continued)

TABLE 6.2. Qualitative studies of social capital and health; key characteristics. (continued)

First author	Year	Setting	Population	Sample size	Methods	Research question	Definition of/ orientation to social capital	Outcomes	Key findings
Altschuler	2004	Oakland, California	Residents and key-informants	49 focus group participants, 9 key informant interviews	Interviews and focus groups	"to understand ways in which residents of diverse neighborhoods in one large Californian city perceived their local communities were affecting health"	A loose generic definition, with the paper centered around Putnam's division between bridging and bonding social capital	"the meaning of neighborhood, neighborhood amenities and liabilities and the mobilization/ activism of neighborhoods"	Bonding social capital is fairly uniform across neighborhoods, but bridging social capital is disproportionately higher in high SES neighborhoods, allowing greater success in mobilization to improve the neighborhood
Campbell	2002	South England Town	African-Caribbeans	25	Interviews	"examine the impact of ethnic identity on the likelihood of peoples' participation in local community networks"	Investigation based on Putnam's formulation encapsulating "civic participation and civic engagement" but interpretation of results based on Bourdieu's emphasis on differential access and reproduction of inequalities	identifying "obstacles that stand in the way of participation of black people in community-level networks and initiatives"	"levels of participation . . . were low". This was ascribed to various factors related to ethnic identity, mainly ongoing socioeconomic exclusion and historical discrimination.

Baum	2002	Adelaide suburbs	Residents	40	Interviews	"examine the features of the study area that were perceived as health-damaging or health promoting"	Bourdieu and his ideas regarding social capital as access to resources, thereby reproducing economic relations.	barriers and facilitators to participation/ use of opportunity structures	Identified need for "third-places", greater community safety, biographical ties or pride related to the neighborhood. Barriers included monopolization, women working and decline in walking, stigma of place
Cattell	2001	Inner-London	Residents and key-informants	100 (approximately)	Interviews and ethnography	"look at aspects of poverty and exclusion, neighborhood and well-being by considering the role of social networks and social capital in the social processes involved."	Various theorists invoked in the introduction (Putnam, Coleman, Jacobs, Portes) though mostly centered on Putnam's/ Coleman's formulation.	Production of social network typologies. Variations in access to and utilization of social capital.	Participation is beneficial, but not adequate to explain deleterious affects on health
Raphael	2001	Toronto, Ontario	Key-informants (service providers and elected representatives) and residents (seniors, youth, low-income and new Canadians.)	102 residents, 17 key informants	Interviews and focus groups	"consider aspects of their community that affected quality of life . . . explore factors seen by participants as influencing health" use the notion of community quality of life	No a priori specification, grounded theory approach	New model indicating various macro, meso and micro level influences on health and well-being	Neighborhood quality of life is largely dependent on macro and meso level factors such as government retrenchment.

(continued)

TABLE 6.2. Qualitative studies of social capital and health; key characteristics. (continued)

First author	Year	Setting	Population	Sample size	Methods	Research question	Definition of/ orientation to social capital	Outcomes	Key findings
Campbell	2001	South England Town	Residents	37	Interviews	"We seek to provide an account of networks and relationships which characterize local community life and critically examine the suitability of the concept of social capital as a tool for characterizing social life in England, in the context of our broader interest in health promotion"	Testing the appropriateness of Putnam's model in a British urban setting	Personal experiences of local community life	Putnam's conceptualization does not fully capture the lived social experience of residents. It is unduly esssentialist and localized

same data, written by some of the same authors. Similarly, the two Australian studies derived from the same data and included some of the same authors.

In total, a ratio of less than two qualitative peer-reviewed papers on social capital and any aspect of human health have been published annually in the first six years of the 21st century, an astonishingly low number in comparison to quantitative studies on the same topic. The remainder of this chapter is devoted to the critical examination of these eleven papers, simultaneously exploring how far they address some of the conceptual and methodological ambiguities raised previously. The papers will be dealt with in chronological order, starting with the least recent. As will become clear during the review, this approach was empirically driven as the studies cluster together chronologically, with natural clefts corresponding with subtle conceptual changes in approaches to social capital and health.

6.1.7. 2000–2002 In the Beginning . . .

As previously noted, no qualitative studies of social capital and health were identified by a 2001 literature review (Mackinko & Starfield, 2001). My own preliminary search corroborated this conclusion. Additionally, no studies were published in the year 2000, with the first peer-reviewed qualitative studies emerging in the literature in 2001. Five studies were published in 2001–2002, three from the UK, one from Canada, and one from Australia. It is interesting to note that, despite social capital's re-discovery by Putnam, an American academic working from a leading American university, the center of gravity for the early studies was the United Kingdom, with outcrops of work occurring in two other Commonwealth countries. This may reflect more favorable funding opportunities for qualitative health research in these environments, which in turn may reflect wider epistemological orientations that value qualitative contributions to public health.

All five of the studies have considerable overlap, conducted as they were at the beginning of the concept's entry into public health. All were conducted in low-income urban or semi-urban neighborhoods. All were exploratory, with deliberately loose research questions designed to examine how the nature of community life influenced health and well-being, from the perspective of study participants. Social capital appeared to provide a convenient entrée into the focused study of urban community life and its affect on health. The developing concept appeared to speak to researchers, funders and policy-makers equally. Authors indicated that in addition to exploring social capital's relationship to health, a parallel aim of their research was to compare the grounded experience of community residents with extant definitions of social capital. This form of corroboration is of course an abiding strength of qualitative research and has been used to some effect by researchers questioning existing concepts and categories.[2] Thus, in true qualitative tradition,

---

[2] Readers are referred to Arthur Kleinman's excellent qualitative studies in Asia showing the cultural biases and conceptual fallacies inherent in extant western psychiatric nosologies (Kleinman, 1986).

concepts such as "social capital", "community" and even "health" were weakly defined a priori, with an aim being to root conceptual development in the lived experience of study participants.

Campbell and Gillies (2001) explicitly set out to critically assess the extent to which Putnam's concept of social capital encompassed the most important elements of local community life in a UK setting. This was done in the context of the authors' (and the British Government's) broader interest in health promotion and community-level interventions. They conducted 37 in-depth interviews in a town in Southern England exploring personal experiences of local community life. They found that Putnam's formulation of social capital failed to capture many important elements of community social activity important in a British setting that may affect health, most notably informal networks and networks extending beyond the locality. Similarly, their data suggested Putnam's concept failed to pay attention to the role of socio-demographic variation *within* the locale. Social capital appeared to interact with age, gender, ethnicity and housing tenure. Taken in the round, this study indicated the limitations of Putnam's emphasis on formal activity and on local norms and networks. It also suggested within-neighborhood variation in levels of social capital, with some sub-groups being privileged over others, this phenomena being a natural corollary of Bourdieu's thesis. This study demonstrated the complexity of social life when considered through an ethnographic lens, this being an important counterfoil to contemporary quantitative studies of social capital and health which generally treated geographical entities as homogenous in nature, and were rather uncritical in their acceptance of Putnam's definition. As a conceptual tool for characterizing local community life in England, social capital as defined by Putnam was inadequate. Measurement of narrowly defined social capital may be missing active ingredients of community life that influence health.

A rather similar conclusion was drawn by Cattell (2001) who conducted approximately 100 interviews with residents and key informants in two low-income neighborhoods in London. Cattell's aim was an open-ended investigation of how social capital and social networks interact with poverty and exclusion to influence grounded notions of health and well-being. Her design and analysis were mostly centered on Putnam's definition of social capital. From the point of view of residents, participation in networks and neighborhood social capital could moderately buffer some of the negative effects of being poor in a poor neighborhood, however overall impact was mild considering the ongoing adverse effects of poverty, unemployment and social exclusion. Overall, this study cautioned against some of the speculative enthusiasm greeting the concept of social capital at the time, strongly suggesting that more concrete socio-economic variables such as poverty, unemployment, lack of opportunity and fear could over-ride any health-enhancing behaviors or affective responses concomitant with a strong sense of community pride or belonging. Like Campbell and Gillies (2001), Cattell found little participation in formal activities and organizations. In contrast, activities within families and informal events were more common. This supports the view that many important elements of British social life are missed by Putnam's definition. The two hitherto considered studies suggested that old-fashioned terms such as "community spirit" may encompass more meaningful components of communal life in the UK setting than social science's vogue jargon- "social capital".

Moving across the Atlantic, Raphael et al. (2001) conducted a qualitative study of social capital and health in a low-income neighborhood of Toronto, Ontario. Rather like the two previous studies, the authors set out to loosely investigate how residents thought about neighborhood life, exploring what was perceived to be health promoting and health damaging. 102 residents and 17 key informants took part in interviews and focus groups designed to elicit opinions on neighborhood-influences on health. Unlike the previous studies, the authors do not set out to test the applicability of Putnam's definition, but instead ground their outcomes in the day-to-day experience of participants, a true grounded-theory bottom-up approach. Like Cattell, they found that participants imputed meso-level and macro-level factors as the most important influences on health, considerably out-weighing any positive effect of micro-level social capital on health. Having said that, participants did value caring and concerned neighbors and local amenities, but effect on health appeared to be minimal in comparison to factors such as ongoing unemployment, deteriorating economic conditions and weakening finan-cial safety nets for low-income people. Based on their results, the authors argue that Putnam is "remarkably myopic" for not considering the role of economic marginalization and macro/ meso level factors. Their data seems to bear out such an assertion.

Baum and Palmer (2002) conducted a similar study in Adelaide, Australia. 40 residents, divided into divided into "high" and "low" Community participators took part in in-depth interviews. Again, they had a loose research question examining which features of the study area were perceived by residents as health-damaging or health-promoting. Safety, community amenities and connectedness to the area were all considered by participants as important aspects of a healthy community. The presence of these factors appeared to encourage participation and the build up of social capital. Unlike the previous studies, the authors embed their analysis in the work of Bourdieu, noting that historic, economic and socio-cultural factors deter-mine the nature of community-spirit in urban districts. Neighborhoods and neigh-borhood characteristics are thus conceptualized as dialectical outcomes of complex historical, economic and socio-cultural phenomena, rather than as static "independ-ent" variables, which some social capital research implicitly assumes.

All the above studies share common components. Firstly they all have loose research questions, aiming to simultaneously explore conceptualizations of social capital as well as potential influence on health and illness. Discussion of social cap-ital was embedded in progressive public health paradigms such as health promotion and the health inequalities literature. Results from the studies converged signifi-cantly. Considering the recent entry of the concept into public health, these studies understandably did not focus on the downsides of social capital, firstly examining its potential use as a heuristic for health-promotion. All of the studies examine urban or semi-urban districts, conceptualizing social capital at a small-area level. All studies invoke Putnam, almost all suggesting that his conceptualization of social capital was missing important elements of community life, notably informal net-work and extra-locale participation. They also agreed that Putnam's focus on micro-level processes obscures investigation of important influences on health in the neighborhood that are dependent upon meso- and macro- level factors (e.g. govern-ment retrenchment). Being the first qualitative studies of social capital and health, the studies dealt with above mostly recruited from the general population of neigh-borhoods under investigation. However the last study to be considered in this sec-tion focused on one specific population sub-groups, perhaps mindful of suggestions from previous research that important socio-demographic sub-groups within the same neighborhood could differentially experience social capital.

Campbell and McClean (2002) interviewed 25 African-Caribbean residents of a South England town in order to examine the impact of ethnic identity on the likelihood of participation in local community networks. This study was mindful of contemporary policy in the UK encouraging greater participation as a source of empowerment and health promotion. Such participation is also considered a defining factor of "high" social capital communities. The authors found low lev-els of participation by African-Caribbeans, with present behavior determined by historical discrimination and ongoing socio-economic exclusion. They concluded that universal calls to participate may lead to further marginalization of socially-excluded groups, as the already privileged may use their entrenched power and capabilities to disproportionately respond to such calls in an assertive and confi-dent manner. Rather than focusing on between-locale differences (a cornerstone of most quantitative studies) this research indicated some of the disproportionate obstacles *within* a neighborhood which act against an ethnic minority's potential participation. The authors correctly frame their interpretation in Bourdieu's con-cept of social capital, indicating how social capital (or lack thereof) can play a role in perpetuating extant social inequalities.

6.1.8. 2003–2006: Growth and Diversification

This section deals with studies published from 2003 to the present. Interestingly, no studies were published in 2003, again indicating the incipient nature of the concept's entry into public health. However two studies a year have been pub-lished from 2004 to 2006, indicating small but steady interest in the impact of social capital on health.

Campbell, Cornish and McClean (2004) continued their study of the same South England town by focusing their attention on African-Caribbean mental health service users and other African-Caribbean community stake-holders. Again this marks an interesting watershed in the literature, as it is the first time participants have been wholly sampled from consumers of a specific health service. 30 service-users and other community stakeholders took part in inter-views or focus groups discussing obstacles to participation in local "partner-ships" and communal initiatives to improve mental health. Like their previous study of African-Caribbeans, they found that obstacles to participation were determined by historical, economic and socio-cultural factors. Again they bring their discussion back to Bourdieu, arguing that marginalized groups such as African-Caribbeans do not have the social, educational, temporal or financial resources necessary to participate in local "partnerships". Trite calls to participate in local networks, unmindful of socio-historical context, are therefore unlikely to be answered by vulnerable groups. In fact, these "acultural" paradigms of participation may accentuate associated marginalization by amplifying African-Caribbean's estrangement from the mainstream. Three years after the first peer-reviewed qualitative study of social capital and health was published, this study is singular in that it is equally centered around the work of Bourdieu as that of Putnam. The ethnographic flow of studies focusing on Putnam's concept of social capital appeared to be receding.

In 2004, Altschuler, Somkin and Adler published the first qualitative study of social capital and health to be conducted in the United States. Like the previous studies, the location for the study was in urban districts, with some data being collected in both higher and lower income neighborhoods. 49 people took part in focus groups and 9 in key informant interviews in Oakland, California, designed to understand ways in which participants felt that their local communities were affecting health. The authors center their analysis on Putnam's division of social capital into "bonding" and "bridging"; bonding referring to intra-neighborhood inwardly-focused trust and cohesion, bridging referring to externally-focused links to other neighborhoods, bodies and organizations. Safety in the neighborhood appeared to be the most prominent theme in terms of well-being, a phenomenon occasionally emerging in previous studies, but not predominant. This may reflect higher-levels of crime and violence in US cities compared to the sites of the studies previously considered (urban areas in Canada, Australia and the UK). The authors also found that stores of bonding social capital were uniform across neighborhoods, however higher-income neighborhoods had greater amounts of bridging social capital than lower-income, allowing them to successfully lobby local leadership and act appropriately to protect neighborhood interests (e.g. preventing city attempts to change lighting or local tax-rates). Though the authors do not embed their discussion in the work of Bourdieu, like the previous study, their analysis suggests that access to elites and collective resources (mainly financial and temporal) are key determinants of a neighborhood's ability to protect its own interests, many of which will be related to health and well-being. This ability seemed to outweigh any positive effect of intra-neighborhood trust and reciprocity when de-contextualized from the wider socio-economic milieu.

Similar results were found in an Australian study (Ziersch, Baum, & MacDougall, 2005), linked to the 2002 Australian paper previously discussed. Again the authors analyzed the same 40 interviews outlined in the 2002 study, further focusing on residents' perceptions of their neighborhood and relationship with health. In this paper, results were triangulated with parallel quantitative findings from a larger epidemiological survey. This is the first instance of a mixed-method design being employed to study social capital and health, with the results demonstrating the potential of such an approach. Like some of the earlier studies, perceptions of safety were linked to health and well-being in both the qualitative and

quantitative analysis. The authors' data also converged with the developing literature, suggesting that socio-economic factors unrelated to social capital have
independent and much stronger effects on health than any of the classical components of Putnam's theory of social capital (trust, connections, reciprocity).

Whitley and Prince (2005) similarly found minimal evidence linking neighborhood trust and reciprocity (bonding social capital) to positive health, in particularly mental health. In a study of a London neighborhood with atypically high
prevalence of anxiety and depression, 32 residents took part in interviews and
focus groups assessing residents' satisfaction with neighborhood trust, amenities
and community life. Half of the residents sampled had an identifiable mental illness (anxiety or depression); the other half being mentally healthy. The aim was
to explore how aspects of social capital were perceived to impact on mental health
and illness, and whether lack of social capital may be an explanatory factor determining high prevalence. Residents expressed satisfaction with almost all aspects
of community life (except fear of crime), regardless of their mental health status,
suggesting high-levels of social capital. Few linked their psychological suffering
to neighborhood-level factors, most attributing their distress to the deleterious
impact of individual-level risk factors such as unemployment, low-income, dys-
functional family dynamics and other forms of life-span insult. This study represents a further diversification of approaches, as it was the first to attempt to link
social capital (or lack thereof) to specific nosological outcomes (anxiety and
depression), rather than the grounded, generic concept of "health and well-being"
used by most previous studies.

Further specialization of the literature is represented in a study conducted by
Boneham and Sixsmith (2006). This was the first study to focus solely on women,
informed by previously discussed theory and research suggesting that social capital could be experienced differentially according to socio-demographic sub-
group. 19 women aged 55–82, living in a North England Town participated in
interviews and focus groups. The aim of the study was to elicit women's accounts
of their health experiences exploring the ways social capital was created, maintained and linked to health. Like the previous British studies, informal support
and information from family and friends was more common and important than
associational involvement. Women also played a significant role in the creation of
social capital, being frequently consulted as "lay health experts" by friends and
family. Like the studies with African-Caribbeans, this paper suggested potential
downsides to social capital; in this case lay leaders felt their involvement was not
valued or rewarded by either professionals or other community members. This
challenges notions that have placed a sole emphasis on the positive aspects of
social capital.

The final study considered in this review (De Silva et al., 2006) is somewhat
atypical in various respects. Firstly, it is the only qualitative study to be conducted
in low-income countries, Peru and Vietnam, some of the participants additionally
coming from rural areas. Furthermore, the research question was dissimilar to
that posed in the other studies; in this case, the authors were principally
concerned with validation of a quantitative screening measure designed to assess

levels of social capital– the short version of the Social Capital Assessment Tool, a tool based mostly on Putnam's notion of social capital. In total 44 open-ended interviews were conducted with caregivers of young children (almost all women) in order to explore how each question on the SCAT was interpreted by study participants. Data was analyzed to test the construct validity of the SCAT. The interviews revealed that participants had varying definitions of "community". Vietnamese participants linked community to the geographically bounded commune, whereas the majority of Peruvians conceptualized community by function rather than geography, i.e. who was providing solace and support, regardless of propinquity. In light of these findings, the authors suggested modifications to the SCAT to improve construct validity of the SCAT in Vietnam and Peru. Whilst the authors' findings were centered on psychometrics rather than health outcomes, this study is interesting in that findings reinforce conclusions from previously considered studies that the nature and scope of social and communal life vary significantly according to the culture under consideration. In this study, the authors decided to use their data to modify the screening tool so that participants could focus more narrowly on Putnam's conceptualization of "social capital". An alternative approach would have been to use the data to expand the concept and stretch the limits of extant definitions.

6.1.9. The Qualitative Contribution

Taken in the round, the qualitative studies considered in this review converge in numerous different areas (see Table 6.3). Almost all studies agree that Putnam's conceptualization of social capital does not capture important aspects of community life, such as informal networks, family support and fear of crime. This finding cautions against the use of the concept of "social capital" as a proxy for diverse neighborhood-level socio-cultural events and processes. Old-fashioned as it may sound, the term "community spirit" may be a more appropriate heuristic

TABLE 6.3. Key findings of qualitative studies.

Key findings
• Putnam's definition of social capital fails to capture important health-impacting dimensions of local community life, most notably informal networks, family support and fear of crime.
• Networks beyond the local community have an important function, but this is neglected in neighborhood-based conceptualizations of social capital.
• Community participation is determined by complex historical and socio-economic variables, naïve calls to participate tend to be ignored by the marginalized giving further power to those with extant hegemony
• Neighborhoods are "downstream" outcomes determined by social, historical and economic factors. Attention must be paid to the idea that neighborhoods are not necessarily upstream "independent" variables.
• Sub-groups within the same neighborhood may experience social capital differently. Race, age and gender appear to be important variables in this regard.
• The mildly positive impact of social capital on health appears to be overwhelmed by more powerful health-damaging factors such as poverty, unemployment and life-span insult.

than "social capital" to encapsulate important elements of neighborhood life influencing health. In fact many of the studies indicate that health research has focused too narrowly on Putnam's "communitarian" conceptualization of social capital, to the detriment of Bourdieu's formulation of social capital as a "credential" by which individuals and groups can buy into positive benefits. The qualitative studies suggest that a further focus on Bourdieu's conceptualization of social capital as an exposure variable may reveal highly-relevant links to health outcomes, especially in terms of health inequalities.

This leads to another key contribution of the qualitative studies, namely the documentation of complex differentials in social capital *within* neighborhoods and between socio-demographic groups. All the qualitative studies emphasize that social capital is not a stand-alone variable shared equally within a population, in isolation from wider contextual variables. For example, the studies with African-Caribbeans suggest that "levels of social capital" may simply be epiphenomena of more influential historical and socio-economic processes, in this case discrimination and marginalization. The studies converge to suggest that social capital varies within the same neighborhoods between sub-groups, with women, older people, and ethnic minorities experiencing social capital in a differential manner. As part of Putnam's miasma-like theory, neighborhood social capital has hitherto generally been treated like ambient air temperature, an area level variable which all residents experience equally. In fact, the qualitative studies suggest that social capital may be more like indoor air temperature, a variable somewhat dependent upon ambient air temperature, but open to manipulation by those who have money, apparatus and know-how, through interventions such as central heating and air-conditioning. In contrast, the marginalized may be at the mercy of "meteorological" processes, whether they like them or not, with few resources available to alter or change events to their advantage.[3] Again, greater application of Bourdieu's theory of social capital may be important in this regard.

By the nature of the in-depth methodological approach, qualitative studies have focused on small neighborhoods as a unit of analysis in social capital. This has led to some interesting findings with regards to the ambiguities over appropriate unit of analysis with regards to social capital. The studies did suggest that small neighborhoods were an appropriate unit of analysis; though they cautioned against the proclivity to treat neighborhoods as independent, exposure variables. Most studies suggested that neighborhoods themselves are "downstream" outcomes, determined by complex historical, political, economic, social and cultural processes and events. In other words, if neighborhoods are to be treated as a unit of analysis, attention must be paid to their contextual complexities. This can be seen in action in the studies of African-Caribbeans in the UK. Long marginalized

---

[3] Hurricane Katrina comes to mind in this regard. Whilst the poor population of New Orleans were left at the mercy of meteorological processes, the rich population effortlessly protected their health and well-being through adaptation to changing ambient conditions (by using their money and cars to leave the city).

and ostracized within their neighborhoods, African-Caribbeans were low community participators, showing a distinct unwillingness to engage with new neighborhood "health partnerships" or "health initiatives". A related point is that almost all of the qualitative studies suggest that networks and relationships beyond the local community play an important role in health and well-being. This fact is negated by a geographical approach to social capital which sometimes assumes an almost "medievalist" position with regards to social and communal life in the modern world.

To conclude this section, it should be noted that whilst the qualitative studies almost unanimously suggest that social capital can play a minor role in protecting some aspects of health and well-being, this pales into relative insignificance when wider socio-economic variables such as employment, income, discrimination and life-span insult are taken into account.

6.2. Conclusion

Table 6.4 indicates principal interstitial terrain with regards to the qualitative study of social capital and public health. Few studies have been conducted in rural locations or in low-income countries. None have focused on the downside of social capital, even though deviant sub-cultures may facilitate the spread and maintenance of health-damaging behaviors (Portes, 1998). With its roots firmly entrenched in the disciplines of anthropology and sociology, qualitative research could be the way forward to address some of these deficits in the literature. Multi-site studies, for example the comparison of rural and urban districts, may be one comparative technique useful for the illumination of differential communal social exposures and related health outcomes.

However to close this paper, a wider question must be asked before researchers are admonished to go forth and collect more qualitative data in the area of social capital and health. Numerous qualitative and quantitative studies have suggested that the social environment undoubtedly affects health and well-being (Frohlich, Corin, & Potvin, 2001; Yen & Syme, 1999). Nevertheless as this review indicates, narrowly focused studies utilizing social capital as a proxy for the social world may be missing important elements of the lived, communal experience influencing health and well-being amongst community members. This review suggests that the social experience of participants has a bearing on their health and well-being; however this social experience is colored by economic, historical, cultural

TABLE 6.4. Gaps in the literature and future research.

Future Research
• Studies examining the downside of social capital
• Studies in non-urban settings
• Studies in low-income countries
• Multi-site Studies

and social factors beyond the predominant definitions of social capital. New studies must advance in a manner commensurate with such knowledge, ensuring experience is appropriately contextualized so that health inequalities are not fallaciously attributed to an absence of social capital, which may simply be an epiphenomena of stronger currents within and around neighborhoods and localities.

References

Almedom, A. M. (2005). Social capital and mental health: an interdisciplinary review of primary evidence. *Social Science and Medicine, 61*, 943—964.

Altschuler, A., Somkin, C. P., & Adler, N. E. (2004). Local services and amenities, neighborhood social capital, and health. *Social Science and Medicine, 59*, 1219–1229.

Baum, F. (2000). Social capital: Is it good for your health? Issues for a public health agenda. *Journal of Epidemiology and Community Health, 53*, 195–196

Baum, F., & Palmer, C. (2002). Opportunity structures: Urban landscape, social capital and health promotion in Australia. *Health Promotion International, 17*, 351–361.

Benoit, C., Carroll, D., & Chaudhry, M. (2003). In search of a healing place: aboriginal women in Vancouver's Downtown Eastside. *Social Science and Medicine, 56*, 821—833.

Boneham, M. A., & Sixsmith, J. A. (2006). The voices of older women in a disadvantaged community: Issues of health and social capital. *Social Science and Medicine, 62*, 269–279.

Bourdieu, P. (1986). The forms of capital. In J. G. Richardson (Ed.), *Handbook of theory and research for the sociology of education* (pp. 241–258). New York: Greenwood.

Campbell, C., & Gillies, P. (2001). Conceptualising 'social capital' for health promotion in small local communities: a micro-qualitative study. *Journal of Community and Applied Social Psychology, 11*, 329–346.

Campbell, C., & McClean, C. (2002). Ethnic identities, social capital and health inequalities: Factors shaping African-Caribbean participation in local community networks in the UK. *Social Science and Medicine, 55*, 643–657.

Campbell, C., Cornish, F., & McClean, C. (2004). Social capital, participation and the perpetuation of health inequalities: obstacles to African-Caribbean participation in 'partnerships' to improve mental health. *Ethnicity and Health, 9*, 313–335.

Cattell, V. (2001). Poor places, poor people, and poor health: the mediating role of social networks and social capital. *Social Science and Medicine, 52*, 1501–1516.

Davey-Smith, G., & Lynch, J. (2004). Commentary: Social capital, social epidemiology and disease aetiology. International *Journal of Epidemiology, 33*, 691–700

Denzin, N. K., & Lincoln, Y. S. (2000). *Handbook of qualitative research*. Thousand Oaks CA: Sage.

De Silva, M. J., Harpham, T., Tuan, T., Bartolini, R., Penny, M. E., Huttly, S. R. (2006). Psychometric and cognitive validation of a social capital measurement tool in Peru and Vietnam. *Social Science and Medicine, 62*, 941–953.

De Tocqueville, A. (1961). *Democracy in America*. New York NY: Schocken Books.

Fadiman, A. (1997). *The spirit catches you and you fall down: A Hmong child, her American doctors, and the collision of two cultures*. New York: Noonday Press.

Frohlich, K. L., Corin, E., & Potvin, L. (2001). A theoretical proposal for the relationship between context and disease. *Sociology of Health and Illness, 23*, 776—797.

Fukuyama, F. (1995). *Trust: The social virtues and the creation of prosperity*. New York NY: The Free Press.

Glaser, B., & Strauss, A. (1967). *The discovery of grounded theory*. Chicago IL: Aldine.

Goffman, E. (1961). *Asylums*. New York: Doubleday.

Graham, H. (1993). *When life's a drag: Women, smoking and disadvantage*. London: HMSO.

Halpern, D. (2004). *Social capital*. Cambridge: Polity Press.

Kleinman, A. (1986). *Social origins of distress and disease: depression, neurasthenia and pain in modern China*. New Haven CT: Yale University Press.

Kunitz, S. (2004). Social capital and health. *British Medical Bulletin, 69*, 61–73.

Mackinko, J., & Starfield, B. (2001). The utility of social capital in research on health determinants. *Milbank quarterly, 79*, 387–427.

Miles, M., & Huberman, A. (1994). *Qualitative data analysis*. Thousand Oaks CA: Sage.

Muntaner, C. (2004). Commentary: Social capital, social class, and the slow progress of psychosocial epidemiology. *International Journal of Epidemiology, 33*, 674–680.

Navarro, V. (2004). Commentary: Is capital the solution or the problem? *International Journal of Epidemiology, 33*, 672—674.

Portes, A. (1998). Social capital: Its origins and applications in modern sociology. *Annual Review of Sociology, 24*, 1–24.

Putnam, R. (1993). *Making democracy work; civic traditions in modern Italy*. Princeton NJ: Princeton University Press.

Raphael, D., Renwick, R., Brown, I. Steinmety, B., Sehder, H., Philliphs, S. (2001). Making the link between community structure and individual well-being: Community quality of life in Riverdale, Toronto, Canada. *Health and Place, 7*, 179–196.

Spradley, J. P. (1980). *Participant observation*. London: Thomas Learning.

Whitley, R., & Prince, M. (2005). Is there a link between rates of common mental disorder and deficits in social capital in Gospel Oak, London? Results from a qualitative study. *Health and Place, 11*, 237–248.

Whitley, R., & Crawford, M. (2005). Qualitative Research in Psychiatry. *Canadian Journal of Psychiatry, 50*, 108–114.

Whitley, R., & McKenzie, K. (2005). Social capital and psychiatry: Review of the literature. *Harvard Review of Psychiatry, 13*, 71–84.

Yen, I. H., & Syme, S. L. (1999). The social environment and health. *Annual Review of Public Health, 20*, 287–308.

Ziersch, A. M., Baum, F. E., & MacDougall, C. (2005). Neighbourhood life and social capital: the implications for health. *Social Science and Medicine, 60*, 71–86.

7
The Economic Approach to Cooperation and Trust
Lessons for the Study of Social Capital and Health

LISA R. ANDERSON AND JENNIFER M. MELLOR

A rapidly growing empirical literature from across the social sciences relates social capital to a diverse array of indicators of well-being, including economic growth (Knack & Keefer, 1997), labor force participation (Aguilera, 2002), violent crime (Galea, Karpati, & Kennedy, 2002), political corruption (La Porta et al., 1997), and even self-reported happiness (Bjornskov, 2003). Of all the phenomena thought to be affected by social capital, health and health-related outcomes have received the greatest attention, evidenced in part by the contributions in this volume. Yet, despite repeated findings of a statistical association between social capital and various health outcomes[1] and risk factors,[2] as well as the existence of plausible causal pathways linking social capital to individual health,[3] many health economists are skeptical of the importance of social capital for health (e.g., Mellor & Milyo, 2005).

---

[1] Selected examples of the many types of health outcomes studied in relation to social capital include mortality (Kawachi, Kennedy, Lochner, & Prothrow-Stith, 1997), self-reported health status (Subramanian, Kim, & Kawachi, 2002), cardiovascular disease (Kaplan et al., 1988), sexually-transmitted diseases (Holtgrave & Crosby, 2003), dementia (Fratiglioni et al., 2000), and the severity of the common cold (Cohen, Doyle, Skoner, Rabin, & Gwaltney, 1997).

[2] Several studies have focused on health-related behaviors, such as binge drinking (Weitzman & Kawachi, 2000), drug use (Lo Sciuto, Rajala, Townsend, & Taylor, 1996), tobacco use (Silvia, Thorne, & Tashjian, 1997), teen childbearing (Gold, Kennedy, Connell, & Kawachi, 2002), child abuse (Saluja, Kotch, & Lee, 2003), handgun ownership (Hemenway, Kennedy, Kawachi, & Putnam, 2001), physical activity (Lindstrom, Hanson, & Ostergren, 2001), and health care utilization (Deri, 2005). Related studies have examined the effects of social capital on access to care (Hendryx, Ahern, Lovrich, & McCurdy, 2002), trust in providers (Ahern & Hendryx, 2003), and health insurance coverage among the elderly (Beiseitov, Kubik, & Moran, 2003).

[3] Theoretical explanations for the influence of social capital on health suggest several distinct potential pathways. For example, social capital may ameliorate the stress of modernity and its concomitant effects on individual health and health-related behaviors (Wilkinson, 1996). Alternatively, social capital may expand the informational resources available to individuals, including information about access to quality health care, or the health consequences of individual behavior. Finally, social capital may lead to increased political support for the provision of public goods and social welfare programs (Kawachi et al., 1997).

117

Part of the skepticism arises from the definition of social capital itself as the attributes of organizations or communities that facilitate mutual cooperation and trust. This leads to the question of which attributes constitute social capital, a subject of some debate. On the one hand, Coleman (1988) and Putnam (2000) argue that social capital is not merely the aggregation of individual attributes of group members, but rather a group-level (or contextual) phenomenon. On the other hand, empirical researchers often quantify social capital as the average level of either individual civic participation or generalized trust in others in a particular community, or even by individual-level measures of trust and participation.[4] While such measures may be viewed as proxies for latent characteristics of the relevant community (e.g., social capital), they may instead proxy for latent individual characteristics. Consequently, statistical evidence of an association between social capital and health may reflect only a spurious relationship driven by omitted individual attributes.

This ambiguity is just one reason that social capital research has been critiqued by economists. However, decades of economic research in the fields of game theory and experimental economics and several recent non-experimental empirical studies all provide substantial guidance as to the determinants of cooperation and trust. One lesson that emerges from the economic literature is that both group attributes and individual-level attributes are determinants of cooperation and trust.

In this essay, we describe several important connections between the existing economic literature on games and experiments and the study of social capital. In the next section, we briefly review some of the more general and non-technical concerns expressed by economists about social capital research. In section 7.2, we describe some important predictions from game theory regarding the determinants of social capital. Section 7.3 summarizes relevant findings from economic analyses of data from surveys and human subject experiments. In the final section, we elaborate on the implications of these findings for the empirical literature on social capital and health, and discuss several challenges for future policy-relevant research in this area.

7.1. Economists and Social Capital

The concept of social capital has been a lightning rod for criticism from economists (e.g., Durlauf 1999, 2002; Glaeser, Laibson, Scheinkman, & Soutter, 2000; Sobel, 2002). Complaints include the vagueness of the definition of social capital, the reliability of survey data for measuring social capital, and the inferences made from statistical associations between social capital and various measures of well-being. However, much of economists' skepticism of social capital is rooted in the

---

[4] Other measures include voting (Putnam, 2000), blood donation (Guiso, Sapienza, & Zingales, 2004), and mail response rates to the 2000 census (Vigdor, 2004).

inherent difficulties of translating across disciplines. Further, social capital remains something of a contested construct, with different disciplines honing in on distinct (albeit related) definitions of the term.[5] For example, among sociologists, social capital may be taken to mean the informational or material resources of social networks, while in political science, the term is most often associated with determinants of mutual cooperation and trust.[6] With different denotations across disciplines, it is not surprising that even sympathetic audiences are sometimes left with the impression that social capital is a nebulous concept (e.g., Hawe & Shiell, 2000).

A more idiosyncratic reason for skepticism among economists stems from the socialization of the discipline itself. By training, economists strive to explain social phenomena as the product of individual motivations and constraints, and are unlikely to be satisfied with group-level explanations. Discussions that define social capital as a group-level attribute are less persuasive, and instead, economic studies of social capital focus on individual-level trust and cooperation (Alesina & La Ferrara, 2000, 2002; Costa & Kahn, 2003a,b).

Economists also tend to distrust "attitudinal" measures from surveys, such as whether an individual expresses generalized trust in others. Questions about attitudes can be highly speculative and subject to interpretation by the respondent, as opposed to questions focused on specific trusting behaviors, such as loaning money to friends, or locking doors. Further, because survey respondents are not compensated for answering in a truthful or thoughtful manner, economists tend to doubt the reliability of their responses, especially in those cases where respondents are asked to make difficult mental calculations or may have self-interested reasons to answer insincerely. Of course, survey responses are the mainstays of social capital measurement (e.g., generalized trust in others and participation in voluntary associations). This has led several economists to study the reliability of attitudinal measures of social capital (e.g., Anderson, Mellor, & Milyo, 2004; Glaeser et al., 2000).

This brief discussion demonstrates that despite the critical reaction of many economists to the concept of social capital research, several economists are actively engaged in research on this subject. Beyond this, however, we argue that there is in fact a long-standing theoretical and empirical tradition in economics that is largely consistent with the concept of social capital as popularized by Robert Putnam. In the following sections we describe some of the key insights from this literature as they pertain to the study of social capital.

---

[5] Economist Glenn Loury (1977) coined the term "social capital" to describe how individuals of different races are affected by social perceptions about their race; however, that particular usage of the term never gained widespread currency.

[6] Among economists, particularly those who study labor markets, education, and household decision making, the potential importance of social networks and peer influences have long been acknowledged, but typically have not been framed as social capital. For recent examples, see Carman (2004) and Cooley (2005).

7.2. Predictions from Game Theory

The concepts of cooperation and trust embedded in the definition of social capital are often modeled by economists using game theory. Broadly speaking, games that highlight the tension between individual self-interest and what is best for a group are classified as social dilemmas. In this section, we will describe the most well-known social dilemma – the prisoner's dilemma. In Section 7.3, we build on this by reviewing findings from economic experiments designed to measure cooperation and the related concept of trust using more complex social dilemma games.

7.2.1. One-Shot Prisoner's Dilemma Games

In a classic prisoner's dilemma game (PD), two players choose simultaneously whether to cooperate or defect and the payoffs to either player are determined by both their own choice and that of the other player. Further, payoffs are structured such that individually rational behavior leads each player to defect and thereby realize a lower payoff than if each player had cooperated (hence the dilemma). However, in repeated prisoner's dilemma games (RPD), even narrowly self-interested players may find it individually rational to cooperate.

To illustrate the logic of the one-shot PD, consider the following payoffs, from largest to smallest: the Temptation (T) is the payoff to a player who chooses to defect when the other player cooperates; the Reward (R) is the payoff to each player when both players choose to cooperate; the Punishment (P) is the payoff to each player when both players choose to defect; and the Sucker payout (S) is the payoff to a player who chooses to cooperate when the other player defects. Given this game structure with payoffs ordered such that T>R>P>S, it is straightforward to prove that rational and self-interested individuals will each choose to defect.

First, notice that both players (I, II) are in similar positions, so the game is symmetric. Second, because the game consists of only two players who must choose simultaneously, there is no opportunity to write an enforceable contract in which both players commit to cooperate. Third, because this game is played only once and choices are made simultaneously, there is no way in which one player's choice to cooperate or defect will influence the other's choice to cooperate or defect.

Now consider the game from Player I's perspective. If Player II chooses to cooperate, then Player I's decision to defect or cooperate is really a choice between a payout of T versus R. Because T>R and there are no future repercussions to defection, self-interest motivates Player I to defect. However, if Player II chooses to defect, then Player I's decision to defect or cooperate is really a choice between P or S. Since P>S, self-interest motivates Player I to defect. Therefore, regardless of Player II's choice, it is in Player I's self-interest to defect. Because the game is symmetric, Player II likewise is motivated to defect regardless of Player I's anticipated behavior. Clearly both players could have realized a higher combined payoff (R, R) versus (P, P) if they had both cooperated.

In the PD, mutual defection is a "Nash equilibrium;" that is, given the strategy of the other player (which in this case is to defect), neither player can do better than to defect. No other pair of actions has this property. For example, if both players choose to cooperate, then Player I could do better changing his strategy to defection (and likewise for Player II). Therefore, mutual cooperation is not a Nash equilibrium in a classic PD.[7]

Further, notice that if the ordering of payoffs is not $T>R>P>S$, then other predictions about the behavior of self-interested players would arise. For instance, if $R>T$, then mutual cooperation is a Nash equilibrium.[8] Therefore, the existence of cooperation is first and foremost a function of the structure of social interactions, which is best viewed as a group-level or an environmental factor.

Thus far we have demonstrated only the absence of cooperation in a PD, but this simple exposition already makes clear the potential importance of real-life phenomena that are not represented in this abstract game: the structure of social interactions (i.e., the game), third-party enforcement of contracts, and other-regarding preferences.

Returning to the classic PD setup (i.e., $T>R>P>S$), next consider what happens if players can write an enforceable contract. In that case, they could credibly commit to cooperate; in fact, each player would be willing to pay as much as (R-P) in order to enter into such a contract. Of course, the efficacy of third-party enforcement of contracts depends on the likelihood that defectors are caught and the severity of punishment in such cases. However, any enforcement regime that imposes a sufficient expected punishment for defection will alter the logic of the PD such that players find it in their narrow self-interest to cooperate (Axelrod, 1984). Therefore, in societies with well-established legal systems one would expect greater collective efficacy because of the ability to enter into formal contracts. But as Axelrod notes, formal contracts are not the only means to gain cooperation; in societies with more vengeful citizens, informal cooperative norms may be more common, because of the willingness of individuals to punish defectors.

Now consider the importance of other-regarding preferences, such as altruism. If Player I cares about both his own payoff and that of Player II, then it is possible that Player I will decide to cooperate even in a classic PD game. However, the existence of altruism alone is not sufficient to guarantee cooperation: Player I must care about Player II enough to overcome his own narrow self-interest. Closely related to altruism is the concept of a "warm glow," a benefit from the act of cooperation alone, and given sufficient warm glow players will cooperate even in a one-shot PD.

Finally, we consider the dark side of other-regarding preferences – some individuals may exhibit animus toward disfavored groups. Social scientists have long

---

[7] The Nash equilibrium concept is a fundamental solution concept employed in non-cooperative games; several refinements exist, but for our purposes the Nash solution is sufficient to illustrate the basic economic theory of cooperation and trust.

[8] If instead $S>P$, then two Nash equilibria exist; in each, one player cooperates and one player defects. This is sometimes known as the "chicken" game.

understood that there may be psychological barriers that make it difficult for people to associate with others who are different from themselves, so group associations may naturally form around common socioeconomic attributes. In economic theory, this phenomenon has been described as either racial or ethnic group loyalty (Luttmer, 2001), or as the existence of a "transaction cost" of dealing with people of a different age, class, ethnicity, or race (Alesina & La Ferrara, 2000). Within the framework of the prisoner's dilemma, this is a deviation from the assumption that the two players are identical; players instead may realize a disutility from cooperating with a member of a disfavored group.

7.2.2. Repeated Prisoner's Dilemmas

It is a common misconception that in repeated prisoner's dilemma games, mutual defection is no longer an equilibrium outcome. Rather, for any finite number of repetitions of the classic PD, mutual defection remains the only Nash equilibrium for rational and self-interested players.[9] But if the game is repeated an infinite number of times, or if the game is repeated with an uncertain ending point, then mutual cooperation may be an equilibrium outcome under certain conditions. Since many real-life social interactions have an indefinite quality to them (e.g., there is some chance you will meet someone again), we continue our exposition using this case.[10]

Consider an indefinitely repeated prisoner's dilemma game (RPD) with the following structure: in each round of the game, two players engage in a classic PD, but after each round there is a positive probability that the game ends. Let (1-q) be the independent probability that the game ends after any given round, where $0 < q < 1$. Given this, we can formulate the expected payoff to each player under different strategies, and in doing so identify the exact conditions under which mutual cooperation might arise as the outcome of Nash equilibrium behavior.

As a simple illustration, assume that Player II uses the following strategy: "cooperate in round one and thereafter cooperate conditional on Player I having cooperated in the last round; but if Player I ever defects, then choose to defect forever." This strategy is known as the "Grim Trigger" (GT), since any instance of defection is met with perpetual defection. We will consider whether Player I finds it in her self-interest to follow a similar strategy or to choose the strategy of

---

[9] To see this, suppose the PD is played for two rounds. In the second round of the game, the players find themselves in a one-shot PD, and so mutual defection is the only Nash equilibrium. However, knowing this, the players realize that in the first round, there can be no future reward for cooperating (since both players will defect in round two).

[10] The logic of indefinitely repeated games also holds in a multiplayer setting even when no two individuals interact more than once; mutual cooperation may be supported as a Nash equilibrium provided every individual's history of play is common knowledge, punishment strategies are conditioned on defection against any person, and players value rewards in the future sufficiently highly.

"always defect." In fact this particular strategy pair (GT, GT)is a Nash equilibrium under the most expansive set of conditions that satisfy the assumptions of the RPD (i.e., T>R>P>S and 0>q>1); we now turn to describing those conditions.[11]

When both players choose the GT strategy, the result is an indefinitely long stream of mutually cooperative play. In this case, Player I receives a payout of R in the first period with certainty, but after that, only a q probability of receiving R in the second round, a q^2 probability of receiving R in the third round, and so on. For individuals who discount future payouts by the probability of ever receiving them, the expected value of mutual cooperation can be defined as $(R + qR + q^2R + ..)$.

Alternatively suppose that Player I decides to defect in the first round and thereafter. Since Player II is assumed to be using the GT strategy, Player I's payoffs will instead be $(T + qP + q^2P + ..)$. Finally notice that in round one, Player I gains from defecting versus cooperating (T-R>0), but this comes at the cost of all potential future cooperation. So the choice of Player I hinges on whether the short-term gains of defection outweigh the longer-term loss.

Given the above, it follows that the strategy pair of (GT, GT) will be a Nash equilibrium whenever: $(T-R) < [q(R-P) + q^2(R–P) + ..]$; that is, when the short-term gains from defection do not outweigh the long term gains from mutual cooperation. Obviously, this condition depends on the particular values of T, R, and P, but a key insight is that cooperation is easier to support for higher values of q; that is, an increased likelihood of repeated interaction facilitates cooperation in RPDs. For this reason, we expect greater cooperation and trust among family members and friends than between strangers, and also in small communities versus large cities, all else constant.

The tradeoff between the immediate benefits of defection and the long-run benefits of cooperation inherent in RPDs makes apparent the importance of an individual's ability to delay gratification for the realization of cooperation. If Player I is very impulsive or short-sighted, then she will discount the potential value of cooperation in the future and more likely succumb to the temptation to defect. Formally, we can incorporate a player's "patience" by adding a per-period discount factor that represents the declining value of future payouts; however, by analogy to q above, the mathematics of this should be fairly intuitive.

This discussion of indefinitely repeated prisoner's dilemmas suggests additional contextual and idiosyncratic determinants of cooperation. Cooperation is facilitated by frequent repeated interactions which are a product of an individual's particular social environment. Repeated interaction may give rise to trust building between players, and the ability to delay immediate gratification to establish a trustworthy reputation may be influenced by social forces, but is undeniably an attribute of the individual.

---

[11] The GT strategy is not the only strategy that can elicit cooperation in RPDs. See, for example, Axelrod's (1984) discussion of the "Tit-for-Tat" strategy.

7.2.3. Some Lessons from Game Theory

The prisoner's dilemma game is a simple and powerful tool for understanding an individual's motives for cooperation in a highly abstract setting. By analyzing individual motives in the anarchical setting of the PD, the functions of the social norms and institutions of civil society become clear. Social institutions are both a means to create environments that facilitate cooperation and build trust, and a force for transforming individual preferences away from narrow self-interested behavior so that people are more than just impetuous creatures bent on immediate gratification. Thus community, education, family and religion may all influence individual preferences in a way that facilitates the realization of greater coopera-tion. At the same time, social groups may create environments with more frequent and repeated interactions, or increase the likelihood of punishment for deviant or anti-social behavior. However, there is a potential dark side of civil society – increased interaction within a particular group or community may come at the expense of interactions with outsiders, leading to segregation and distrust across groups.

7.3. Evidence from Economic Analysis of Surveys and Experimental Data

Game theoretic analysis of the prisoner's dilemma suggests that social capital researchers must consider cooperation to be associated with group-level attrib-utes, as well as determined by individual characteristics. Recent studies by econ-omists have reinforced this conclusion with findings from survey data on memberships in voluntary organizations and generalized trust. These measures are widely used to quantify social capital, and are closely related to the economic construct of cooperation.

In this section, we briefly summarize results from several key studies in this area, and we note some important considerations regarding measures of social capital derived from survey responses. This discussion sets the stage for describ-ing the literature from experimental economics, a field that offers a unique approach to the measurement of social capital and the analysis of social capital determinants.

7.3.1. Economic Analyses of Survey Data

Several economists have undertaken studies of social capital which focus on individual-level trust and participation in group organizations. Two widely-cited studies are those by Alesina and La Ferrara (2000, 2002), which employed data from the General Social Survey. Both studies reported results from a mixed-level analysis of the determinants of an individual-specific measure of social capital, with the former focusing on membership in voluntary associations, and the latter examining generalized trust. Both studies found evidence that individual-specific measures of social capital are influenced by individual traits (such as age, educational attainment, income, and race), as well as contextual factors. In the former study, median metropolitan area income was found to be strongly and positively associated with membership, while several measures of metropolitan area heterogeneity (income inequality, and racial and ethnic "fragmentation" were significantly likely to reduce membership in voluntary organizations. Alesina and La Ferarra (2002) found that income inequality and racial fragmentation have similar effects on trust, but neither ethnic nor religious heterogeneity are significant determinants of trust.

Further support for a negative relationship between population heterogeneity and social capital has been reported by Costa and Kahn (2003a,b), who conducted mixed-level analyses of the determinants of individual trust and participation using several different survey datasets.[12] Costa and Kahn also demonstrated that much of the recent decline in social capital in the U.S. can be attributed to increasing female labor force participation and increasing community heterogeneity.[13]

Like many studies linking social capital to health and other outcomes, the studies cited above are subject to the concern that responses to survey questions on trust and other attitudes may not be reliable measures of social capital. This critique is often associated with a study by Glaeser et al. (2000), which cautioned that survey respondents may have different interpretations of generalized trust. For example, if a respondent indicates a general lack of trust in others, does that mean the respondent does not trust familiar acquaintances, or does this mistrust apply only to random strangers? Different persons with identical trust in others may offer different responses to an open-ended question about generalized trust. Glaeser et al. (2000) suggested that questions about specific trusting behaviors, such as whether a person locks their door at night, might better indicate the degree to which a person trusts others.

7.3.2. Economic Analyses of Experimental Data

Another important contribution of Glaeser et al. (2000) was the pairing of survey questions on trust with a series of real-life exercises designed to measure subject behaviors in controlled laboratory settings. The design and methods of the particular exercises were developed decades ago by researchers in the field of experimental economics, but in pairing well-known experimental designs with survey-based measures of trust, the Glaeser et al. study illustrated another important economic contribution to the study of social capital.

A defining characteristic of economic experiments is that subjects are paid based on their actions within the experiment and apart from any compensation for

---

[12] See Vigdor (2002) for a more critical take on these findings.
[13] Also, see Vigdor's (2004) study of community-level response rates to the 2000 Census, and Costa and Kahn's (2003c) study of acts of cowardice and desertion in the Union Army.

merely showing up to participate. This allows researchers to observe subjects making choices with monetary consequences. For this reason, economic experiments may better reveal the determinants of genuine cooperation and trust, as opposed to survey instruments which may be subject to both recall bias and self-serving response bias. Another advantage of experimental studies of the determinants of trust and cooperation is that the researcher can observe subjects in well-defined treatment and control groups and thereby limit the problems of omitted variable bias that can plague studies of survey responses. Experiments have been designed to test theoretical predictions about various economic decisions, from market interactions to retirement savings; here we focus on several experiments pertaining to social capital components, namely trust and cooperation.

7.3.3. Trust Experiments

One of the experiments employed in the Glaeser et al., (2000) study was the trust experiment, first designed by Berg, Dickhaut, and McCabe (1995). In this experiment, one subject (the first mover) is given some amount of money and offered the opportunity to pass some, all, or none to a partner (the second mover). All passed money is multiplied by some predetermined amount ($k>1$) before being received by the second mover. Finally, the second mover has the opportunity to pass some, all, or none of the money she receives back to the first mover. In the discussion that follows, we focus on the amount sent by the first mover, which is commonly interpreted as trusting behavior by the subject.

A notable finding from the Glaeser et al. study was that responses to survey questions about generalized trust were not related to trusting behavior. In contrast, survey questions that address whether subjects engage in specific trusting behaviors were significantly correlated with decisions in trust experiments. Numerous follow-up studies have found inconsistencies between survey-based measures of trusting behaviors in experimental settings, including Anderson, Mellor, and Milyo (2006), Burks, Carpenter, and Verhoogan, (2003) and Fehr, Fischbacher, von Rosenbladt, Schupp, and Wagner (2003).

Taken together, experimental economics studies offer two important implications for the study of social capital. First, their findings suggest that some caution is in order, particularly when employing survey-based generalized trust as a measure of social capital. A second and arguably more important implication is that trust experiments can allow researchers to test the statistical importance of various factors associated with trusting behavior. The Nash equilibrium for this game is that no money will be passed in the first stage since second movers have no incentive to return money in the second stage. However, Berg et al. (1995) found that on average first movers sent around half of their endowment. This finding has been replicated numerous times, although the exact amounts sent by subjects vary across studies (Ostrom & Walker, 2003).

The widespread existence of non-Nash behavior has motivated studies on how behavior in the trust game is affected by both individual-specific and context-specific characteristics. The effect of gender has been examined in several studies, but with mixed results. Several studies have found that the amount sent in trust games does not differ by gender (e.g., Croson & Buchan, 1999; Glaeser et al., 2000). However, using a novel design to capture different motives for trusting behavior, Ashraf, Bohnet, and Piankov (2006) found that expectations of return mattered more for women than men. Among men, preferences for fairness were more strongly aligned with trust than were expectations of return. Anderson, Mellor, and Milyo (2005) examined the effects of religious affiliation and political ideology in separate studies, but found neither individual trait to have a significant effect on trust.

In terms of contextual determinants of trust, numerous studies have explored whether the difference between game theoretic predictions and observed trust behavior can be accounted for by culture, making the trust game one of the most well-traveled economics experiments.[14] The majority of these studies conclude that there are few differences in behavior in trust experiments across cultures or nationalities. For example, Croson and Buchan (1999) found no significant differences in trust comparing subjects from China, Japan, Korea and the United States. For a more comprehensive collection of studies that examines various social influences on trust, see Ostrom and Walker (2003).

Looking at how individuals from different cultures or nationalities interact provides another means of identifying the effects of contextual factors on trust. Glaeser et al. (2000) found a small negative, but statistically insignificant, effect on amount sent when players interacted face-to-face with a partner of a different nationality. This type of interaction also produced a negative, and in this case significant, effect on the amount returned by second movers. Fershtman and Gneezy (2001) conducted a trust game with Israeli college students, in which subjects were told the last name of their partner as a means of revealing their ethnicity. In this study, significantly less money was transferred to Eastern origin players by partners from both the East and the West, a finding that held for males but not females. Bouckaert and Dhaene (2004) conducted a similar experiment using businessman of Turkish or Belgian origin, but they reported no evidence of ethnic differences in the amount sent or returned. Finally, Willinger, Keser, Lohmann, and Usunier (2003) paired French and German students and found no difference in behavior when subjects knew they were playing with someone from a country other than their own. Thus, half of these studies provided evidence that heterogeneity in the players' ethnicity or national origin reduces trusting behavior.

---

[14] Trust experiments have been conducted in Belgium (Bouckaert & Dhaene, 2004), Brazil (Csukas, Fracalanza, Kovacs, & Willinger,2003), Bulgaria (Koford, 2001), China (Buchan & Croson, 2004; Croson & Buchan, 1999), France (Willinger et al., 2003), Germany (Fehr et al., 2003; Willinger et al., 2003), Greece (Csukas et al., 2003), Hungary (Csukas et al., 2003), Israel (Fershtman & Gneezy, 2001), the Netherlands (Bellemare & Kroger, 2003), Russia (Ashraf et al., 2006; Gächter, Herrmann, & Thöni, 2003; Csukas et al., 2003), South Africa (Ashraf et al., 2006), Tanzania (Danielson & Holm, 2004), Turkey (Bouckaert & Dhaene, 2002) and Zimbabwe (Barr, 1999, 2003).

Related to these studies is recent work by Anderson, Mellor, and Milyo (2006) which induces heterogeneity in a trust experiment by awarding subjects different amounts for showing up to participate. Heterogeneity did not influence trust behavior uniformly for all subjects in the group. One contextual factor that had a large impact on trusting behavior was the manner in which heterogeneity was induced (privately so that subjects only knew their own payments, or publicly so that subjects knew the payments received by everyone in the group). In addition, subject-specific motives, such as guilt or entitlement, also appeared to influence trusting behavior.

7.3.4. Public Goods Experiments

In addition to trust experiments, there are a number of experimental designs that capture cooperative play in games with simultaneous moves. These range from a simple two-person one-shot prisoner's dilemma to experiments involving repetition and multiple players. One of the first economic experiments examining behavior in a prisoner's dilemma was reported by Flood (1952); the key finding in this and subsequent studies was that human subjects do not always defect even in a one-shot game. A common variation of the simple PD experiment is known as the voluntary contribution mechanism or public goods experiment. This game is essentially a multi-person prisoner's dilemma used to explore the extent to which people "free ride" when resources are shared within a group.

In a simple public goods game, each person in a group of N-persons is given an endowment of tokens and offered the opportunity to contribute (simultaneously and anonymously) to a group account. The sum of all tokens contributed by the group (G) is then multiplied by some factor, w, and the resulting amount (w*G) is divided equally among all subjects regardless of the amount that each contributed. Tokens not contributed to the group account have a value $v>w$ to the individual; this gives subjects an incentive to forego group contributions (i.e., free ride). When $N^*w>v$, this is a prisoner's dilemma game; the Nash equilibrium prediction is that all subjects will free ride (or defect), even though the group is better off when everyone contributes to the group account (or cooperates).

This particular version of the PD was first examined by two sociologists, Marwell and Ames (1981), and a vast literature has developed from replications and extensions conducted by economists in the last twenty-five years. Our summary highlights only a few of the empirical findings from this literature relevant to the study of social capital, and interested readers are advised to consult several systematic reviews in Anderson (2001) and Ledyard (1995).

A frequent result in public goods experiments is that subjects contribute about half their tokens to the group account the first time they play the game. As subjects play the game repeatedly, contributions fall to 20% to 40% of the token endowment (Isaac, Walker, & Thomas, 1984). The drop in contributions with finite repetition is typically attributed to subject learning, and Isaac, Walker, and Thomas (1984) also found that subjects with prior experience with experiments contributed less than inexperienced subjects (also see Andreoni, 1988). Nevertheless, lack of familiarity with the game is not the sole cause of cooperation; across hundreds of similar experimental studies, rates of cooperation remain significantly greater than zero.

These findings suggest that individuals possess a taste for cooperation that drives them to cooperate when narrow self-interest would dictate otherwise. Whether the taste for cooperation is purely altruistic or motivated by warm glow has been examined in several studies. Support for altruism comes from the finding that contributions increase with the size of the group, since contributions to the group account benefit more individuals (Isaac, Walker, & Williams, 1984). Another possibility is that subjects are motivated to cooperate because of a warm glow benefit, that is, the utility subjects experience from contributing regardless of the degree to which others benefit. In an attempt to isolate altruism from warm glow motives, Palfrey and Prisbrey (1997) had the same subjects participate in public goods experiments in which payoffs to group account contributions (w) were varied. The authors found that contributions were not sensitive to w, and so concluded that the warm glow motive is the more important determinant of cooperation.

A related study by Goeree, Holt, and Laury (2002) decomposed the value of the group account into an internal return that an individual gets from the tokens she puts into the group account and an external return that everyone else gets from her contributions to the group account. They found that contributions increased with group size and the external return, which suggests that warm glow alone does not explain cooperation in this context. Goeree, Holt, and Laury (2002) also estimated an individual-specific altruism parameter and found that it varies widely, especially for men.

Although the relative importance of altruism versus warm glow remains contested, a consistent finding across these studies is that individual-specific tastes or attitudes influence cooperation for some persons and not others. As was the case with trust experiments, this repeated finding has led naturally to questions about what kinds of whether people are more or less likely to cooperate. Gender differences in public goods games appear to be modest and inconsistent across studies; for example, a recent study utilizing a classic one-shot prisoner's dilemma reported no significant differences in cooperation by men and women (Branas-Garza & Morales, 2003). In contrast, Brown-Kruse and Hummels (1993) explored the importance of gender composition of groups; counter to popular stereotypes, they found that groups of males achieved significantly higher rates of cooperation than groups of females.

Anderson, Mellor, and Milyo (2004) found that individuals who self-report greater generalized trust in others or greater participation in voluntary groups are significantly more likely to contribute in a public goods game, in contrast to the findings from trust experiments reported in Glaeser et al. (2000). However, other characteristics that might seem intuitively related to cooperation are not. For example, neither liberal political ideology nor religious affiliation are strongly related to contribution rates (Anderson, Mellor, & Milyo 2005).

These examples illustrate the challenge of linking specific, quantifiable individual characteristics to cooperation.

Some support for the importance of contextual factors comes from studies that report differences in rates of cooperation across countries. Anglo-Americans appear to free ride more than Italian or German subjects (Burlando & Hey, 1997), and Japanese and American subjects behave differently in a two-stage public goods game (Cason, Saijo, & Yamato, 2002). A review of behavior in public goods games conducted in more than a dozen small, developing societies revealed significant cross-cultural differences (Henrich et al., 2001).

Our discussion of the theoretic predictions from infinitely repeated prisoner's dilemma games made the point that the structure of the game may matter greatly in determining cooperation. Anonymity among players in the public goods game appears to have little effect on contributions (Laury, Walker, & Williams, 1995), although when communication is permitted among subjects, contributions do increase (Isaac & Walker, 1988).

Another contextual factor that has been shown to influence play in public goods games is group heterogeneity. Building on survey-based studies that relate individual social capital to various measures of population heterogeneity (e.g., Alesina & La Ferarra, 2000, 2002; Costa & Kahn, 2003a,b), Anderson, Mellor, and Milyo (forthcoming) examined the effects of induced heterogeneity on behavior in a public goods game. The authors induced inequality in their treatment groups by varying the "show-up" payments made to subjects for participating. Because these payments were independent of subject choices in the game, this source of variation was not expected to alter subjects' behavior according to economic theory. Compared to those in a control group, participants in the inequality treatment contributed about 20% fewer tokens to the public account regardless of whether their own show-up payment was large or small.

7.4. Lessons for the Study of Social Capital and Health

A consistent theme throughout this essay is that economic theory and evidence offer support for modeling cooperation and trust as a function of both contextual and individual determinants. This has immediate and important implications for empirical studies on social capital and well-being, particularly those studies that measure social capital by aggregating survey responses to questions about generalized trust or participation in voluntary membership organizations.

The primary lesson for empirical studies on social capital is the importance of controlling for individual-level attributes, including factors associated with altruistic preferences and warm-glow motives. Failing to do so may result in observed associations between indicators of well-being and aggregate measures of social capital that are uninformative about the importance of contextual versus compositional factors. Unfortunately, many empirical studies examine only ecological associations between social capital and well-being, with few or even no control variables.[15] As shown in Mellor and Milyo (2005), the inclusion of relevant explanatory variables lessened the magnitude of the observed association between state-level social capital and self-reported health status.

While numerous studies of trust experiments and public goods experiments have suggested the importance of altruism or warm glow in decision making, we should acknowledge the difficulty of measuring these individual traits. At the same time, readily observable traits like gender, political ideology and religiosity have had limited success in predicting cooperation or trusting behaviors. For these reasons, empirical researchers may find great advantages from employing panel data on social capital, which allows for the control of unobservable fixed individual effects.

A second implication for the empirical study of social capital pertains to the treatment of social capital as exogenous. To illustrate the problems associated with this, consider the case where individual participation in voluntary associations is a function of the individual's health because healthy individuals find it easier to meet and greet other folks. In this circumstance, ordinary least squares regression estimates of the effects of social capital on health will be biased upward due to simultaneity bias (i.e., reverse causality).

Because the two most common indicators of social capital employed in empirical studies are themselves aggregations of individual attributes (trust and membership in voluntary associations), they are by definition determined by the behavior and circumstances of individuals. Suppose the researcher measures state-level social capital by average responses within a state to survey questions about generalize social trust, then observes that state-level social capital is associated with individual health status. Further suppose that some unobserved individual-level factor (e.g., household wealth) determines both individual health status and individual responses about trust in others. In this case it is impossible to determine whether the association between state social capital and individual health status reflects a true causal relationship or is merely a spurious correlation driven by the fact that state social capital is a proxy for unobserved individual household characteristics.

This problem is compounded if there is also a contextual effect of state household wealth on health status, as will be the case if state wealth influences political support for public health programs. We are unsure whether the observed association between social capital and health reflects a true causal link, proxies for individual unobserved factors, or proxies for unobserved contextual factors. These concerns are only amplified when one takes into account that social capital is not itself directly observed in empirical studies, but instead measured by proxies that are determined by a number of individual, social and contextual factors.

---

[15] Subramanian et al. (2002) and Subramanian, Lochner, and Kawachi (2003) are noteworthy studies in that they examine the effects of aggregate and individual-level measures of social capital on health.

Of course, the failure to deal adequately with the methodological challenges described above is not unique to the social capital literature. The identification of social influences on individuals is well understood by economists to be fraught with perils (Brock & Durlauf, 2001; Durlauf, 2001; Manski, 1993, 1995, 2000; Moffit, 2000). In general, social effects and other contextual factors cannot be separately identified and estimated absent strong assumptions about the precise structural system of causal relationships relating individual, contextual and social influences. Nonetheless, the endogeneity problem is an important reason that all researchers, and not just economists, should be more cautious in evaluating the efficacy of social capital research.

A third lesson we offer for the study of social capital regards the interpretation of results for a public policy audience. Suppose there is indeed a strong causal link from cooperation and trust to health outcomes. The interpretation of this finding depends a great deal on whether social capital is the product of contextual or compositional factors. For example, policies that attempt to create community interaction, through zoning or subsidization of community events, may be seen as attempts to generate repeated interaction. However, if diversity breeds distrust, then creating greater community interaction may actually reduce social capital. Also, if the primary driver of cooperation and trust in communities is the prevalence of individual community members who are patient and altruistic, then such policies may prove ineffectual. Instead, policymakers would need to focus on actions that shape individual preferences; perhaps this would involve greater indoctrination in civic virtues in schools.

These speculations illuminate our main point: social capital researchers must take seriously the methodological challenges presented by the existence of both contextual and compositional determinants of cooperation and trust and strive to develop rigorous tests of the substantive importance of social capital for health. Beyond providing better evidence on the importance of causal links from social capital and health, researchers also must attempt to distinguish which determinants of social capital matter most, and how amenable these factors are to policy manipulation.

References

Aguilera, M. B. (2002). The impact of social capital on labor force participation: Evidence from the 2000 Social Capital Benchmark Survey. *Social Science Quarterly, 83*(3), 853–874.

Ahern, M. M., & Hendryx, M. S. (2003). Social capital and trust in providers. *Social Science and Medicine, 57*(1), 1195–1204.

Alesina, A., & La Ferrara, E. (2000). Participation in hetergeneous communities. *Quarterly Journal of Economics, 115*(3), 847–904.

Alesina, A., & La Ferrara, E. (2002). Who trusts others? *Journal of Public Economics, 85*(2), 207–234.

Anderson, L. R. (2001). Public choice as an experimental science. In W. Shughart & L. Razzolini (Ed.), *The Elgar companion to public choice*. Northampton, MA: Edward Elgar Publishing.

Anderson, L. R., Mellor J. M., & Milyo J. (2004). Social capital and contributions in a public goods experiment. *American Economics Review Papers and Proceedings, 94*(2), 373–376.

Anderson, L. R., Mellor J. M., & Milyo, J. (2005). Do liberals play nice? The effects of political party and ideology in public goods and trust games. In J. Morgan (Ed.), *Advances in applied microeconomics: Experimental and behavioral economics*. Stamford, Connecticut: JAI Press.

Anderson, L. R., & Mellor J. M. (2006). Did the Devil make them do it? The effects of religion in public goods and trust games. Working Paper Number 20, Department of Economics, The College of William and Mary.

Anderson, L. R., Mellor J. M., & Milyo, J. (forthcoming). Inequality, group cohesion and public goods provision: An experimental analysis. The Journal of Socio-Economics.

Anderson, L. R., Mellor J. M., & Milyo, J. (2006). Induced heterogeneity in trust experiments. *Experimental Economics, 9*(3), 223–235.

Andreoni, J. (1988). Why free ride? Strategies and learning in public goods experiments. *Journal of Public Economics, 37*, 291–304.

Ashraf, N., Bohnet, I., & Piankov, N. (2006). Decomposing trust and trustworthiness. *Experimental Economics, 9*(3), 193–208.

Axelrod, R. (1984). *The evolution of cooperation*. New York, NY: Basic Books.

Barr, A. (1999). Familiarity and trust: An experimental investigation. The Center for the Study of African Economies Working Paper Series, Paper 107.

Barr, A. (2003). Trust and expected trustworthiness: Experimental evidence from Zimbabwean villages. *The Economic Journal, 113*, 614–630.

Beiseitov, E., Kubik, J. D., & Moran, J. R. (2003). Informal informational sharing and the demand for health insurance among elderly. Robert Wood Johnson Scholars Working Paper WP-24, Boston University (Boston, MA).

Bellemare, C.,, & Kroger, S. (2003). On representative trust. Tilberg University, CentER Discussion Working Paper No. 2003–47.

Berg, J., Dickhaut J., & McCabe, K. (1995). Trust, reciprocity, and social history. *Games and Economic Behavior, 10*, 122–142.

Bjornskov, C. (2003). The happy few: Cross-country evidence on social capital and life satisfaction. *Kyklos, 59*(1), 3–16.

Bouckaert, J., & Dhaene, G. (2004). Inter-ethnic trust and reciprocity: Results of an experiment with small business entrepreneurs. *European Journal of Political Economy, 20*(4), 869—886.

Branas-Garza, P., & Morales, A. (2003). Gender differences in prisoners' dilemma. manuscript, Centro de Estudios Andaluces (Seville, Spain).

Brock, W., & Durlauf, S. (2001). Interactions-based models. In Heckman & Leamer (Eds.), *Handbook of econometrics*, (Elsevier Science B.V.)

Brown-Kruse, J., & Hummels, D. (1993). Gender effects in laboratory public goods contributions: Do individuals put their money where their mouth is? *Journal of Economic Behavior and Organization, 22*, 355–267.

Buchan, N., & Croson, R. (2004). The boundaries of trust: Own and other's actions in the US and China. *Journal of Economic Behavior and Organization, 55*(4), 485–504.

Burks, S. V., Carpenter, J. P., & Verhoogan, E. (2003). Playing both roles in the trust game. *Journal of Economic Behavior and Organization, 51*(2), 195–216.

Burlando, R., & Hey, J. D. (1997). Do Anglo-Saxons free-ride more? *Journal of Public Economics, 64*, 41–60.

Cason, T., Saijo, T., & Yamato, T. (2002). Voluntary participation and spite in public good provision experiments: An international comparison. *Experimental Economics*, 5, 133–153.

Carman, K. G. (2004). Social influences and the private provision of public goods: Evidence from charitable contributions in the workplace, manuscript. Cambridge, MA: Harvard University).

Cohen, S., Doyle, W., Skoner, D., Rabin, B., & Gwaltney, J. (1997). Social ties and susceptibility to the common cold. *JAMA*, 227(24), 1940–1944.

Coleman, J. S. (1988). Social capital in the creation of human capital. *American Journal of Sociology*, 94, S95–S120.

Cooley, J. (2005). Desegregation and the acheivement gap; Do diverse peers help? manuscript. Durham, NC: Duke University.

Costa, D. L., & Kahn, M. E. (2003a). Understanding the decline in American social capital. *Kyklos*, 56(1), 17–46.

Costa, D. L., & Kahn, M. E. (2003b). Civic engagement and community heterogeneity: An economists perspective. *Perspectives on Politics*, 1(1), 103–112.

Costa, D. L., & Kahn, M. E. (2003c). Cowards and heroes: Group loyalty in the American civil war," *Quarterly Journal of Economics*, 118(2), 519–548.

Croson, R., & Buchan, N. (1999). Gender and culture: International experimental evidence from trust games. *American Economic Review Papers and Proceedings*, 89(2), 386–391.

Csukas, C., Fracalanza, P., Kovacs, T., & Willinger, M. (2003). Stated trust versus trusting behavior in an intercultural experiment. Working Paper 2003–25, Technical University of Budapest, Department of Finance and Accounting.

Danielson, A. J., & Holm, H. (2004). Do you trust your brethren? Eliciting attitudes and trust behavior in a Tanzanian congregation. Working Paper 2004:2. Economics Department, University of Lund.

Deri, C. (2005). Social networks and health service utilization. *Journal of Health Economics*, 24, 1076–1107.

Durlauf, S. (1999). The case against social capital. *Focus*, 20, 1–5.

Durlauf, S. (2001). A Framework for the study of individual behavior and social interactions. University of Wisconsin Working Paper.

Durlauf, S. (2002). On the empirics of social capital. *Economic Journal*, 112(483), 459–479.

Fehr, E., Fischbacher, U., von Rosenbladt, B., Schupp, J., & Wagner, G. G. (2003). A Nation-wide laboratory: Examining trust and trustworthiness by integrating behavioral experiments into representative surveys. IZA Discussion Paper No. 715.

Fershtman, C., & Gneezy, U. (2001). Discrimination in a segmented society: An experimental approach. *Quarterly Journal of Economics*, 116(1), 351–377.

Flood, M. (1952). Some experimental games. Research Memorandum RM-789, RAND Corporation.

Fratiglioni, L., Wang, H.X., Ericsson, K., Maytan, M., & Winblad, B. (2000). Influence of social network on occurence of dementia: a community-based longitudinal study. *Lancet*, 355, 1315–1319.

Gächter, S., Herrmann, B., & Thöni, C. (2003). Trust, voluntary cooperation, and socioeconomic background: Survey and experimental evidence. *Journal of Economic Behavior and Organization*, 55(4), 505–531.

Galea, S., Karpati, A., & Kennedy, B. (2002). Social capital and violence in the United States, 1974–1993. *Social Science and Medicine*, 55, 1373–1383.

Glaeser, E. L., Laibson, D. I., Scheinkman, J. A., & Soutter, C. L. (2000). Measuring trust. *Quarterly Journal of Economics*, *115*(3), 811–846.

Goeree, J., Holt, C., & Laury, S. (2002). Private costs and public benefits: Unraveling the effects of altruism and noisy behavior. *Journal of Public Economics*, *83*(2), 257–278.

Gold, R., Kennedy, B. P., Connell, F., & Kawachi, I. (2002). Teen births, income inequality and social capital: developing an understanding of the causal pathway. *Health and Place*, *8*, 77–83.

Guiso, L., Sapienza, P., & Zingales, L. (2004). The role of social capital in financial development. *American Economic Review*, *94*(3), 526–556.

Hawe, P., & Shiell, A. (2000). Social capital and health promotion: A review. *Social Science and Medicine*, *51*, 871–875.

Hemenway, D., Kennedy, B. P., Kawachi, I., & Putnam, R. (2001). Firearm prevalence and social capital. *Annals of Epidemiology*, *11*(7): 484–490.

Hendryx, M. S., Ahern, M. M., Lovrich, N. P., & McCurdy, A. H. (2002). Access to health care and community social capital. *Health Services Research*, *37*(1), 87–103.

Henrich, J., Boyd, R., Boyd, S., Camerer, C., Fehr, E., Gintis, H. et al. (2001). In search of homo economicus: Behavioral experiments in 15 small-scale societies. *American Economic Review*, *91*, (2), 73–78.

Holtgrave, D. R., & Crosby, R. A. (2003). Social capital, poverty, and income inequality as predictors of gonorrhoea, syphilis, chlamydia and AIDS case rates in the United States. *Sexually Transmitted Infections*, *79*(1), 62–65.

Isaac, R. M., & Walker, J. M. (1988). Communication and free riding behavior: The voluntary contribution mechanism. *Economic Inquiry*, *26*, 585–608.

Isaac, R. M., Walker, J. M., & Thomas, S. (1984). Divergent evidence on free riding: An experimental examination of some possible explanations. *Public Choice*, *43*(2), 113–149.

Kaplan, G. A., Salonen, J. T., Cohen, R. D., Brad, R.J., Syme, S.L., & Puska, P. (1988). Social connections and mortality from all causes and from cardiovascular disease: Prospective evidence from Eastern Finland. *American Journal of Epidemiology*, *128*, 370–380.

Kawachi, I., Kennedy, B. P., Lochner, K., & Prothrow-Stith, D. (1997). Social capital, income inequality and mortality. *American Journal of Public Health*, *87*, 1491–1498.

Knack, S., & Keefer, P. (1997). Does social capital have an economic payoff? A cross-country investigation. *Quarterly Journal of Economics*, *112*(4), 1251–1288.

Koford, K. (2001). Trust and reciprocity in Bulgaria: A replication of Berg, Dickhaut and McCabe. Working paper, University of Delaware.

La Porta, R., Lopez-de-Silanes, F., Shleifer, A., & Vishny, R. (1997). Trust in large organizations. *American Economic Review Papers and Proceedings*, *87*(2), 333–338.

Laury, S. K., Walker, J. M., & Williams, A. W. (1995). Anonymity and the voluntary provision of public goods. *Journal of Economic Behavior and Organization*, *27*, 365–380.

Ledyard, J. O. (1995). Public goods: A survey of experimental research. In J. Kagel & A. Roth (Eds.), *The handbook of experimental economics*. Princeton, NJ: Princeton University Press.

Lindstrom, M., Hanson, B., & Ostergren, P.-O. (2001). Socioeconomic differences in leisure-time physical activity: The role of social participation and social capital in shaping health related behaviors. *Social Science and Medicine*, *52*(3), 441–451.

Lo Sciuto, L, Rajala, A., Townsend, T. N., & Taylor, A. S. (1996). An outcome evaluation of across ages: An intergenerational mentoring program to drug prevention. *Journal of Adolescent Research*, *11*, 116–129.

Loury, G. C. (1977). A dynamic theory of racial income differences. In P. Wallace & A. M. La Monde (Eds.), *Women, minorities and employment discrimination*. Heath (Lexington, MA).

Luttmer, E. F.P. (2001). Group loyalty and the taste for redistribution. *Journal of Political Economy, 109*(3), 500–528.

Manski, C. (1993). Identification of endogenous social effects: The reflection problem. *Review of Economic Studies, 60*(3), 531–542.

Manski, C. (1995). *Identification problems in the social sciences*. Cambridge, Massachusetts: Harvard University Press.

Manski, C. (2000). Economic analysis of social interactions. *Journal of Economic Perspectives, 14*, 115–136.

Marwell, G., & Ames, R. (1981). Economists free ride: Does anyone else? Experiments on the provision of public goods IV. *Journal of Public Economics, 15*, 295–310.

Mellor, J. M., & Milyo, J. (2005). State social capital and individual health status. *Journal of Health Politics, Policy and Law, 30*(6), 1101–1130.

Moffit, R. (2000). Policy interventions, low-level equilibria and social interactions. Johns Hopkins Working Paper.

Ostrom, E., & Walker, J. (2003). *Trust and reciprocity: Interdisciplinary lessons from experimental research*. New York: Russell Sage Foundation.

Palfrey, T. R., & Prisbrey, J. R. (1997). Anomalous behavior in public goods experiments: How much and why? *American Economic Review, 87*, 829–846.

Putnam, R. D. (2000). *Bowling alone: The collapse and revival of American community*. New York: Simon and Schuster.

Saluja, G., Kotch, J., & Lee, L. (2003). Does social capital really matter? *Archives of Pediatric and Adolescent Medicine, 157*, 681–686.

Silvia, E. S., Thorne, J., & Tashjian, C. A. (1997). School-based drug prevention programs: A longitudinal study in selected school districts. Research Triangle Part, NC: Research Triangle Institute and U.S. Department of Education.

Sobel, J. (2002). Can we trust social capital? *Journal of Economic Literature, 40*, 139–154.

Subramanian, S. V., Kim, D. J., & Kawachi, I. (2002). Social trust and self-rated health in U.S. communities: A multilevel analysis. *Journal of Urban Health, 79*(4), S21–S34.

Subramanian, S. V., Lochner, K. A., & Kawachi, I. (2003). Neighborhood differences in social capital: A compositional artifact or a contextual construct? *Health & Place, 8*, 33–44.

Vigdor, J. (2002). Interpreting ethnic fragmentation effects. *Economic Letters, 75*(2), 271–276.

Vigdor, J. (2004). Community composition and collective action: Analyzing initial mail response to the 2000 census. *Review of Economics and Statistics, 86*(1), 303–312.

Weitzman, E. R., & Kawachi, I. (2000). Giving means receiving: The protective effect of social capital on binge drinking on college campuses. *American Journal of Public Health, 90*(12), 1936.

Wilkinson, R. G. (1996). *Unhealthy societies: The afflictions of inequality*. New York: Routledge.

Willinger, M., Keser, C., Lohmann, C., & Usunier, J.-C. (2003). A comparison of trust and reciprocity between France and Germany: Experimental investigation based on the investment game. *Journal of Economic Psychology, 24*, 447–466.

Part II
Empirical Evidence

8
Social Capital and Physical Health
A Systematic Review of the Literature

DANIEL KIM, S.V. SUBRAMANIAN, AND ICHIRO KAWACHI

In this chapter, we describe the key findings from a systematic review of empirical studies linking social capital to physical health outcomes. As noted in the Introduction, as well as the chapters by van der Gaag and Webber (chapter 2), and Lakon and colleagues (chapter 4), much of the public health literature has focused on the health effects of *social cohesion*. That is, both ecological and multilevel studies have sought to examine the health impacts of group cohesion measured at different scales (e.g., neighborhoods, states, nations). In turn, a number of individual-level studies have sought to test the relationships between individual perceptions of social cohesion (e.g., trust of others) and health outcomes. Accordingly, our systematic review of the literature focuses on empirical studies of social cohesion and physical health outcomes. There is a huge body of literature describing the linkages between social integration, social networks, social support, and health (Berkman & Glass, 2000); however, the authors of these studies do not typically classify their investigations under the heading of "social capital", and indeed a substantial portion of this literature pre-dates the recent explosion of interest in social capital within the public health field.[1] Similarly, there have been a number of empirical investigations in the health field using sociometric analysis. These studies have tended to focus on the "dark side" of social capital e.g., the contagion of high risk behaviors within networks – such as the spread of suicidal ideation (Bearman & Moody, 2004), injection drug use (Friedman & Aral, 2001), or alcohol and other drug use among adolescents (Valente, Gallaher, & Mouttapa, 2004). The authors of chapter 4 would no doubt argue that these are studies of social capital. However, since they did turn up in our search strategy for "social capital and health" (described further below), we shall not discuss them here (except to agree with the authors of chapter 4 that more studies of this type should be encouraged).

---

[1] Outside the public health field, scholars seem happy to mix them up. Thus in his chapter on social capital and health (chapter 20) in the book *Bowling Alone* (2000), Robert Putnam cites evidence from every type of study, including not only social cohesion, but also social networks and social support.

8.1. Systematic Literature Review

We conducted a systematic literature review of all studies in English that have examined social capital in relation to measures of physical health, including all-cause mortality, self-rated health, and major chronic diseases or conditions (e.g., cardiovascular disease, cancer, obesity, and diabetes), as well as acute infectious diseases. Citations were searched using the US National Library of Medicine's PubMed database (which provides electronic citations from MEDLINE and other life science journals for biomedical articles) for the period between 1966 and November 1, 2006, corresponding to the keyword combinations of "social capital" with each of the following: "life expectancy", "mortality", "cardiovascular disease", "cancer", "diabetes", "obesity", and "infectious diseases". Articles were then obtained and reviewed. Reference sections of retrieved articles were searched to identify additional potential articles for inclusion. Tables 8.1 through 8.6 display the key characteristics and findings from these studies, stratified by the type of study design (ecological, multilevel, individual-level) and the highest spatial level of social capital (country, state/region, neighborhood/community), and are listed chronologically by year of publication within each grouping. From each study, we abstracted the study authors and year of publication, sample size and population/setting, age range for social capital and health outcome measures, type of study design (cross-sectional versus prospective/longitudinal), measures of social capital and health/disease, factors included as covariates in statistical models (or stratified on), and individual-level and area-level effect estimates for social capital. For studies that only analyzed individual-level measures of social capital, our keyword search excluded a much more established body of literature that has focused on social networks and social support (which we would argue conceptually belong to social capital). Nevertheless, our review identifies studies that have used indicators of social cohesion such as individual perceptions of trust and reciprocity, as well as reports of civic engagement and social participation. For the outcome of self-rated health, to facilitate comparison and discussion of the findings across studies in which the outcome was dichotomous (fair/poor health versus excellent/very good/good health), all odds ratios and 95% confidence intervals presented in Table 8.2 for social trust and associational memberships correspond to associations between *higher* social capital and the relative odds of *fair/poor* self-rated health. These estimates were then plotted on the same graph for the same indicators at each of the individual and contextual levels.

8.2. Social Capital, All-Cause Mortality, and Life Expectancy

Table 8.1 provides details of the 15 studies of social capital and life expectancy or all-cause mortality that met our inclusion criteria. Of these, only three studies conducted multilevel analyses (two of which were prospective; Blakely et al., 2006; Mohan, Twigg, Barnard, & Jones, 2005), while the remaining studies were ecological (only one of which was prospective; Milyo & Mellor, 2003).

TABLE 8.1. Social capital, life expectancy, and all-cause mortality.

Authors, year	Sample size, population/ setting	Age range	Social capital measure	Health outcome measure	Covariates	Individual-level effect estimate	Area-level effect estimate
ECOLOGICAL STUDIES: *Country level* Lynch et al., 2001	16 countries	Social capital measures: 18+y Health outcome measures: All ages	Social mistrust, organizational memberships, trade union memberships, volunteering	Life expectancy, all-cause mortality rates	GDP per capita; stratified by gender	—	*1) Social mistrust:* Life expectancy $r = -0.14$, $p = 0.65$ (men) $r = 0.45$, $p = 0.12$ (women) All-cause mortality rates $r = -0.06$, $p = 0.84$ (men) $r = -0.33$, $p = 0.27$ (women) *2) Organizational memberships:* Life expectancy $r = -0.07$, $p = 0.82$ (men) $r = -0.33$, $p = 0.29$ (women) All-cause mortality rates $r = 0.17$, $p = 0.59$ (men) $r = 0.20$, $p = 0.53$ (women) *3) Trade union memberships:* Life expectancy $r = 0.13$, $p = 0.68$ (men) $r = -0.31$, $p = 0.30$ (women) All-cause mortality rates $r = 0.25$, $p = 0.42$ (men) $r = 0.36$, $p = 0.23$ (women) *4) Volunteering:* Life expectancy $r = 0.28$, $p = 0.40$ (men) $r = 0.41$, $p = 0.20$ (women)

(Continued)

TABLE 8.1. (*Continued*).

Authors, year	Sample size, population/ setting	Age range	Social capital measure	Health outcome measure	Covariates	Individual-level effect estimate	Area-level effect estimate
							All-cause mortality rates r = −0.53, p = 0.09 (men) r = −0.59, p = 0.06 (women)
Kennelly et al., 2003	19 OECD countries	Social capital measures: 18+y Health outcome measures: All ages	Social trust, associational memberships, volunteering	Gender-specific life expectancy, infant mortality rates, perinatal mortality rates	GDP per capita, Gini coefficient, physicians per capita, proportion of public expenditure in total health expenditure, fruit and vegetable consumption per capita, tobacco consumption per capita, alcohol consumption per capita, country of Japan; analyses stratified by gender and account for survey wave	—	*1) Social trust:* Life expectancy ß > 0, p = 0.47 (men) ß > 0, p = 0.25 (women) Infant mortality rates ß < 0, p = 0.31 Perinatal mortality rates ß < 0, p = 0.14 *2) Associational memberships:* Life expectancy ß > 0, p = 0.14 (men) ß > 0, p = 0.32 (women) Infant mortality rates ß < 0, p = 0.65 Perinatal mortality rates ß > 0, p = 0.22 *3) Volunteering:* Life expectancy ß > 0, p = 0.76 (men) ß > 0, p = 0.48 (women) Infant mortality rates ß > 0, p = 0.46 Perinatal mortality rates ß > 0, p = 0.15

State or regional level

Study	Sample	Measures	Social capital measure	Health outcome	Control variables		Results
Kawachi et al., 1997	39 US states	Social capital measures: 18+y Health outcome measure: all ages	Social mistrust, lack of helpfulness, voluntary group memberships	Age-standardized all-cause mortality rates	State prevalence of poverty	–	1) Social mistrust: β > 0, p < 0.01 2) Lack of helpfulness: β > 0, p < 0.01 3) Voluntary group memberships: β < 0, p < 0.01
Wilkinson et al., 1998	39 US states	Social capital measures: 18+y Health outcome measure: all ages	Social mistrust	Age-standardized all-cause mortality rates	–	–	r = 0.76, p < 0.05
Siahpush & Singh, 1999	7 states/ territories in Australia in each of seven years (n=49)	Social capital measures: 15+y Health outcome measure: all ages	Percentage of labor force with union memberships	Age-standardized all-cause mortality rates	Calendar year	–	β > 0, p < 0.05
Milyo & Mellor, 2003	2 samples: 48 US states; 39 US states	Social capital measures: 18+y Health outcome measures: All ages	Putnam social capital index (derived from 14 indicators), social mistrust	Age-standardized all-cause mortality rates	Proportion of population in poverty	–	1) Putnam social capital index: β < 0, p < 0.01 2) Social mistrust: β > 0, p < 0.01
Veenstra, 2002	29 health districts in the province of Saskatchewan, Canada	Social capital measure: 18+y Health outcome measures: All ages	Social capital index (associational memberships, social involvement, electoral participation)	Age-standardized all-cause mortality rates	Income inequality, gender composition, total crime	–	β > 0, p = 0.81
Kennedy et al., 1998	40 regions in Russia	Social capital measure: 16+y Health outcome measures: All ages	Mistrust in local and in regional government, lack of social cohesion at	Life expectancy, age-standardized all-cause mortality rates	Per capita income, proportion in poverty, perceived economic hardship in	–	1) *Mistrust in local government:* Life expectancy β < 0, p = 0.02 (men) β < 0, p = 0.053 (women) All-cause mortality rates

(Continued)

TABLE 8.1. (Continued).

Authors, year	Sample size, population/ setting	Age range	Social capital measure	Health outcome measure	Covariates	Individual-level effect estimate	Area-level effect estimate
			work, lack of interest in politics		region, per capita crime rate; analyses stratified by gender		$\beta > 0$, p = 0.01 (men)
							$\beta > 0$, p = 0.06 (women)
							2) Mistrust in regional government:
							Life expectancy
							$\beta < 0$, p = 0.15 (men)
							$\beta < 0$, p = 0.24 (women)
							All-cause mortality rates
							$\beta > 0$, p = 0.0497 (men)
							3) Lack of social cohesion at work:
							Life expectancy
							$\beta < 0$, p = 0.01 (men)
							$\beta < 0$, p = 0.04 (women)
							All-cause mortality rates
							$\beta > 0$, p = 0.02 (men)
							4) Lack of interest in politics:
							Life expectancy
							$\beta < 0$, p = 0.02 (men)
							$\beta < 0$, p = 0.06 (women)
							All-cause mortality rates
							$\beta > 0$, p = 0.10 (men)
							$\beta > 0$, p < 0.10 (women)
Skrabski et al. 2003	20 counties in Hungary	Social capital measure: 16+y Health outcome measures: 45–64 y	Social mistrust, reciprocity, received help from civic organizations	Age-specific (ages 45–64) and gender-specific all-cause mortality rates	GDP per capita, income, education, prevalence of smoking, average alcohol consumption, unemployment rate;	—	1) Social mistrust:
							$\beta > 0$, p < 0.01 (men)
							$\beta > 0$, p < 0.01 (women)
							2) Reciprocity:
							$\beta < 0$, p < 0.01 (men)
							$\beta < 0$, p < 0.01 (women)

Reference	Study population	Measures	Social capital measures	Health outcome	Follow-up	Covariates	Results
						analyses stratified by gender	3) *Received help from civic organizations:* β > 0, p < 0.01 (men)
Skrabski et al., 2004	150 subregions in Hungary	Social capital measures: 18+y; Health outcome measures: 45–64 y	Social mistrust, reciprocity, membership in civic organizat-ions, religious group involvement	Age-specific (ages 45–64) and gender-specific all-cause mortality rates	—	Income per capita, mean years of education, preva-lence of smoking, average alcohol consumption, collective efficacy; analyses stratified by gender	1) *Social mistrust:* β > 0, p < 0.01 (men); β > 0, p < 0.01 (women) 2) *Reciprocity:* β < 0, p < 0.01 (men); β < 0, p < 0.01 (women) 3) *Membership in civic organizations:* β < 0, p < 0.01 (men); β < 0, p < 0.01 (women) 4) *Religious group involvement:* β > 0, p < 0.01 (men); β < 0, p < 0.01 (women)
Turrell et al., 2006	Persons aged 25–74 years in 41 statis-tical local areas in the state of Tas-mania, Australia	Social capital meas-ures: 18+y; Health outcome measures: 25–74 y	Social trust, social cohesion, politi-cal participation	All-cause age-standardized mortality rates	—	*Area:* age, gender, socioeconomic disadvantage, geographic remoteness, neighborhood safety	1) *Social trust:* β > 0, p > 0.05 2) *Political participation:* β > 0, p > 0.05 3) *Trust in public and private institutions:* β > 0, p > 0.05 4) *Neighborhood integration:* β < 0, p > 0.05 5) *Neighborhood isolation:* β > 0, p > 0.05
Neighborhood level							
Lochner et al., 2003	342 neighborhoods in Chicago in the US	Social capital meas-ures: 18+y; Health outcome measures: 45–64 y	Trust, reciprocity, associational memberships	All-cause mortality rates (ages 45–64)	—	Socioeconomic dep-rivation; analyses stratified by	1) *Trust:* White women β < 0, p < 0.01; White men

(Continued)

TABLE 8.1. (*Continued*).

Authors, year	Sample size, population/ setting	Age range	Social capital measure	Health outcome measure	Covariates	Individual-level effect estimate	Area-level effect estimate
					race/ethnicity and gender		ß < 0, p < 0.01 Black women
							ß < 0, p < 0.05 Black men
							ß < 0, p > 0.05
							2) *Reciprocity:* White women
							ß < 0, p < 0.01 White men
							ß < 0, p < 0.05 Black women
							ß < 0, p > 0.05 Black men
							ß < 0, p < 0.05
							3) *Associational memberships:* White women
							ß < 0, p < 0.01 White men
							ß < 0, p < 0.01 Black women
							ß < 0, p > 0.05 Black men
							ß < 0, p < 0.01

MULTILEVEL STUDIES:
Neighborhood- or regional-level social capital

| Wen et al., 2005 | 12,672 adults diagnosed and hospitalized with one of 13 serious illnesses in 51 zip codes in Chicago | Social support, social network density, participation in local organizations, voluntary associations | Social capital measures: 18+y Health outcome measures: 67+years | All-cause mortality (dichotomous) | *Individual level:* age, gender, race/ ethnicity, Medicaid recipient, co-morbidity *Zip code level:* socioeconomic status | — | *1) Social support:* HR = 0.996, p > 0.05 *2) Social network density:* HR = 1.02, p > 0.05 *3) Local organizations:* HR = 3.994, p > 0.05 *4) Voluntary associations:* HR = 1.005, p > 0.05 |
| Mohan et al., 2005 | 7,578 adults in 396 electoral wards in England | *Individual level:* Belonging to community, reliable friends, frequency of feeling lonely *Ward level:* Volunteering, participation in social activities, altruistic activities, political activities, electoral participation, importance of local friends, attitudes towards belonging to neighborhood, willingness to work to improve neighborhood, talking to neighbors, frequency of meeting local people, perceived | Social capital and health outcome measures: 18–94 y | All-cause mortality | Age, gender, social class, household tenure, smoking, alcohol consumption, exercise, diet | 1) Perceived belonging to community: OR = 1.11, 95% CI = 0.93–1.32 2) Reliable friends: OR = 1.05, 95% CI = 0.63–1.78 3) Frequency of feeling lonely: OR = 1.30, 95% CI = 0.98–1.72 | *Lowest levels of:* 1) Any volunteering: OR = 1.35, 95% CI = 1.06–1.71 2) Volunteering (11+ *days over past year*): OR = 1.31, 95% CI = 1.03–1.67 3) Participation in social organizations: OR = 1.36, 95% CI = 1.37–1.73 4) Participation in altruistic organizations: OR = 1.27, 95% CI = 1.00–1.57 5) Political activities: OR = 1.27, 95% CI = 1.01–1.60 6) Electoral participation: OR = 1.03, 95% CI = 0.81–1.29 7) Importance of local friends: OR = 1.20, 95% CI = 0.96–1.51 8) Attitudes towards belonging to neighborhood: OR = 0.93, 95% CI = 0.73–1.18 9) Willingness to work to improve neighborhood: OR = 1.09, 95% CI = 0.86–1.38 10) Talking to neighbors: OR = 1.04, 95% CI = 0.83–1.30 |

(Continued)

TABLE 8.1. (*Continued*).

Authors, year	Sample size, population/ setting	Age range	Social capital measure	Health outcome measure	Covariates	Individual-level effect estimate	Area-level effect estimate
			friendliness of area, blood donation				11) Frequency of meeting local people: OR = 0.80, 95% CI = 0.63 – 1.02 12) Perceived friendliness of area: OR = 0.84, 95% CI = 0.67 – 1.06 13) Blood donation: OR = 1.05, 95% CI = 0.83 – 1.32
Blakely et al., 2006	All 25–74 year-olds in 1,683 Census area units in New Zealand	Social capital measure: 15+ y Health outcome measures: 25–74 y	*Census area unit level:* volunteering	All-cause mortality, stratified by gender	*Individual level:* age, race/ ethnicity, marital status, income, education, car access, employment status, urban residence *Neighborhood level:* socioeconomic deprivation	—	Low volunteerism: RR = 0.95, 95% CI = 0.89 – 1.02 (men) RR = 0.96, 95% CI = 0.88 – 1.04 (women)

Among ecological studies, the unit of analysis for social cohesion varied widely, from the country level down to the neighborhood level, whereas multi-level studies assessed social capital at the regional or neighborhood, but not country levels. In the country-level ecological studies, nations that were included consisted primarily of OECD nations, and excluded developing nations. Within-country ecological studies analyzed population samples in the US, Canada, Australia, as well as Russia and Hungary, while the multilevel analyses employed samples in the US, England, and New Zealand.

The vast majority of studies focused on a single indicator of social capital, such as social trust, associational memberships, and reciprocity, and were derived by aggregating survey responses among adults to the area level, while one study (Milyo & Mellor, 2003) applied the Putnam social capital index (based on 14 state-level social capital indicators), and another study (Siahpush & Singh, 1999) investigated the association for the percentage of the labor force with union memberships. Most ecological studies examined all-cause mortality rates as the health outcome across *all* age groups, including children and adolescents (appropriately summarized through age-standardization), but without stratification by age. A small subset of studies confined the examination of mortality to those of middle age (45–64 years) (Lochner, Kawachi, Brennan, & Buka, 2003; Skrabski, Kopp, & Kawachi, 2003, 2004). Two of the three multilevel analyses analyzed the risk of all-cause mortality among adults in most age groups, while the other analysis (Wen, Cagney, & Christakis, 2005) was restricted to an elderly population (67+ years), and estimated the relative hazards of dying among those diagnosed and hospitalized with serious illnesses.

Adjustment for potential confounders In ecological studies was variable, with some studies limiting control to gender and area-level deprivation (e.g., Lynch et al., 2001), and other studies controlling for ecological factors expectedly correlated with health behaviors, that could plausibly mediate the effects of social capital (Kennelly, O'Shea, & Garvey, 2003; Skrabski et al., 2003, 2004). In multilevel studies, suitable control was made for several individual-level factors including demographic characteristics (e.g., age, gender, and race/ethnicity) and socioeconomic status (e.g., income or education), through adjustment in statistical models or stratification. Nonetheless, control at the area level was confined to area-level socioeconomic deprivation (Blakely et al., 2006; Wen et al., 2005), or was absent altogether (Mohan et al., 2005), so that residual confounding bias due to effects of other area-level factors such as racial/ethnic heterogeneity cannot be excluded.

Social cohesion was fairly consistently associated in a protective direction with mortality outcomes at the state, regional, and/or neighborhood levels in the US, Russia, and Hungary, whereas the relationships were statistically non-significant in other countries including Canada, Australia, and New Zealand as well as in cross-national studies. Among the three multilevel studies, findings were more mixed, with only one study (Mohan et al., 2005) observing significant associations for selected social capital measures (volunteering, organizational participation, and non-electoral political participation, but not informal socializing domains) after adjustment for individual-level social capital indicators.

8.3. Social Capital and Self-Rated Health

Altogether 32 studies met our inclusion criteria for social capital and self-rated health (Table 8.2). Only one of these studies was ecological, while 24 were multi-level (with higher-level units ranging from the country level to the state and neighborhood or community level), and seven were conducted at the individual level. Only two studies (both multilevel; Mellor & Milyo, 2005; Zimmerman & Bell, 2006) were prospective, while all other studies were cross-sectional.

As with studies involving mortality, studies of self-rated health have predominantly analyzed single indicators of social cohesion such as trust, associational membership, and reciprocity. Studies that incorporated a large number of indicators combined indicators either through factor analysis or by taking the mean of standardized values for multiple indicators, with one such study measuring both community- and individual-level bonding and bridging social capital (Kim, Subramanian, & Kawachi, 2006a). In nine of the 25 multilevel studies, individual and collective social capital were simultaneously examined, with individual-level social capital being measured via the same survey items (without aggregation) as at the area level.

Most studies dichotomized the outcome of self-rated health into fair/poor versus excellent/very good/good health, though some studies analyzed the outcome as a continuous or ordinal variable.

The sole ecological study (Lynch et al., 2001) was conducted with countries as the unit of analysis, and adjusted for gross domestic product (GDP) per capita. The majority of multilevel studies adjusted for key individual-level covariates including age, gender, race/ethnicity, and income or education. Meanwhile, adjustment for potential confounders at the area level ranged widely, with some studies making no adjustment at all, and other studies controlling for multiple potential confounders (see for e.g., Browning & Cagney, 2003).

In multilevel studies, measures of social capital at the individual level were for the most part significantly associated with better self-rated health. By contrast, the association between area social cohesion and self-rated health was more mixed, especially after adjustment for individual-level covariates (Table 8.2). These contrasts between the individual and area level are apparent in Figures 8.1 through 8.4, which plot the odds ratios and 95% confidence intervals for the associations between higher social trust and associational memberships and fair/poor self-rated health (Figures 8.1 and 8.3 at the individual level, and Figures 8.2A and 8.4A at the area level after adjustment for individual-level social capital, respectively).

There was also evidence of attenuation of the odds ratios with the addition of individual-level social capital indicators, in some instances to statistical non-significance: Figures 8.2B and 8.4B show the odds ratio estimates for area-level social trust and associational memberships in the multilevel analyses *without* adjustment for individual-level social capital. All of these studies were cross-sectional in design. Here, a general pattern emerges of stronger inverse and statistically significant odds ratios prior to multivariate adjustment, compared to the

TABLE 8.2. Social capital and self-rated physical and general health.

Authors, year	Sample size, population/ setting	Age range	Social capital measure	Form of self-rated health measure	Covariates	Individual-level effect estimate	Area-level effect estimate
ECOLOGICAL STUDIES: *Country-level social capital*							
Lynch et al., 2001	16 countries	Social capital measure & health outcome measure: 18+ y	Social mistrust, organizational memberships, trade union memberships, volunteering	Proportion reporting fair/ poor health	GDP per capita	—	1) Social mistrust: r = 0.47, p = 0.11 2) Organizational memberships: r = −0.36, p = 0.25 3) Trade union memberships: r = −0.17, p = 0.58 4) Volunteering: r = −0.80, p = 0.003
MULTILEVEL STUDIES: *Country-level social capital*							
Helliwell & Putnam, 2004	83,520 adults in 49 countries	Social capital measure & health outcome measure: 18+ y	*Individual level:* social trust (general, in police) associational memberships, *National level:* social trust, associational memberships	Continuous (higher = better health)	*Individual level:* age, gender, marital status, employment status, importance of God/religion, frequency of attending religious service *National level:* median income, importance of God/religion,	1) General social trust: β > 0, p < 0.01 2) Trust in police: β > 0, p < 0.01 3) Associational memberships: β > 0, p < 0.05	1) General social trust: β > 0, p < 0.01 2) Associational memberships: β > 0, p < 0.01

(Continued)

TABLE 8.2. (Continued)

Authors, year	Sample size, population/ setting	Age range	Social capital measure	Form of self-rated health measure	Covariates	Individual-level effect estimate	Area-level effect estimate
Poortinga, 2006a	42,358 adults in 22 European countries	Social capital measure & health outcome measure: 15+ y	*Individual level:* social trust, associational memberships *National level:* social trust, associational memberships	Dichotomous	governance quality *Individual level:* age, gender, education, income	1) High social trust: OR = 0.66, 95% CI = 0.62–0.70 2) High associational memberships: OR = 0.76, 95% CI = 0.70–0.82	1) High social trust: OR = 0.91, 95% CI = 0.73–1.14 2) High associational memberships: OR = 0.91, 95% CI = 0.71–1.17
State-level social capital							
Kawachi et al., 1999	167,259 adults in 39 US states	Social capital measure & health outcome measure: 18+ y	*State level:* social trust, reciprocity, group memberships	Dichotomous	*Individual level:* age, gender, race/ ethnicity, income, marital status, smoking, obesity, health insurance coverage, health checkup in last two years	–	1) High social trust: OR = 0.71, 95% CI = 0.67–0.75 2) High reciprocity: OR = 0.68, 95% CI = 0.64–0.71 3) High group memberships: OR = 0.82, 95% CI = 0.76–0.88
Subramanian et al., 2001	144,692 adults in 39 US states	Social capital measure & health outcome measure: 18–98 y	*State level:* social mistrust (continuous %)	Dichotomous	*Individual level:* age, gender, race/ethnicity, marital status, income, smoking, health insurance coverage, health	–	Higher social trust: OR = 0.99; 95% CI = 0.98–0.996

Study	Sample	Measures	Outcome type	Covariates	Results
				checkup in last year *State level:* median household income, income inequality *State-individual interaction:* state income inequality x individual income interactions	—
Mellor & Milyo, 2005	2 samples: ~68,000 adults in 39 US states; ~76,000 adults in 48 US states	Social capital measure: 18+y Health outcome measure: 16+y *State level:* social mistrust, group memberships, Putnam social capital index (derived from 14 indicators)	Ordinal (five categories; higher = better health)	*Individual level:* age, gender, race/ethnicity, marital status, income, education, health insurance coverage, central city/ MSA residence, *State level:* median household income	1) Social mistrust: β < 0, p < 0.05 2) Group memberships: β > 0, p > 0.05 3) Putnam social capital index: β > 0, p < 0.05
Neighborhood- or community-level social capital					
Subramanian et al., 2002	21,456 adults in 40 US communities	Social capital measure & health outcome measure: 18–89 y *Community level:* social trust (general; trust in neighbors, coworkers, fellow congregants, store employees, local police)	Dichotomous	*Individual level:* age, gender, race/ ethnicity, marital status, income, education	High social trust: OR = 0.55, 95% CI = 0.50-0.61 High social trust: OR = 0.87, 95% CI = 0.62-1.21 Interaction models: significant positive interaction between high community social trust and high individual social trust

(Continued)

TABLE 8.2. (*Continued*)

Authors, year	Sample size, population/ setting	Age range	Social capital measure	Form of self-rated health measure	Covariates	Individual-level effect estimate	Area-level effect estimate
Browning & Cagney, 2003	2,218 adults in 333 neighborhoods in the city of Chicago, US	Social capital measure & health outcome measure: 18+y	*Neighborhood level:* friendship social support and networks	Dichotomous	*Individual level:* age, gender, race/ ethnicity, marital status, income, education, household tenure, years in neighborhood, foreign-born status, interview year *Neighborhood level:* total population, residential stability, immigrant concentration, prior neighborhood health, disorder, anomie, tolerance of risk behavior, collective efficacy	–	High social support and networks: OR = 0.89, 95% CI = 0.78-1.02
Wen et al., 2003	3,459 adults in 275 neighborhood clusters in Chicago	Social capital measure & health outcome measure: 18+y	*Neighborhood level:* social resources (reciprocity, density of social networks, social cohesion, informal social control)	Ordinal (four categories; higher = better health)	*Individual level:* age, gender, race/ ethnicity, marital status, income, education, smoking, hypertension, interview year	–	Higher social resources: OR = 1.19 p < 0.05

Study	Sample	Social capital measure & health outcome measure	Variables	Results
Drukker et al., 2003	3,401 adolescents in 36 neighborhoods in Maastricht, Netherlands	Social capital measure: 20–65 y Health outcome measure: ~10–12 y *Neighborhood level:* social cohesion and trust Continuous	*Neighborhood level:* poverty, affluence, income inequality, education, health-enhancing services, crime exposure, prior health *Individual level:* gender, grade retention *Household level:* occupational status, education, family welfare status, single parent *Neighborhood level:* socioeconomic deprivation, residential instability	– ß < 0, p > 0.05
Lindström et al., 2004	3,602 adults in 75 neighborhoods in Malmö, Sweden	Social capital measure & health outcome measure: 20–80 y *Individual level:* social participation Dichotomous	*Individual level:* age, gender, country of origin, education	High social participation: OR = 0.34, 95% CI = 0.27–0.43
Helliwell & Putnam, 2004	28,766 adults in 40 US communities	Social capital measure & health outcome measure: 18–99 y *Individual level:* associational memberships, social trust (general, in neighbors, police) *Community level:* associational Continuous (higher = better health)	*Individual level:* age, gender, marital status, employment status, importance of God/religion, frequency of attending religious	1) Associational memberships: ß > 0, p < 0.01 2) General trust: ß > 0, p < 0.01 3) Trust in neighbors: ß > 0, p < 0.01
				1) Associational memberships: ß > 0, p > 0.05 2) Social trust: ß > 0, p < 0.01

(Continued)

TABLE 8.2. (*Continued*)

Authors, year	Sample size, population/ setting	Age range	Social capital measure	Form of self-rated health measure	Covariates	Individual-level effect estimate	Area-level effect estimate
			memberships, social trust		service, commute time to work *Community level:* median income, importance of God/religion	4) Trust in police: ß > 0, p < 0.01	
Veenstra, 2005a	1,184 adults in 25 communities in the province of British Columbia, Canada	Social capital measures & health outcome measure: 18+y	*Individual level:* social trust, political trust, social participation	Dichotomous	*Individual level:* age, gender, foreign-born, income, education	*Social trust:* OR = 0.73, 95% CI = 0.56–0.97 p = 0.03 *Political trust:* OR = 0.57, 95% CI = 0.44–0.75 p < 0.01 *Participation in voluntary associations:* OR = 0.96, 95% CI = 0.84–1.10 p = 0.58	—
Ziersch et al., 2005	2,400 adults in sub-urban neighbor-hoods in Adelaide, Australia	Social capital measure & health outcome measure: 18+y	*Neighborhood level:* social trust, social connections/cohesion	Self-reported physi-cal health (continuous)	*Individual level:* age, gender, income, education, house-hold tenure, years at address *Neighborhood level:* pollution, safety	—	1) *Neighborhood trust:* ß > 0, p > 0.05 2) *Neighborhood connections/ cohesion:* ß > 0, p > 0.05

Steptoe & Feldman, 2001	654 adults in 37 neighborhoods in London, England	Social capital measure & health outcome measure: 18–94 y	*Neighborhood level:* social cohesion	Self-reported physical function (dichotomous)	*Individual level:* age, sex, socioeconomic deprivation *Neighborhood level:* socioeconomic deprivation	–	Low social cohesion: OR = 2.31, 95% CI = 1.16-6.63
Kavanagh et al., 2006b	15,112 adults in 41 statistical local areas in the state of Tasmania, Australia	Social capital measure & health outcome measure: 18–97 y	*Area level:* social trust, social cohesion, political participation	Dichotomous	*Individual level:* age, marital status, income, education, indigenous status, smoking *Area level:* socioeconomic disadvantage, geographic remoteness, neighborhood safety	–	*Men:* 1) Social trust: $\beta < 0$, $p = 0.01$ 2) Political participation: $\beta > 0$, $p = 0.88$ 3) Trust in public and private institutions: $\beta > 0$, $p = 0.92$ 4) Neighborhood integration: $\beta < 0$, $p = 0.53$ 5) Neighborhood alienation: $\beta < 0$, $p = 0.02$ *Women:* 1) Social trust: $\beta < 0$, $p = 0.01$ 2) Political participation: $\beta > 0$, $p = 0.91$ 3) Trust in public and private institutions: $\beta > 0$, $p = 0.96$ 4) Neighborhood integration: $\beta < 0$, $p = 0.30$ 5) Neighborhood alienation: $\beta < 0$, $p = 0.31$

(Continued)

TABLE 8.2. (Continued)

Authors, year	Sample size, population/ setting	Age range	Social capital measure	Form of self-rated health measure	Covariates	Individual-level effect estimate	Area-level effect estimate
Zimmerman & Bell, 2006	4,817 adults in 855 US counties and 45 states	Social capital measure: 18+y Health outcome measure: 40–45 y	*State level:* social capital index (derived from nine indicators of social trust, civic engagement, and anomie)	Dichotomous	*Individual level:* gender, race/ ethnicity, marital status, urban residence, region, education, poverty status, employment status, health insurance status *County level:* proportion wealthy, unskilled wages, housing affordability, crime rate, proportion unemployed, proportion Black, proportion Hispanic, mean income, mean years of education, index of availability of psychiatric services, index of availability of health services *State level:* generosity of state spending	–	OR = 1.09, 95% CI = 0.56–2.12

Study	Sample	Age of measures	Social capital measure	Measurement	Covariates	Results	Results
Drukker et al., 2005	801 adolescents in 343 neighborhoods in Chicago; 533 adolescents in 36 neighborhoods in Maastricht, Netherlands	Social capital measure: 18+y Health outcome measure: 12 y (Chicago); 10–13 y (Maastricht)	Neighborhood level: social cohesion and trust	Continuous (higher = better health)	Individual level: gender, age/grade retention, race/ethnicity, Household level: occupational status, education, family welfare status, single parent Neighborhood level: socioeconomic deprivation	–	Maastricht: β < 0, p > 0.05 Chicago, non-Hispanics: β > 0, p > 0.05 Chicago, Hispanics: β > 0, p > 0.05
Poortinga, 2006d	7,394 adults in 4,332 households in 720 postal code sectors in the UK	Social capital measure & health outcome measure: 16+y	Individual level: Social support, social trust, civic participation Community level: reciprocity	Dichotomous	Individual level: age, gender, physical activity Household level: social class, household tenure	1) Severe lack of social support: OR = 2.17, 95% CI = 1.72-2.73 2) High social trust: OR = 0.69, 95% CI = 0.58-0.82 3) High civic participation: OR = 0.62, 95% CI = 0.51-0.76	Reciprocity: OR = 0.52, 95% CI = 0.33-0.83
Kim et al., 2006a	24,835 adults in 40 US communities	Social capital measure & health outcome measure: 18–99 y	Individual level: formal bonding social capital, trust in members of one's race/ethnicity; formal bridging, informal bridging, social trust	Dichotomous	Individual level: age, gender, race/ethnicity, marital status, income, education Community level: mean age, percent low income, state community	1) High formal bonding social capital: OR = 0.77, 95% CI = 0.66-0.88 2) High trust in members of one's race/ethnicity: OR = 0.88, 95% CI = 0.79-0.98	1-SD* higher bonding social capital: OR = 0.86, 95% CI = 0.80-0.92 1-SD* higher bridging social capital: OR = 0.95, 95% CI = 0.88-1.02 Interaction models: significantly weaker bonding social capital associations among Blacks and those in the "Other"

(Continued)

TABLE 8.2. (Continued)

Authors, year	Sample size, population/ setting	Age range	Social capital measure	Form of self-rated health measure	Covariates	Individual-level effect estimate	Area-level effect estimate
			Community level: bonding social capital, bridging social capital			3) High formal bridging: OR = 1.07, 95% CI = 0.87-1.31 4) High informal bridging: OR = 0.99, 95% CI = 0.91-1.08 5) High social trust OR = 0.54, 95% CI = 0.49-0.59	racial/ethnic category than among Whites
Kim et al., 2006b	24,835 adults in 40 US communities	Social capital measure & health outcome measure: 18–99 y	*Individual level:* social trust, informal social interactions, diversity of friendship networks, electoral political participation, non-electoral political participation, formal group involvement/religious group involvement/ giving and volunteering *Community level:* three social capital subscales based on same	Dichotomous	*Individual level:* age, gender, race/ethnicity, marital status, income, education, proximity to core urban areas *Community level:* mean age, proportion with low income, proportion with low income, state community	1) Social trust: OR = 0.56, 95% CI = 0.52-0.62 2) Informal social interactions: OR = 0.96, 95% CI = 0.88-1.05 3) Electoral participation: OR = 0.78, 95% CI = 0.71-0.86 4) Diversity of friendships: OR = 0.98, 95% CI = 0.90-1.07 5) Non-electoral participation OR = 1.18, 95% CI = 1.06-1.31	*Subscale 1* (social trust, informal social interactions, electoral political participation): OR = 1.00, 95% CI = 0.93-1.06 *Subscale 2* (formal group participation, religious group participation, giving and volunteering): OR = 0.94, 95% CI = 0.89-0.99 *Subscale 3* (diversity of friendships, non-electoral political participation): OR = 0.91, 95% CI = 0.85-0.98 *High on all three subscales:* OR = 0.82, 95% CI = 0.69-0.98

Author, year	Sample	Social capital measure & health outcome	Indicators	Type	Covariates	Results (sample 1)	Results (sample 2)
			8 indicators as at individual level			6) Formal group involvement/religious group involvement/giving and volunteering OR = 0.68, 95% CI = 0.62–0.75	
Poortinga, 2006c	2 UK samples: 1) 7,988 adults in 4,787 households in 360 sampling points/postal code sectors 2) 7,394 adults in 4,332 households in 720 postal code sectors	Social capital measure & health outcome measure: 16+y	*Individual level:* social support, social trust, civic participation *Community level:* social trust, civic participation, reciprocity	Dichotomous	*Individual level:* age, gender, physical activity *Household level:* social class, household tenure	1) Severe lack of social support: OR = 2.21, 95% CI = 1.76–2.78 2) High social trust: OR = 0.75, 95% CI = 0.62–0.90 3) High civic participation: OR = 0.62, 95% CI = 0.51–0.77	1) High social trust: OR = 0.39, 95% CI = 0.22–0.71 2) High civic participation: OR = 0.90, 95% CI = 0.53–1.54 3) High reciprocity: OR = 0.52, 95% CI = 0.33–0.83
Poortinga, 2006b	14,836 adults in 720 postal code sectors in the UK	Social capital measure & health outcome measure: 16+y	*Individual level:* social support, social trust, civic participation, reciprocity	Dichotomous	*Individual level:* age, gender, marital status, social class, unemployment status, household tenure, access to amenities, presence of local social problems, urban residence	1) Severe lack of social support: OR = 1.64, 95% CI = 1.42–1.90 2) High social trust: OR = 0.74, 95% CI = 0.67–0.82 3) High social participation: OR = 0.67, 95% CI = 0.60–0.76 4) High reciprocity: OR = 0.82, 95% CI = 0.73–0.93	–
Franzini et al., 2005	3,151 adults in 100 neighborhoods in Texas	Social capital measure & health	*Neighborhood level:* social capital	Continuous	*Individual level:* age, gender, race/	–	$\beta > 0$, $p < 0.05$

(Continued)

TABLE 8.2. (*Continued*)

Authors, year	Sample size, population/setting	Age range	Social capital measure	Form of self-rated health measure	Covariates	Individual-level effect estimate	Area-level effect estimate
			(based on 2 sub-scales of social trust, reciprocity)		ethnicity, family income-to-needs ratio *Neighborhood level:* collective efficacy, child-related processes, disorder, fear, racism		
Yip et al., in press	1,218 adults in 48 villages in the Shandong province, China	Social capital measure & health outcome measure: 16-80 y	*Individual level:* Social trust, party memberships, voluntary organization memberships *Village level:* Social trust, party memberships, voluntary organization memberships	Dichotomous	*Individual level:* age, gender, marital status, occupation, education *Household level:* income, assets, size	1) Social trust: OR = 0.71, 95% CI = 0.61-0.83 2) Party memberships: OR = 0.62, 95% CI = 0.43-0.90 3) Voluntary organization memberships: OR = 0.81, 95% CI = 0.50-1.32	1) Social trust: OR = 0.76, 95% CI = 0.51-1.13 2) Party memberships: OR = 0.96, 95% CI = 0.13-7.10 3) Voluntary organization memberships: OR = 1.15, 95% CI = 0.04-35.30
INDIVIDUAL-LEVEL STUDIES: Rose, 2000	1,904 adults in the Russian Federation	Social capital measure & health outcome measures: 18+ y	General social trust, social support	Self-rated physical health (continuous; higher = better health)	Age, gender, income, education, subjective social status	1) General social trust: β > 0, p < 0.05 4) Social support: β > 0, p < 0.05	—

(Continued)

					Selected outcomes	

| Veenstra, 2000 | 534 adults in the province of Saskatchewan, Canada | Social capital measure & health outcome measure: 18+y | Civic participation, participation in clubs; political trust, trust in neighbors, trust in community members, trust in members of part of province, general social trust; frequency of socialization with co-workers, willingness to turn to co-worker in time of need, religious service attendance | Dichotomous | income, education | Civic participation: ß not reported, p > 0.05 Participation in clubs: ß not reported, p > 0.05 Political trust, trust in neighbors, trust in community members, trust in members of part of province, general social trust: ß not reported, p > 0.05 *Also adjusted for income, education:* Frequency of socialization with co-workers: ß < 0, p > 0.05 Willingness to turn to co-worker in time of need: ß < 0, p > 0.05 Religious service attendance: ß < 0, p < 0.05 |
| Hyyppä & Mäki, 2001 | 2,000 adults in municipalities in Finland | Social capital measure & health outcome measure: 16+y | Social mistrust, associational participation, religious group | Dichotomous | Age, income, smoking, body mass index, urban residence, migration, | 1) 1–SD* higher social trust: OR = 0.69, 95% CI = 0.43–1.16 (men); |

TABLE 8.2. (*Continued*)

Authors, year	Sample size, population/ setting	Age range	Social capital measure	Form of self-rated health measure	Covariates	Individual-level effect estimate	Area-level effect estimate
			participation, community participation		comorbidity; analyses stratified by gender	OR = 0.64, 95% CI = 0.39–1.06 (women) 2) 1–SD* higher associational participation: OR = 0.74, 95% CI = 0.47–1.17 (men); OR = 0.80, 95% CI = 0.54–1.19 (women) 3) 1–SD* higher religious group participation: OR = 0.42, 95% CI = 0.21–0.85 (men); OR = 0.68, 95% CI = 0.41–1.13 (women) 4) 1–SD* higher community participation: OR = 1.02, 95% CI = 0.55–1.88 (men) OR = 0.83, 95% CI = 0.44–1.59 (women)	

Hyyppä & Mäki, 2003	2,000 adults in municipalities in Finland	Social capital measure & health outcome measure: 16–65 y	Associational participation, friendship networks, religious group participation, hobby group participation	Dichotomous	Age, gender, language, migration, education, income, employment status, smoking, drinking, body mass index, comorbidity	1) 1–SD* higher associational participation: OR = 0.84, 95% CI = 0.71–1.00 2) 1–SD* higher friendship network: OR = 0.80, 95% CI = 0.69–0.92 3) Religious group participation: OR = 0.75, 95% CI = 0.64–0.89 4) Hobby group participation: OR = 1.09, 95% CI = 0.89–1.33	–
Pollack & Knesebeck, 2004	608 adults in the US and 682 adults in Germany	Social capital measure & health outcome measure: 60+y	Social trust, reciprocity, associational memberships	Dichotomous	Age, gender, income, education	1) High social trust: OR = 0.5, 95% CI = 0.3–0.8 2) High reciprocity OR = 0.4, 95% CI = 0.2–0.6 3) High associational memberships OR = 0.7, 95% CI = 0.4–1.2	–
Veenstra et al., 2005b	1,504 adults in the city of Hamilton, Canada	Social capital & health outcome measures: 18+y	Membership/involvement in voluntary associations	Dichotomous	Age, gender, income, education, neighborhood	Higher voluntary association involvement: OR = 0.92, p = 0.20	–

(Continued)

TABLE 8.2. (*Continued*)

Authors, year	Sample size, population/ setting	Age range	Social capital measure	Form of self-rated health measure	Covariates	Individual-level effect estimate	Area-level effect estimate
Rojas & Carlson, 2006	1,794 adults in Taganrog, Russia	Social capital measure & health outcome measure: 20+ y	Membership in trade union/ political organizations, in other organizations, contact with neighbors	Continuous (higher = better health)	Age, gender, marital status, income, education	1) Membership in trade union/ political organizations: ß > 0, p < 0.01 2) Membership in other organizations: ß > 0, p = 0.01 3) Contact with neighbors: ß > 0, p = 0.10	–

* 1–SD = l–standard deviation.

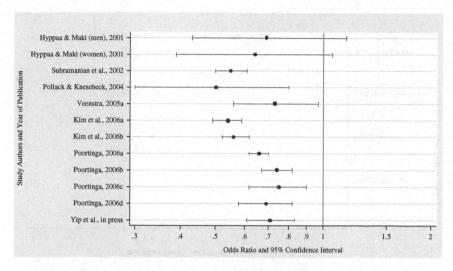

FIGURE 8.1. Studies of Individual-Level Trust and Fair/Poor Self-Rated Health
(Dichotomous)

odds ratios *after* adjustment for individual-level social capital indicators. Since
perceptions of social cohesion among individuals are arguably shaped by social
cohesion at higher spatial levels, the contextual effect of social cohesion after
adjustment for individual-level variables may be considered "lower bound" estimates for the odds ratios and confidence intervals.

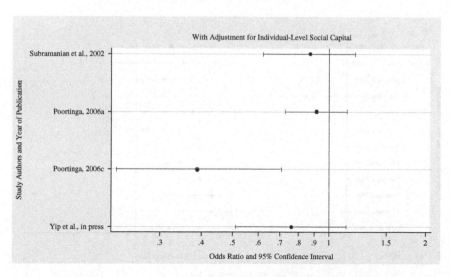

FIGURE 8.2A. Studies of Area-Level Trust and Fair/Poor Self-Rated Health
(Dichotomous)

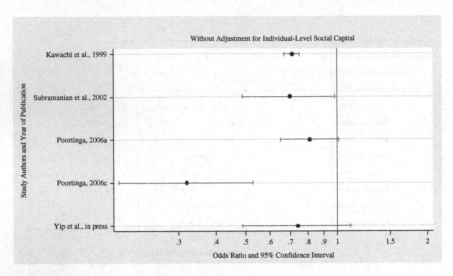

FIGURE 8.2B. Studies of Area-Level Trust and Fair/Poor Self-Rated Health (Dichotomous)

In the multilevel studies, it is also noteworthy that the studies that were null (i.e., with 95% confidence intervals that included the null value) were mainly based on study samples in relatively more egalitarian countries (for individual-level social trust, in Finland; and for individual-level associational memberships, in Finland, China, and Canada) (Figures 8.1 and 8.3). In the two studies that used

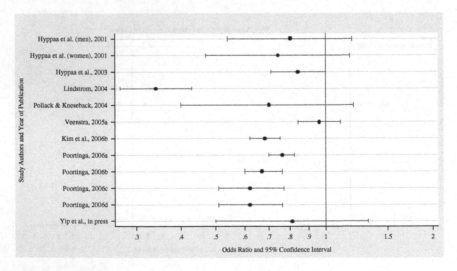

FIGURE 8.3. Studies of Individual-Level Associational Memberships and Fair/Poor Self-Rated Health (Dichotomous)

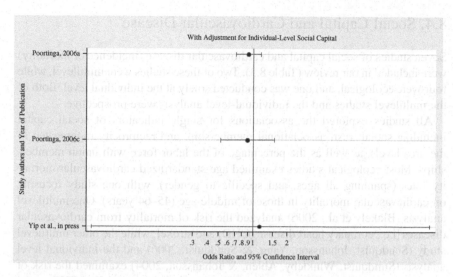

FIGURE 8.4A. Studies of Area-Level Associational Memberships and Fair/Poor Self-Rated Health (Dichotomous)

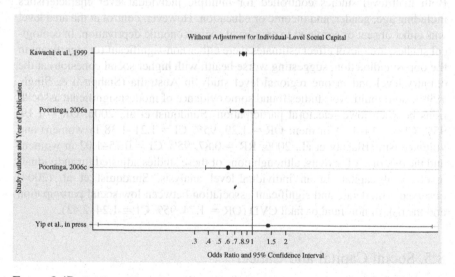

FIGURE 8.4B. Studies of Area-Level Associational Memberships and Fair/Poor Self-Rated Health (Dichotomous)

composite indices constructed from multiple social capital indicators (Kim & Kawachi, 2006b; Mellor & Milyo, 2005), significant associations were found, and were stronger than for any given subscale in the study by Kim & Kawachi (2006b), suggesting that measurement error in studies that utilized single-item measures of social cohesion may have downwardly biased the effect estimates.

8.4. Social Capital and Cardiovascular Disease

Seven studies of social capital and cardiovascular disease (incidence or mortality) were included in our review (Table 8.3). Two of these studies were multilevel, while four were ecological, and one was conducted solely at the individual level. Both of the multilevel studies and the individual-level analysis were prospective.

All studies explored the associations for single indicators of social capital including social trust, associational membership, and reciprocity (aggregated to the area level), as well as the percentage of the labor force with union memberships. Most ecological studies examined age-standardized cardiovascular mortality rates (spanning all ages, and specific to gender), with one study focusing on cardiovascular mortality in those of middle age (45–64 years). One multilevel analysis (Blakely et al., 2006) analyzed the risk of mortality from cardiovascular diseases [i.e., coronary heart disease (CHD) and stroke], while the other multilevel study (Sundquist, Johansson, Yang, & Sundquist, 2006) and the individual-level analysis (Sundquist, Winkleby, Ahlen, & Johansson, 2004) examined the risk of first incident non-fatal CHD events requiring hospitalization and fatal CHD.

Adjustment for key potential confounders in ecological studies was variable. Both multilevel studies controlled for multiple individual-level characteristics including age, gender, and income or education. However, control at the area level was either absent or confined to area-level socioeconomic deprivation. In ecological studies, area-level effect estimates were either non-significant (or significant in the opposite direction, suggesting worse health with higher social cohesion) at the country level and in one regional-level study in Australia (Siahpush & Singh, 1999). Both multilevel studies found some evidence of modest significant associations between lower electoral participation (Sundquist et al., 2006; OR = 1.19, 95% CI = 1.14–1.24 in men; OR = 1.29, 95% CI = 1.21–1.38 in women) and volunteerism (Blakely et al., 2006; RR = 0.87, 95% CI = 0.75–1.02 in women) and the risk of CVD events, although none of these studies adjusted for individual-level social capital. In an individual-level analysis, Sundquist et al. (2004) observed a moderate and significant association between low social participation and the risk of non-fatal or fatal CVD (OR = 1.74, 95% CI = 1.24–2.43).

8.5. Social Capital and Cancer

Four studies of social capital and cancer met our inclusion criteria (Table 8.4), and overlapped with studies that looked at cardiovascular disease. Only one of these studies was multilevel (and was additionally prospective) (Blakely et al., 2006), with volunteering measured through aggregation of individual-level measures to the neighborhood level, while the remaining studies were ecological and cross-sectional, investigating social capital in relation to age-standardized cancer mortality rates at the country, state, and regional levels. One of these studies (Lynch et al., 2001) examined mortality rates for cancer at specific sites (lung, prostate, and breast).

TABLE 8.3. Social capital and cardiovascular disease.

Authors, year	Sample size, population/ setting	Age range	Social capital measure	Health outcome measure	Covariates	Individual-level effect estimate	Area-level effect estimate
ECOLOGICAL STUDIES: *Country level*							
Lynch et al., 2001	16 countries	Social capital measures: 18+ y Health outcome measures: All ages	Social mistrust, organizational memberships, trade union memberships, volunteering	Gender-specific age-standardized mortality rates for each of heart disease and stroke	GDP per capita; analyses stratified by gender	—	*1) Social mistrust:* Heart disease r = −0.63, p = 0.02 (men) r = −0.61, p = 0.03 (women) Stroke r = −0.29, p = 0.33 (women) r = −0.15, p = 0.62 (men) *2) Organizational memberships:* Heart disease r = 0.30, p = 0.35 (women) r = 0.36, p = 0.25 (men) Stroke r = 0.02, p = 0.95 (women); r = −0.08, p = 0.81 (men) *3) Trade union memberships:* Heart disease r = 0.46, p = 0.11 (women) r = 0.53, p = 0.06 (men) Stroke r = 0.31, p = 0.29 (women); r = 0.31, p = 0.30 (men) *4) Volunteering:* Heart disease r = −0.14, p = 0.67 (women) r = −0.11, p = 0.74 (men)

(Continued)

TABLE 8.3. (*Continued*)

Authors, year	Sample size, population/ setting	Age range	Social capital measure	Health outcome measure	Covariates	Individual-level effect estimate	Area-level effect estimate
							Stroke: $r = -0.55$, $p = 0.08$ (women) $r = -0.60$, $p = 0.05$ (men)
State or regional level							
Siahpush & Singh, 1999	7 states/territories in Australia in each of 7 years (n = 49)	Social capital measures: 15+y Health outcome measures: All ages	Percentage of labor force with union memberships	Age-standardized mortality rates for each of heart disease and stroke	Calendar year	–	Heart disease: $\beta > 0$, $p < 0.05$ Stroke: $\beta > 0$, $p < 0.05$
Kennedy et al., 1998	40 regions in Russia	Social capital measure: 16+y Health outcome measures: All ages	Mistrust in local and in regional government, lack of social cohesion at work, lack of interest in politics	Gender-specific age-standardized cardiovascular disease mortality rates	Per capita income, proportion in poverty, perceived economic hardship in region, per capita crime rate; analyses stratified by gender	–	1) Mistrust in local government $\beta > 0$, $p < 0.01$ (men) $\beta > 0$, $p = 0.02$ (women) 2) Mistrust in regional government $\beta > 0$, $p = 0.01$ (men) $\beta > 0$, $p = 0.04$ (women) 3) Lack of social cohesion at work $\beta > 0$, $p = 0.58$ (men) $\beta > 0$, $p = 0.72$ (women) 4) Lack of interest in politics $\beta > 0$, $p = 0.046$ (men) $\beta > 0$, $p = 0.10$ (women)
Neighborhood level							
Lochner et al., 2003	342 neighborhoods in Chicago in the US	Social capital measures: 18+y	Trust, reciprocity, associational memberships	Gender and race/ ethnicity specific	Socioeconomic deprivation; analyses	–	1) *Trust:* White women $\beta < 0$, $p < 0.05$

		Health outcome measures: 45–64 y	heart disease mortality rates	stratified by race/ethnicity and gender	White men β < 0, p < 0.01 Black women β < 0, p > 0.05 Black men β < 0, p > 0.05 2) *Reciprocity:* White women β < 0, p > 0.05 White men β < 0, p < 0.05 Black women β > 0, p > 0.05 Black men β < 0, p > 0.05 3) *Associational memberships:* White women β < 0, p < 0.01 White men β < 0, p < 0.01 Black women β < 0, p > 0.05 Black men β < 0, p > 0.05
MULTILEVEL STUDIES: *Neighborhood- or regional-level social capital* Sundquist et al., 2006	1,358,932 men and 1,446,747 women aged 45–74 years in 9,667 small	Social capital measure: 18+y Health outcome measures: 45–74 y *Area level:* local electoral participation	First hospitalization for a fatal or non-fatal coronary heart disease event	*Individual level:* age, country of birth, marital status, education, housing tenure; –	Low electoral participation: OR = 1.19, 95% CI = 1.14–1.24 (men) OR = 1.29, 95% CI = 1.21–1.38 (women)

(Continued)

TABLE 8.3. (*Continued*)

Authors, year	Sample size, population/ setting	Age range	Social capital measure	Health outcome measure	Covariates	Individual-level effect estimate	Area-level effect estimate
	area market sta- tistics in Sweden				analyses stratified by gender		
Blakely et al., 2006	All 25–74 year-olds in 1,683 Census area units in New Zealand	Social capital measure: 15+y Health outcome measure: 25–74 y	Volunteering	Cardiovascular mortality	*Individual level:* age, race/ ethnicity, marital status, income, education, car access, employ- ment status, urban residence *Neighborhood level:* socioeconomic deprivation Analyses stratified by gender	–	Low volunteerism: RR = 1.00, 95% CI = 0.90–1.12 (men) RR = 0.87, 95% CI = 0.75–1.02 (women)
INDIVIDUAL- LEVEL STUDIES:							
Sundquist et al., 2004	6,861 men and women in Sweden	Social capital & health outcome measures: 35–74 y	Social participation (derived from 18 items on informal social interactions and associational memberships)	Death due to coro- nary heart disease or first hospital- ization for a non- fatal coronary heart disease event	Age, sex, education, housing tenure	Low social participation: HR = 1.74, 95% CI = 1.24–2.43	–

TABLE 8.4. Social capital and cancer.

Authors, year	Sample size, population/ setting	Age range	Social capital measure	Health outcome measure	Covariates	Individual-level effect estimate	Area-level effect estimate
ECOLOGICAL STUDIES: *Country level* Lynch et al., 2001	16 countries	Social capital measure: 18+y Health outcome measures: All ages	Social mistrust, organizational memberships, trade union memberships, volunteering	Age-standardized mortality rates for each of lung, prostate, and breast cancer	GDP per capita; analyses stratified by gender	–	*1) Social mistrust:* Lung cancer r = −0.07, p = 0.83 (men) r = −0.44, p = 0.13 (women) Prostate cancer (men) r = −0.16, p = 0.60 Breast cancer (women) r = −0.21, p = 0.49 *2) Organizational memberships:* Lung cancer r = 0.33, p = 0.30 (men) r = 0.17, p = 0.59 (women) Prostate cancer (men) r = 0.48, p = 0.12 Breast cancer (women) r = 0.37, p = 0.23 *3) Trade union memberships:* Lung cancer r = −0.34, p = 0.26 (men) r = −0.06, p = 0.84 (women) Prostate cancer (men) r = 0.52, p = 0.07 Breast cancer (women) r = 0.20, p = 0.50 *4) Volunteering:* Lung cancer r = 0.27, p = 0.43 (men)

(Continued)

TABLE 8.4. (Continued)

Authors, year	Sample size, population/ setting	Age range	Social capital measure	Health outcome measure	Covariates	Individual-level effect estimate	Area-level effect estimate
							$r = 0.53$, $p = 0.10$ (women) Prostate cancer (men) $r = 0.07$, $p = 0.84$ Breast cancer (women) $r = -0.22$, $p = 0.51$

State or regional level

Authors, year	Sample size, population/ setting	Age range	Social capital measure	Health outcome measure	Covariates	Individual-level effect estimate	Area-level effect estimate
Siahpush & Singh, 1999	7 states/territories in Australia in each of 7 years ($n = 49$)	Social capital measures: 15+y Health outcome measures: All ages	Percentage of labor force with union memberships	Age-standardized cancer mortality rates	Calendar year	–	$\beta > 0$, $p < 0.05$
Kennedy et al., 1998	40 regions in Russia	Social capital measure: 16+y Health outcome measures: All ages	Mistrust in local and in regional government, lack of social cohesion at work, lack of interest in politics	Age-standardized cancer mortality rates	Per capita income, proportion in poverty, perceived economic hardship in region, per capita crime rate	–	1) Mistrust in local government $\beta > 0$, $p = 0.06$ (men) $\beta > 0$, $p = 0.23$ (women) 2) Mistrust in regional government $\beta > 0$, $p = 0.18$ (men) $\beta > 0$, $p = 0.70$ (women) 3) Lack of social cohesion at work $\beta > 0$, $p = 0.13$ (men) $\beta > 0$, $p = 0.89$ (women) 4) Lack of interest in politics $\beta > 0$, $p = 0.29$ (men) $\beta > 0$, $p = 0.91$ (women)

MULTILEVEL STUDIES: *Neighborhood-level social capital*					
Blakely et al., 2006	All 25–74 year-olds in 1,683 Census area units in New Zealand	Social capital measure: 15+y Health outcome measures: 25–74 y	Volunteering	Gender-specific all-cancer mortality	*Individual level:* age, race/ ethnicity, marital status, income, education, car access, employ- ment status, urban residence *Neighborhood level:* socioeconomic deprivation Analyses stratified by gender	Low volunteerism: RR = 0.98, 95% CI = 0.88–1.10 (men) RR = 1.00, 95% CI = 0.89–1.12 (women)

As with the health outcomes already reviewed, all studies in this group analyzed associations for single indicators of social cohesion (trust, associational membership, and reciprocity), as well as the percentage of the labor force with union memberships. With the exception of one study that was confined to adults (Blakely et al., 2006), studies examined cancer mortality rates across all age groups (summarized through age-standardization).

Adjustment for key potential confounders in ecological studies was variable. The single multilevel analysis controlled for multiple individual-level characteristics including age, gender, income, and education, as well as neighborhood-level socioeconomic deprivation.

As observed for cardiovascular disease, area-level effect estimates were non-significant or significant in the opposite direction (i.e., suggesting increased harm from social cohesion) at the country level (e.g., for prostate cancer in Lynch et al., 2001), and at the regional level in Australia (Siahpush & Singh, 1999). However, in contrast to the findings in the regional-level ecological study on social capital and cardiovascular disease in Russia, associations between social cohesion (e.g., mistrust in local and regional government) and cancer mortality rates in the same study were predominantly non-significant. Likewise, the sole multilevel analysis (Blakely et al., 2006) showed null associations between low neighborhood-level volunteerism and individual risk of cancer mortality in women (RR = 1.00, 95% CI = 0.89–1.12), whereas for cardiovascular disease as earlier indicated, it was marginally non-significant for women.

8.6. Social Capital and Obesity and Diabetes

We identified only four studies of social capital and obesity or diabetes to date (Table 8.5). One study that examined US state-level social capital in relation to adult obesity and diabetes prevalence rates was ecological (Holtgrave & Crosby, 2006), while the remaining studies [one of which was prospective (Kim, Subramanian, Gortmaker, & Kawachi, 2006c)] applied multilevel analysis and examined social capital in relation to individual-level obesity status (body mass index, BMI, $\geq$30 kg/m^2).

Studies ranged from those investigating single indicators of social capital, to those applying indices or scales which combined multiple social capital indicators. All studies were based on primarily adult populations.

The only ecological study (Holtgrave & Crosby, 2006) adjusted for the state proportion in poverty, and found statistically significant inverse associations between the Putnam state-level social capital index and obesity and diabetes prevalence rates (the latter which were not explicitly age-standardized). The multilevel analyses controlled for several individual-level characteristics including age, gender, and income and/or education, although only one of these studies (Kim et al., 2006c) controlled for multiple potential contextual confounders. That study found a modest marginally significant association between higher state-level social capital and lower individual risk of obesity (OR = 0.93, 95% CI = 0.85–1.00), but no association for county-level social capital (OR = 0.98,

TABLE 8.5. Social capital, obesity, and diabetes.

Authors, year	Sample size, population/ setting	Age range	Social capital measure	Health outcome measure	Covariates	Individual-level effect estimate	Area-level effect estimate
ECOLOGICAL STUDIES: *State level*							
Holtgrave & Crosby, 2006	48 US states	Social capital & health outcome measures: 18+ y	Putnam social capital index (derived from 14 indicators)	Obesity and diabetes prevalence rates	Proportion in poverty	—	Obesity: ß < 0, p = 0.02 Diabetes: ß < 0, p < 0.01
MULTILEVEL STUDIES: *State- or county-level social capital*							
Kim et al., 2006c	2 samples: 101,198 adults in 413 counties in 48 US states/ District of Columbia; 181,200 adults in 48 US states/ District of Columbia	Social capital & health outcome measures: 18+ y	*County level:* 2 subscales (based on five indicators) corresponding to formal group and attitudinal/informal socializing forms	Obesity (dichotomous)	*Individual level* (both sets of analyses): age, gender, race/ ethnicity, marital status, income, education *County-level analysis:* State-level Gini coefficient and proportion of Black residents; county-level mean household income	—	*County-level analysis:* High in social capital on at least one (vs. neither) of the 2 subscales: OR = 0.98, 95% CI = 0.93-1.03 *State-level analysis:* High in social capital on at least one (vs. neither) of the 2 subscales: OR = 0.93, 95% CI = 0.85-1.00

(Continued)

TABLE 8.5. (*Continued*)

Authors, year	Sample size, population/ setting	Age range	Social capital measure	Health outcome measure	Covariates	Individual-level effect estimate	Area-level effect estimate
			State level: 2 subscales (based on 10 indicators) corresponding to attitudinal/ informal socializing/formal group and formal civic and political participation forms		*State-level analysis:* State-level Gini coefficient, mean household income, proportion of Black residents		
Neighborhood- or regional-level social capital							
Poortinga, 2006b	14,836 adults in 720 postal code sectors in the UK	Social capital & health outcome measure: 16+y	*Individual level:* social support, social trust, civic participation, reciprocity	Obesity (dichotomous)	*Individual level:* age, gender, marital status, social class, unemployment status, household tenure, access to amenities, presence of local social problems, urban residence	1) Severe lack of social support: OR = 1.01, 95% CI = 0.88–1.17 2) High social trust: OR = 0.86, 95% CI = 0.78–0.95 3) High social participation: OR = 1.01, 95% CI = 0.90–1.14 4) High reciprocity: OR = 1.07, 95% CI = 0.95–1.19	–
Veenstra et al., 2005b	1,504 adults in the city of Hamilton, Canada	Social capital & health outcome measures: 18+y	Membership/ involvement in voluntary associations	Body mass index >27 kg/m2 (dichotomous)	Age, gender, income, education, neighborhood	Higher voluntary association involvement: OR = 0.91, p = 0.03	–

95% CI = 0.93–1.03). Evidence from the two other studies that applied a multilevel framework was somewhat mixed, with one study observing high individual-level social trust to be significantly inversely associated with obesity risk (OR = 0.86, 95% CI = 0.78–0.95), but no associations for other social capital measures (social support, social participation, and reciprocity) (Poortinga, 2006b). Meanwhile, the other study (Veenstra et al., 2005b) found higher voluntary association involvement to be significantly associated with a 9% lower risk of a higher body weight (BMI > 27 kg/m^2).

8.7. Social Capital and Infectious Diseases

We identified three studies of social capital and infectious diseases, all of which were ecological (Table 8.6). One of these studies was cross-national and cross-sectional (Lynch et al, 2001), while the other two studies were conducted at the US state level and were prospective (Holtgrave & Crosby, 2003, 2004).

The cross-national study (Lynch et al., 2001) applied single indicators of social capital including social trust, organization and trade union membership, and volunteering (based on surveys among adults), while the two state-level studies employed the Putnam social capital index. All studies included individuals of all ages in the calculation of case rates and mortality rates.

The cross-national study (Lynch et al., 2001) adjusted for GDP per capita, stratified the analyses by gender, and controlled for age composition through age-standardization of the mortality rates. Findings from this study were mixed, with non-significant weak to moderate correlations between each of country-level social mistrust and trade union memberships in the anticipated direction with age-standardized mortality rates from all infectious diseases in men and in women. Associations for organizational memberships in both sexes were null, and there were weak to moderate positive correlations between volunteering and infectious disease mortality rates in men and women, respectively. By contrast, associations in the two studies that examined the Putnam state social capital index in relation to state case rates from each of gonorrhea, syphilis, Chlamydia, AIDS, and tuberculosis (controlling for income inequality for the latter two outcomes) were all significantly inverse, although neither of these studies controlled for area-level socioeconomic deprivation (Holtgrave & Crosby, 2003, 2004).

8.8. Summary and Synthesis

8.8.1. Summary of Findings

Our review of the literature found fairly consistent associations between trust as an indicator of social cohesion and better physical health. The evidence for trust was stronger for self-rated health than for other physical health outcomes, and stronger for individual-level perceptions than for area-level trust. Associational

TABLE 8.6. Social capital and infectious diseases.

Authors, year	Sample size, population/ setting	Age range	Social capital measure	Health outcome measure	Covariates	Individual-level effect estimate	Area-level effect estimate
ECOLOGICAL STUDIES:							
Country level							
Lynch et al., 2001	16 countries	Social capital measure: 18+y; Health outcome measures: All ages	Social mistrust, organizational memberships, trade union memberships, volunteering	Gender-specific, age-standardized mortality rates for all infectious diseases	GDP per capita; analyses stratified by gender	–	1) Social mistrust: r = 0.30, p = 0.32 (men) r = 0.26, p = 0.39 (women) 2) Organizational memberships: r = −0.06, p = 0.85 (men) r = 0.01, p = 0.96 (women) 3) Trade union memberships: r = −0.42, p = 0.16 (men) r = −0.39, p = 0.19 (women) 4) Volunteering: r = 0.24, p = 0.48 (men) r = 0.33, p = 0.32 (women)
State level							
Holtgrave & Crosby, 2003	48 US states	Social capital measure: 18+y Health outcome measures: All ages	Putnam social capital index (derived from 14 indicators)	Gonorrhea, syphilis, chlamydia, AIDS case rates	Income inequality (for analysis of AIDS case rates only)	–	Gonorrhea case rates: r = −0.67, p < 0.01 Syphilis case rates: r = −0.59, p < 0.01 Chlamydia case rates: r = −0.53, p < 0.01 AIDS case rates: β < 0, p = 0.01
Holtgrave & Crosby, 2004	48 US states	Social capital measure: 18+y Health outcome measures: All ages	Putnam social capital index (derived from 14 indicators)	Tuberculosis case rates	Income inequality	–	β < 0, p < 0.01

membership as an indicator of cohesion was also consistently associated with better self-rated health at the individual level, although reverse causation cannot be excluded (see discussion below). On the other hand, the evidence was weak that associational membership at the area level is associated with self-rated health (in either direction).

8.8.2. Social Cohesion in Egalitarian versus Inegalitarian Social Contexts

In a recent systematic review of forty-two published studies, Islam, Merlo, Kawachi, Lindstrom, & Gerdtham, (2006a) found that an association between social capital and health was much more consistently reported in inegalitarian countries i.e., countries with a high degree of economic inequality; whereas an association was either not observed or was much weaker in more egalitarian societies. Economic inequality was assessed by the country's Gini coefficient (based on disposable income) and by the country's public share of social expenditure. Regardless of the type of study (individual, ecological, or multilevel) or the country's degree of egalitarianism, the authors found generally significant positive associations between social capital and better health outcomes.

Moreover, from the multilevel studies that were identified in this review by Islam et al. (2006a), there was also evidence to suggest that the *between-area* variation *in health* (i.e., the random effect) was considerably lower in more egalitarian countries (such as Canada and Sweden) as compared to more unequal countries (such as the United States). For example, the intraclass correlation (ICC, corresponding to the percent of variation in health explained at the area level) was approximately 7.5% in a US study of neighborhood influences on violent crime and homicide, whereas the ICCs ranged from 0–2% for studies in Canada and Sweden (Islam et al., 2006a). Likewise, a recent multilevel analysis of 275 Swedish municipalities found a modest fixed effect association between voting participation and health-related quality of life, with 98% of variation in health attributed to the individual level, and only 2% to the municipality level (Islam et al., 2006b).

One potential explanation for this pattern (of generally null findings from multilevel studies of social capital and self-rated health in more egalitarian countries) is that in egalitarian societies characterized by strong provision of safety nets and spending on public goods (such as health care, education, unemployment insurance), social capital may be less salient for the health of its residents, by contrast to highly unequal and segregated societies such as the United States.

8.8.3. Limitations of Studies

Our review of the literature has highlighted increasing methodological sophistication in study design over time, progressing from the earlier ecological studies of social cohesion and health, to the more recent multilevel study designs. Nonetheless, our review also points to a number of gaps in the existing literature. As the tables demonstrate, many studies continue to rely on secondary sources of data to construct "indicators" of social cohesion. As pointed out by Harpham in chapter 3, proxy indicators of social cohesion – such as trade union membership, volunteering, and social participation – can be construed as either precursors or consequences of social capital, but they are not part of social capital *per se*. Accordingly, there is an urgent need to incorporate direct measures of social cohesion into existing national surveys, taking care to specify the scale of measurement (e.g., neighborhoods) as well as making sure to include relevant distinctions such as bonding versus bridging capital, or cognitive versus behavioral measures (see chapter 3 for further tips).

Virtually none of the studies have distinguished between the effects of bonding versus bridging capital, and few studies have explicitly sought to examine the deleterious consequences of social cohesion through careful analyses of cross-level interactions between community cohesion and individual characteristics. As the multilevel analysis by Subramanian, Kim, and Kawachi, (2002) suggests, community cohesion can be beneficial for some groups, yet can be harmful to the health of others. Studies have also been inconsistent with respect to controlling for potential confounding variables at both the individual and area levels.

Aside from the threat of omitted variable bias, one of the biggest challenges for establishing causality in this area remains the paucity of longitudinal data. Cross-sectional data are less than ideal for establishing causality. For example, at the individual level, one could argue that being in good health is a precursor of having trusting opinions of others, or participating in civic associations (i.e., reverse causation). Ideally, what is needed are data with repeated assessments of both social cohesion and health outcomes; in other words, data of the type that would lend itself to analytical strategies such as "difference-in-difference" (DiD) estimators (Ashenfelter, 1978; Ashenfelter & Card, 1985). The other major criticism of the research to date is that no studies have adequately dealt with the potential problem that community cohesion is endogenous (Kawachi, 2006). For example, some people are likely to choose the communities they live in based on their preferences for social interactions with neighbors. To the extent that such preferences are also correlated with health, we have an endogeneity problem. Solving the endogeneity problem will require study designs in which the exposure (social capital) can be manipulated through either natural experiments (instruments) or randomization (e.g., cluster community trials) (Oakes, 2004) (see also chapter 7 fur further discussion of these issues).

8.8.4. Examining Social Capital in Diverse Populations

While many existing studies have sampled populations across a wide range of ages, the investigation of specific effects among elderly populations (e.g., persons over age 65) and among children and adolescents (for which behaviors may be more malleable; Dietz & Gortmaker, 2001) has been sparse (Drukker, Kaplan, Feron, & van Os, 2003; Drukker, Buka, Kaplan, McKenzie,& van Os, 2005; Wen et al., 2005).

Populations in developing countries further represent an uncharted territory of investigation of the physical health effects of social capital, for which the associations might potentially differ due to vastly different political economies, sociocultural contexts, and patterns of disease than in developed nations.

8.8.5. Mechanisms Linking Social Capital to Physical Health

Although few studies have sought to directly assess the mechanisms linking social capital to health, a variety of hypothesized pathways have been proposed by which cohesion may affect health, including the diffusion of knowledge about health promotion, maintenance of healthy behavioral norms through informal social control, promotion of access to local services and amenities, and psychosocial processes which provide affective support and mutual respect (Kawachi & Berkman, 2000). These mechanisms could broadly be categorized into local behaviorally-mediated mechanisms, and more upstream policy-mediated mechanisms.

On the behavioral front, drawing on the diffusion of innovations theory (Rogers, 2003), we may posit that residents of high social capital neighborhoods or regions in which healthy behaviors (e.g., engagement in exercise and avoidance of foods high in saturated fats) are practiced among some residents may be more likely to adopt these behaviors through diffusion of knowledge about the behaviors.

At larger geographical scales (e.g., the county, state, or regional level), social capital might also conceivably affect physical health through policy-related mechanisms. In his seminal work *Making Democracy Work* (Putnam, 1993) the political scientist Robert Putnam lends empirical credence to the notion that prosperous democracies are tied to the presence of civic engagement and social capital. Within the health context, it has been hypothesized that more cohesive societies are more apt to cooperate in the provision of health-promoting public goods for its residents, such as health care (see also Introduction and chapter 7). Social cohesion at other scales might have contextual effects on individual levels of social capital through attitudinal/cognitive mechanisms. For instance, transparency and the absence of corruption increase public confidence in governmental institutions, which in turn may raise levels of interpersonal trust (Brehm & Rahn, 1997; Levi, 1996).

A number of behavioral risk factors have been established for chronic diseases such as cardiovascular diseases (coronary heart disease and stroke), selected cancers (e.g., colon cancer, lung cancer, breast cancer), and diabetes. Several of these risk factors (e.g., dietary intakes, smoking, and physical inactivity) have themselves been linked to community cohesion (see chapter 10 by Lindström). Psychosocial factors (e.g., depression, anxiety) may also affect disease risk, either through direct pathways (e.g., through psycho-neuro-immune effects) or indirect pathways (e.g., mediated by behavioral changes), and are putative risk factors for heart disease (Kubzansky & Kawachi, 2000; Kuper, Marmot, & Hemingway, 2002), and to a lesser extent, for cancers and infectious diseases (Cohen, Alper, Doyle, Treanor, & Turner,

2006; Kroenke et al., 2005; Leonard, 2000). Of course, social cohesion can also plausibly contribute to *greater* transmission of infectious diseases through higher person-to-person contact (Holtgrave & Crosby, 2003).

8.9. Conclusions

The past decade has borne witness to a flourishing epidemiologic and public health interest in the investigation of the effects of social capital on physical health outcomes. This inquiry has broadened from an emphasis on overall mortality and self-rated health to include more specific disease diagnoses. Our review of the literature to date suggests several points of convergence – for example, the more consistent associations between social cohesion and health in unequal societies with weak safety nets compared to egalitarian countries with a strong tradition of public goods provision; the stronger associations between health and trust (as an indicator of cohesion) compared to associational membership; and stronger associations for the same indicator at the individual compared to collective level. At the same time, our review also points to several gaps that the next generation of research needs to address, in particular, stronger study designs that address questions of causality, and deepen our understanding of causal mechanisms.

References

Ashenfelter, O. (1978). Estimating the effect of training programs on earnings. *Review of Economics and Statistics, 60*, 47–57.

Ashenfelter, O., & Card, D. (1985). Using the longitudinal structure of earnings to estimate the effect of training programs. *Review of Economics and Statistics, 67*, 648–660.

Bearman, P., & Moody, J. (2004). Suicide and friendships among American adolescents. *American Journal of Public Health, 94*, 89–95.

Berkman, L. F., & Glass, T. (2000). Social integration, social networks, social support, and health. In L. F. Berkman & I. Kawachi (Eds.), *Social Epidemiology* (pp. 137–173). New York, NY: Oxford University Press.

Blakely, T., Atkinson, J., Ivory, V., Collings, S., Wilton, J., & Howden-Chapman, P. (2006). No association of neighbourhood volunteerism with mortality in New Zealand: a national multilevel cohort study. *International Journal of Epidemiology, 35*, 981–989.

Brehm, J., & Rahn, W. (1997). Individual-level evidence for the causes and consequences of social capital. *American Journal of Political Science, 41*, 999–1023.

Browning, C. R., & Cagney, K. A. (2003). Moving beyond poverty: neighborhood structure, social processes, and health. *Journal of Health & Social Behavior, 44*, 552–571.

Cohen, S., Alper, C. M., Doyle, W. J., Treanor, J. J., & Turner, R. B. (2006). Positive emotional style predicts resistance to illness after experimental exposure to rhinovirus or influenza a virus. *Psychosomatic Medicine, 68*, 809–815.

Dietz, W. H., & Gortmaker, S. L. (2001). Preventing obesity in children and adolescents. *Annual Review of Public Health, 22*, 337–353.

Drukker, M., Kaplan, C., Feron, F., & van Os, J. (2003). Children's health-related quality of life, neighborhood socioeconomic deprivation and social capital. A contextual analysis. *Social Science & Medicine, 7*, 825–841.

Drukker, M., Buka, S. L., Kaplan, C., McKenzie, K., & van Os, J. (2005). Social capital and young adolescents' perceived health in different sociocultural settings. *Social Science & Medicine*, *61*, 185–198.

Franzini, L., Caughy, M., Spears, W., & Fernandez Esquer, M. E. (2005). Neighborhood economic conditions, social processes, and self-rated health in low-income neighborhoods in Texas: A multilevel latent variables model. *Social Science & Medicine*, *61*, 1135–1150.

Friedman, S. R., & Aral, S. (2001). Social networks, risk-potential networks, health, and disease. *Journal of Urban Health*, *78*, 411–418.

Helliwell, J. F., & Putnam, R. D. (2004). The social context of well-being. *Proceedings of the Royal Society B: Biological Sciences*, *359*, 1435–1446.

Holtgrave, D. R., & Crosby, R. A. (2003). Social capital, poverty, and income inequality as predictors of gonorrhoea, syphilis, chlamydia and AIDS in the United States. *Sexually Transmitted Infections*, *79*, 62–64.

Holtgrave, D. R., & Crosby, R. A. (2004). Social determinants of tuberculosis case rates in the United States. *American Journal of Preventive Medicine*, *26*, 159–162.

Holtgrave, D. R., & Crosby, R. (2006). Is social capital a protective factor against obesity and diabetes? Findings from an exploratory study. *Annals of Epidemiology*, *16*, 406–408.

Hyyppä, M. T., & Mäki, J. (2001). Individual-level relationships between social capital and self-rated health in a bilingual community. *Preventive Medicine*, *32*, 148–155.

Hyyppä, M. T., & Mäki, J. (2003). Social participation and health in a community rich in stock of social capital. *Health Education Research*, *18*, 770–779.

Islam, M. K., Merlo, J., Kawachi, I., Lindstrom, M., & Gerdtham, U-G. (2006a). Social capital and health: Does egalitarianism matter? A literature review. *International Journal for Equity in Health*, *5*, 3. doi:10.1186/1475–9276–5–3.

Islam, M. K., Merlo, J., Kawachi, I., Lindstrom, M., Burstrom, K., & Gerdtham, U-G. (2006b). Does it really matter where you live? A panel data multilevel analysis of Swedish municipality level social capital on individual health-related quality of life. *Health Economics, Policy and Law*, *1*, 209–235.

Kavanagh, A. M., Turrell, G., & Subramanian, S. V. (2006). Does area-based social capital matter for the health of Australians? A multilevel analysis of self-rated health in Tasmania. *International Journal of Epidemiology*, *35*, 607–613.

Kavanagh, A. M., Bentley, R., Turrell, G., Broom, D. H., & Subramanian, S. V. (2006b). Does gender modify associations between self rated health and the social and economic characteristics of local environments? *Journal of Epidemiology & Community Health*, *60*, 490–495.

Kawachi, I., Kennedy, B., Lochner, K., & Prothrow-Stith, D. (1997). Social capital, income inequality, and mortality. *American Journal of Public Health*, *87*, 1491–1498.

Kawachi, I., Kennedy, B., & Glass, R. (1999). Social capital and self-rated health: A contextual analysis. *American Journal of Public Health*, *89*, 1187–1193.

Kawachi, I., & Berkman, L. F. (2000). Social cohesion, social capital, and health. In L.F. Berkman & I. Kawachi (Eds.), *Social Epidemiology* (pp. 178–190). New York, NY: Oxford University Press.

Kawachi, I. (2006). Commentary: Social capital and health – making the connections one step at a time. *International Journal of Epidemiology*, *35*, 989–993.

Kennedy, B., Kawachi, I., & Brainerd, E. (1998). The role of social capital in the Russian mortality crisis. *World Development*, *26*, 2029–2043.

Kennelly, B., O'Shea, E., & Garvey, E. (2003). Social capital, life expectancy and mortality: a cross-national examination. *Social Science & Medicine*, *56*, 2367–2377.

Kim, D., Subramanian, S. V., & Kawachi, I. (2006a). Bonding versus bridging social capital and their associations with self-rated health: a multilevel analysis of 40 U.S. communities. *Journal of Epidemiology & Community Health*, *60*, 116–122.

Kim, D., & Kawachi, I. (2006b). A multilevel analysis of key forms of community- and individual-level social capital as predictors of self-rated health in the United States. *Journal of Urban Health*, *83*, 813–826.

Kim, D., Subramanian, S. V., Gortmaker, S. L., & Kawachi, I. (2006c). US state- and county-level social capital in relation to obesity and physical inactivity: a multilevel, multivariable analysis. *Social Science & Medicine*, *63*, 1045–1059.

Kroenke, C.H., Bennett, G.G., Fuchs, C., Giovannucci, E., Kawachi, I., Schernhammer, E., Holmes, M.D., & Kubzansky, L.D., (2005). Depressive symptoms and prospective incidence of colorectal cancer in women. *American Journal of Epidemiology*, *162*, 839-48.

Kubzansky, L., & Kawachi, I. (2000). Affective states and health. In L. F. Berkman & I. Kawachi (Eds.), *Social epidemiology* (pp. 213–41). New York, NY: Oxford University Press.

Kuper, H., Marmot, M., & Hemingway, H. (2002). Systematic review of prospective cohort studies of psychosocial factors in the etiology and prognosis of coronary heart disease. *Seminars in Vascular Medicine*, *2*, 267–314.

Leonard, B. (2000). Stress, depression and the activation of the immune system. *World Journal of Biology & Psychiatry*, *1*, 17–25.

Levi, M. (1996). Social and unsocial capital: A review essay of Robert Putnam's Making Democracy Work. *Politics and Society*, *24*, 45–55.

Lindström, M., Moghaddassi, M., & Merlo, J. (2004). Individual self-reported health, social participation and neighborhood: A multilevel analysis in Malmö, Sweden. *Preventive Medicine*, *39*, 135–141.

Lynch, J. W., Davey Smith, G., Hillemeier, M. M., Shwa, M., Raghunathan, T., & Kaplan, G. A. (2001). Income inequality, the psychosocial environment and health: comparisons of wealthy nations. *Lancet*, *358*, 194–200.

Lochner, K., Kawachi, I., Brennan, R. T., & Buka, S. L. (2003). Social capital and neighborhood mortality rates in Chicago. *Social Science & Medicine*, *56*, 1797–1805.

Mellor, J. M., & Milyo, J. (2005). State social capital and individual health status. *Journal of Health Politics, Policy & Law*, *30*, 1101–1130.

Milyo, J., & Mellor, J. M. (2003). On the importance of age-adjustment methods in ecological studies of social determinants of mortality. *Health Services Research*, *38*, 1781–1790.

Mohan, J., Twigg, L., Barnard, S., & Jones, K. (2005). Social capital, geography and health: a small-area analysis for England. *Social Science & Medicine*, *60*, 1267–1283.

Oakes, J. M. (2004). The (mis)estimation of neighborhood effects: Causal inference for a practicable social epidemiology. *Social Science & Medicine*, *58*, 1929–1952.

Pollack, C. E., & von dem Knesebeck, O. (2004). Social capital and health among the aged: comparisons between the United States and Germany. *Health & Place*, *10*, 383–391.

Poortinga, W. (2006a). Social capital: An individual or collective resource for health? *Social Science & Medicine*, *62*, 292–302.

Poortinga, W. (2006b). Perceptions of the environment, physical activity, and obesity. *Social Science & Medicine*, *63*, 2835–2846.

Poortinga, W. (2006c). Social relations or social capital? Individual and community health effects of bonding social capital. *Social Science & Medicine*, *63*, 255–270.

Poortinga, W. (2006d). Do health behaviors mediate the association between social capital and health? *Preventive Medicine, 43*, 488–493.

Putnam, R. D. (1993). *Making democracy work.* Princeton, NJ: Princeton University Press.

Putnam, R. D. (2000). *Bowling alone: The collapse and revival of American community.* New York: Simon and Schuster.

Rojas, Y., & Carlson, P. (2006). The stratification of social capital and its consequences for self-rated health in Taganrog, Russia. *Social Science & Medicine, 62*, 2732–2741.

Rogers, E. M. (2003). *Diffusion of innovations* (5th ed.). New York: The Free Press.

Rose, R. (2000). How much does social capital add to individual health? A survey of Russians. *Social Science & Medicine, 51*, 1421–1435.

Siahpush, M., & Singh, G. K. (1999). Social integration and mortality in Australia. *Australia & New Zealand Journal of Public Health, 23*, 571–577.

Skrabski, A., Kopp, M., & Kawachi, I. (2003). Social capital in a changing society: Cross sectional associations with middle aged female and male mortality. *Journal of Epidemiology & Community Health, 57*, 114–119.

Skrabski, A., Kopp, M., & Kawachi, I. (2004). Social capital and collective efficacy in Hungary: Cross sectional associations with middle aged female and male mortality rates. *Journal of Epidemiology & Community Health, 58*, 340–345.

Steptoe, A., & Feldman, P. J. (2001). Neighborhood problems as sources of chronic stress: development of a measure of neighborhood problems, and associations with socioeconomic status and health. *Annals of Behavioral Medicine, 23*, 177–185.

Subramanian, S. V., Kawachi, I., & Kennedy, B. P. (2001). Does the state you live in make a difference? Multilevel analysis of self-rated health in the US. *Social Science & Medicine, 53*, 9–19.

Subramanian, S. V., Kim, D. J., & Kawachi, I. (2002). Social Trust and Self-Rated Health in US Communities: A Multilevel Analysis. *Journal of Urban Health: Bulletin of the New York Academy of Medicine, 79*, S21–S34.

Sundquist, K., Winkleby, M., Ahlen, H., & Johansson, S. E. (2004). Neighborhood socioeconomic environment and incidence of coronary heart disease: a follow-up study of 25,319 women and men in Sweden. *American Journal of Epidemiology, 159*, 655–662.

Sundquist, J., Johansson, S. E., Yang, M., & Sundquist, K. (2006). Low linking social capital as a predictor of coronary heart disease in Sweden: a cohort study of 2.8 million people. *Social Science & Medicine, 62*, 954–963.

Turrell, G., Kavanagh, A., & Subramanian, S. V. (2006). Area variation in mortality in Tasmania (Australia): The contributions of socioeconomic disadvantage, social capital and geographic remoteness. *Health & Place, 12*, 291–305.

Valente, T. W., Gallaher, P., & Mouttapa, M. (2004). Using social networks to understand and prevent substance use: A transdisciplinary perspective. *Substance Use & Misuse, 39*, 1685–1712.

Veenstra, G. (2000). Social capital, SES and health: An individual-level analysis. *Social Science & Medicine, 50*, 619–629.

Veenstra, G. (2002). Social capital and health (plus wealth, income inequality and region health governance). *Social Science & Medicine, 54*, 849–868.

Veenstra, G. (2005a). Location, location, location: Contextual and compositional health effects of social capital in British Columbia, Canada. *Social Science & Medicine, 60*, 2059–2071.

Veenstra, G., Luginaah, I., Wakefield, S., Birch, S., Eyles, J., & Elliott, S. (2005b). Who you know, where you live: social capital, neighborhood and health. *Social Science & Medicine, 60*, 2799–2818.

Wanless, D. (2004). *Securing good health for the whole population*. London, UK: Crown.

Wen, M., Browning, C. R., & Cagney, K. A. (2003). Poverty affluence and income inequality: neighborhood economic structure and its implications for health. *Social Science & Medicine, 57*, 843–860.

Wen, M., Cagney, K. A., & Christakis, N. A. (2005). Effect of specific aspects of community social environment on the mortality of individuals diagnosed with serious illness. *Social Science & Medicine, 61*, 1119–1134.

Wilkinson, R. G., Kawachi, I., & Kennedy, B. P. (1998). Mortality, the social environment, crime and violence. *Sociology of Health & Illness, 20*, 578–597.

Yip, W., Subramanian, S. V., Mitchell, A. D., Lee, D. T., Wang, J., & Kawachi, I. (In press). Does social capital enhance health and well-being? Evidence from rural China. *Social Science & Medicine, 64*, 35–49.

Ziersch, A. M., Baum, F. E., Macdougall, C., & Putland, C. (2005). Neighborhood life and social capital: the implications for health. *Social Science & Medicine, 60*, 71–86.

Zimmerman, F. J., & Bell, J. F. (2006). Income inequality and physical and mental health: testing associations consistent with proposed causal pathways. *Journal of Epidemiology & Community Health, 60*, 513–521.

9
Social Capital and Mental Health
An Updated Interdisciplinary Review of Primary Evidence

ASTIER M. ALMEDOM AND DOUGLAS GLANDON

Social capital is a compound and complex construct, an umbrella term under which social cohesion, social support, social integration and/or participation are often lumped together. Beyond its growing appeal to policy makers, practitioners and researchers in public health in general and mental health in particular, social capital is now also an integral part of broad-based discussions on social-ecological resilience, ecosystem sustainability, and the collective management of natural resources (see for instance, Adger et al., 2005; Hardin, 1968; Pretty, 2003). This chapter revisits and updates the analysis presented in an earlier interdisciplinary review of primary evidence linking social capital and mental health (Almedom, 2005). The aim is to identify key areas where progress has been made in the quest for understanding both theoretical and empirical associations between social capital and mental health and well-being.

Both social capital and mental health remain difficult to define categorically and measure precisely. Research evidence also suggests that both defy institutional appropriation while remaining open to manipulation by formal and/or informal means of social engineering. Academic researchers continue to contribute to the debate that is fuelled by these inherent characteristics of both constructs. Concerning social capital, Putnam's *communitarian* definition continues to be widely used with reference to the types – *bonding* (horizontal) and *bridging/linking* (vertical or horizontal or diagonal) – of social group interactions evident in civic participation; while Bourdieu's "forms of social capital" (human/economic and cultural) also continues to underlie discussions of individual, family and community access to social capital in relation to health and well-being. The earlier evaluation of the published literature had suggested that the various types and/or forms of social capital may have both *structural* and *cognitive* components operating at micro and/or macro levels. However, questions remained as to how availability and/or access to social capital or lack thereof influenced mental well-being, particularly when only quantitative methods of investigation and analysis were employed (Almedom, 2005). The dozen studies reviewed earlier pointed in the general direction of the need for interdisciplinary, multi-method and multi-level research design. An additional four studies identified since are considered below, three of which turn out to be qualitative. All four investigations focus on the structural and cognitive components of social capital.

9.1. Method of Literature Review

Our literature review used exactly the same methods as the earlier one: main electronic bibliographic databases (including "Global Health") were searched for "social capital and mental health"; "social capital and psychosocial" and "social capital and depression" appearing in the summary/abstract, text and/or list of key words in peer-reviewed journal articles published and indexed between January 2004 and April 2006. Items resulting from the electronic search were hand-sifted in order to follow-up cited references and contact authors when necessary, and the same inclusion/exclusion criteria applied. A final short list of four studies reporting primary data on primary indicators of social capital and mental health were added to the results of the earlier review and incorporated in the thematic discussion of social capital and mental health across the life course and with reference to mental health care services conducted by Almedom (2005).

9.2. Findings and Interpretation

The sixteen studies discussed below reflect the general trend of theoretical and empirical advances made in recent years. As expected, due to the compound and complex nature of both "social capital" and "mental health", multiple definitions and measurement scales/assessment tools have been employed. Indicators of "metal health" range from externalizing and/or internalizing behavior problems in children and young people (Beyers, Bates, & Pettit, 2003; Caughy, O'Campo, & Muntaner, 2003; Drukker et al., 2003; Moffitt et al., 2002; van der Linden et al., 2003); to social withdrawal, anxiety and depression (non-clinical, non-referred) in adolescents and young adults (Harpham, Grant, & Rodriguez, 2004; Stevenson, 1998); coping with "refugee trauma" (Weine et al., 2005) and "maternal depression and symptoms of antisocial personality disorder" (Moffitt et al., 2002; Mulvaney & Kendrick, 2005); "emotional well-being" (Cotterill & Taylor, 2001; Rose, 2000a) and "psychological distress" (Mitchell & La Gory, 2002) in adults and senior citizens. Measurement scales and tools of assessment employed include the Child Behavior Check List (CBCL); Child Health Questionnaire (CHQ-CF87); interviews with children, adolescents, and/or their teachers, and/or parents/primary carers; Revised Rutter Scale; Diagnostic & Statistical Manual of Mental Disorders (DSM-IV); Short form Multiscore Depression Index (SMDI); Teacher Report Form (TRF); Self-report Questionnaire (SRQ-20); Diagnostic Interview Schedule (DIS-IV); Short Michigan Alcoholism Screening Test (SMAST); General Health Questionnaire (GHQ-12); CES-D scale; Mirowsky & Ross' psychological scale; and also semi-structured interviews, focus group discussions and observations. Each study is examined in relation to itself *vis a vis* contemporary social capital and mental health debates and dilemmas, and in relation to other studies under review only with reference to policy and/or practice implications of the findings, if any.

Indicators of social capital used include a Dutch translation and adaptation of Informal Social Control (ISC) and Social Cohesion and Trust (SC&T) scales; Neighborhood Social Capital scale (NSC), Kinship Social Support (KSS) and Fear of Calamity scale (FOC); Adapted Social Cohesion and Trust scale (A-SCAT); interviews with youth, teachers and parents; Psychological Sense of Community (PSOC); and Putnam's Community Social Capital Benchmark Survey. A number of the studies reviewed measure two or more types and components of social capital, namely, the structural and/or cognitive components of bonding and bridging social capital measured in geographically delineated urban areas. However, notions of "the shared social environment" are inconsistent across these studies. For example, "neighborhood" can mean "census block" (Caughy et al., 2003) or "census tract" (Beyers et al., 2003; Mitchell & La Gory, 2002) or "postcode" (Steptoe & Feldman, 2001). Only one study uses the term neighborhood in an "ecologically meaningful" way, and recognizes that "perceived neighborhood" (according to the study participants) differs in meaning from the researchers' use of the term (Drukker et al., 2003).

The significance of access to and use of different types, components and levels of social capital varies across the life course. Geographical area-based social cohesion and informal social control translates into a sense of freedom and safety that is conducive to healthy cognitive and emotional development and socialization of children and adolescents (Davis, 1998; Ross, Reynolds, & Geis, 2000; Sampson, Stephen, & Earls, 1997). This is important for the physical safety, emotional security and well-being of senior citizens as well (Klinenberg, 2002; Lindström, Merlo, & Östergren, 2003). Residential social capital may be more critical to families (specifically women) with young children and to the elderly than to relatively young adults without dependants. Therefore empirical links between social capital and mental health are considered below with reference to specific stages of the lifecourse. The sub-grouping of studies in Tables 9.1–9.4 is however fluid, as some studies belong in more than one sub-group. For example, Harpham et al.'s study includes adolescents and young adults (15–25 year olds), Moffitt et al. report on young mothers and their twin children, and Steptoe and Feldman's sample has a very wide age range: 18–94 years, with a mean of 52 and SD of 18 years). Rather than listing these studies twice in Tables 9.1 and 9.2, their "dual" focus is discussed in the text only.

9.3. Social Capital and Mental Health and/or Social Behavior of Children and Youth

Family and neighborhood social capital are evidently important determinants of children's and adolescents' development, health and well-being. Both individual and ecological factors are at play, warranting plurality of methods and levels of investigation and analysis. Stevenson (1998) defines social capital as *"the sum total of positive relationships including families and neighbors that serve as buffers to the negative influences within one's immediate environment."* (p. 48)

Table 9.1. Studies with primary data linking social capital and mental health of adolescents and young children.

Author (year), location of study site(s)	Study design, sample size & unit(s) of analysis	Indicator of social capital & scale(s) used	Indicator of mental health & scale(s) used	Key findings	Policy/practice implications & remarks
Stevenson (1998) Anonymous city, USA	Cross-sectional N = 160 African American youth in an unnamed city in the north-east; correlations and multiple regression, mixed models	Neighborhood Social Capital (NSC) scale, Kinship Social Support (KSS) scale and Fear of Calamity (FOC) scale	Emotional adjustment/ mental health (guilt, cognitive difficulty, sad mood, irritability, low self esteem, instrumental helplessness, social introversion, low energy, pessimism, learned helplessness); MDI (short form)	↑fear of potential violent calamity and ↓ symptoms of global depression in girls compared to boys. Gender differences in access to neighborhood social capital and use of emotionally adaptive strategies, including social introversion. Supportive and watchful neighborhoods (↑ social capital) can make up for lower levels of family social support.	Author argues in favor of building and strengthening structural components of social capital. His recommendation that families and social networks to which a child belongs need to be connected to larger networks of 'fictive kin' resonates with progressive education, social welfare and health policies.
Beyers et al., (2003) Nashville (TN) Knoxville (TN), (IN) USA	Longitudinal, two cohort study of children aged 5 followed into adolescence, age 13 (N = 440) evenly distributed among 3 southern cities; multi-level	structural disadvantage, residential instability, concentrated affluence (census-based measures); parental monitoring and involvement (interview with youth and with parents, parental monitoring and activity scores)	Externalizing behavior (e.g. 'gets into fights', 'disobedient at school') as reported by teachers (grades 6–8); TRF (34 items including aggression and delinquency scales)	Neighborhood structure contributed to socialization of adolescents by moderating the effects of parental monitoring or lack thereof.	Authors point out that their findings may not be generalized to African American families or disadvantaged youth as the majority of the sample consisted of white and middle-class families.

Study/Location	Design	Measures	Findings	Implications
Caughy et al. (2003) Baltimore city(MD), USA	Cross-sectional N=200 African American mothers/care givers of 3–4.5 year olds in 39 neighborhoods; single-level regression models	Parental sense of community (interview with mothers/care givers PSOC-G (general) and PSOC-K ('knows neighbors') scales	Child behavior problems; CBCL scores for internalizing (anxiety, depression, withdrawal), externalizing (aggression) and total problem behavior score.	Contradictory evidence: $\uparrow$ wealth in residential area = $\downarrow$ social capital/ level of attachment with/ sense of community in mothers/carers = $\downarrow$ behavioral/mental health problems among 3–4 year olds; and yet $\downarrow$ levels of neighborhood impoverishment and $\downarrow$ maternal social capital also = $\uparrow$ child behavior/mental health problems.	Potentially harmful policy and practice implications as children as young as 3 and 4 may be labeled 'aggressive' or 'depressed'. No information on how the African American mothers/care givers' interviewed define their own communities; and whether or not they problematize their young children's behavior.
Drukker et al. (2003) Maastricht, The Netherlands	Longitudinal cohort study of 11–12 year old children (N=3401) living in 36 "ecologically meaningful" neighborhoods, to be followed into adulthood; multilevel regression models.	Neighborhood informal social control, social cohesion and trust; translated and adapted ISC and SC&T scales (with 5 site/culture-specific questions added).	General mental health and behavior (aggression, delinquency, hyperactivity, impulsivity and social withdrawal), self esteem; CHQ-CF87	Children's mental health and behavioral problems specifically associated with neighborhood levels of informal social control.	Promising prospects for a sound evidence-base for mental health policy and practice as authors are aware of and responsive to the limitations of epidemiological survey research..
Weine et al. (2004), USA	Multi-site ethnographic study, N = 30, refugee Bosnian adolescents & their families in the Bosnian community of Chicago; interviews and participant observation, thematic analysis.	"cultural capital" – 9 identified mechanisms in emic terms: using our language, obliging family, sticking together, returning to religion, going ghetto, building a future, taking pride in tradition, critiquing America, seeking freedom.	Sadness, isolation, confusion, degradation, dissatisfaction, & anomie (interview coding).	No cultural capital mechanism operates in isolation from others. Families are a critical component of converting cultural capital. More research is needed to determine whether these coping strategies are associated with positive mental health outcomes.	Preventive mental health services may be able to assist in "converting" cultural capital to facilitate effective coping to stress and adversity. Such efforts would need to focus on the attitudes, beliefs, and information among and between teens, parents, school, and other community programs.

TABLE 9.2. Studies with primary data linking social capital and mental health of youth, adults (including mothers with young children).

Author (year), location of study site(s)	Study design, sample size & unit(s) of analysis	Indicator of social capital & scale(s) used	Indicator of mental health & scale(s) used	Key findings	Policy/practice implications & remarks
Rose (2000) Russian Federation	Cross-sectional, multi-stage randomly strati-fied sample, N=1904 adults age 18 and up; Multiple regressions.	Multiple indicators of social integration and individuals' cumulative use of networks includ-ing church attendance, trust in people, sense of control over one's life. New Russia Barometer (NRB) surveys.	Emotional wellbeing (12 months recall) 5 point lickert scale: "in the past year, would you say your emotional health has been very good, good, average, poor or very poor?" NRB surveys.	Social capital increases physical and emotional health more than human capital; Human and social capital together can easily raise the indi-vidual's self-reported health from just below average on the scale to approaching good health.	Author argues that public policy intervention to increase household incomes coupled with autonomy of social capi-tal networks from government would secure emotional and physical health benefits for Russians across all age groups.
Steptoe & Feldman (2001) London, UK	Cross-sectional N=658 postal questionnaire survey respondents in the London area; Multilevel regression models.	Collective efficacy: social cohesion (SC), informal social control (ISC); Neighborhood problem scale	Feeling unhappy and depressed (GHQ-12, 4-point scale)	Neighbourhood problems (including litter in the streets, air pollution, noise, vandalism and disturbance by neighbors or youngsters) correlated with poor self-rated health, psychological distress and impaired physical function inde-pendent of age, sex, neighbourhood SES, individual deprivation, and social capital.	Authors point out that the cross-sectional design and low response rate make it difficult to go beyond recommenda-tions for further research.
Moffitt et al. (2002) England & Wales, UK	Longitudinal, N=1116 women who became mothers of twins in	Neighborhood social cohe-sion and Trust, informal social control.	Mother's mental health his-tory, symptoms of antiso-cial personality disorder, maternal depression;	'Personality traits' suggestion that younger mothers were less 'conscientious' and with more 'problematic'	Authors make explicit pol-icy recommendations for prevention of teen child-bearing, and support for

	1994–95; 562 of whom were < 20 yrs old at the time of their twins' birth.	SMAST; DIS-IV; Children's cognitive ability and prosocial behavior; TRF; DSM-IV.	mother-child relationships; Mother and teacher reports show ↑'inattention-hyperactivity' in children of younger mothers; equal participation in prosocial activity.	teenage mothers to gain access to child care, education, housing, employment and mental health services. They call for comprehensive, 'multimodal' interventions.
Mitchell & LaGory (2002) Birmingham (AL) USA	Cross-sectional N = 222 households (30 Census-blocks)	Individual's extent of participation in the community (*bonding*) and strength of trust and *bridging* ties (Social capital community Benchmark survey)	Strong bonding ties within group; weak bridging ties with other groups;↑ participation = ↑ mental distress due to increased demands on time & resources; ↑'mastery' more important than social capital in mitigating mental distress.	Findings concerning 'mastery' are potentially useful for designing support interventions to promote individual mastery (and by implication collective resilience) in cohesive inner-city African American communities.
Harpham *et al.* (2004), Colombia	Cross-sectional N = 1168 young people in Cali; factor analysis and logistic regression models	Social cohesion and Trust (thick and thin); A-SCAT scale	anxiety and depression in females; low levels of education and employment are more significant risk factors for mental ill health than social capital. In the presence of violence (as a variable), social capital has no statistical effect on mental health variables.	Guarded policy and practice recommendations. More research in progress.
Fram (2005), USA	Qualitative, focus groups N = 21; parents in a family support program	{n/a}	Most family support center relationships seem to be "bonding." However,	Social support needs to be evaluated in context to determine which relationships are helpful, which

(Continued)

TABLE 9.2. (Continued)

Author (year), location of study site(s)	Study design, sample size & unit(s) of analysis	Indicator of social capital & scale(s) used	Indicator of mental health & scale(s) used	Key findings	Policy/practice implications & remarks
	in a suburb of a major West Coast City; analyzed using iterative categorical coding method.	Social relationships (interview coded "core category").		"getting ahead" goals of parents also led to "bridging" social capital.	are harmful, etc. Family support centers need to attract diverse groups of parents to foster bridging social capital.
Mulvaney & Kendrick (2005), UK	Nested case-control N=846 mothers of young children living in deprived areas of Nottingham; random effects logistic regression, likelihood ratio tests.	Neighborhood social capital & stress (questions from 1992 Health & Lifestyles Survey).	Depressive symptoms (CES-D Scale).	Neighborhood-level deprivation, receiving means-tested benefits, lack of social support, and high stress were associated with greater depressive symptoms. Individual-level assessment of neighborhood social capital not associated with depressive symptoms.	Need further research to assess causality between social support, social capital, and maternal mental health. Need both contextual & individual measures of soc. cap. Seems to be a large unmet need for mental health services among mothers of young children in deprived areas.

TABLE 9.3. Study with primary data linking social capital and mental health
with reference to senior citizens.

Author (year), location of study site(s)	Study design, sample size & method(s) of analysis	Instrument used to assess social capital & mental health	Key findings	Policy/practice implications & Remarks
Cotterill & Taylor (2001) Plymouth, UK	Cross-sectional, N=95 participants of Plymouth HAZ-funded Age Well Project in six locations; N=10 non-project participants and N= 10 staff from voluntary organizations involved in AW Project.	Study assessed reported "social health": in terms of social participation, social networks and interpersonal interaction.	Housebound elderly people benefited from opportunities for social interaction, but did not want to spoil the atmosphere of social gatherings by "talking about what was wrong with them"; health information generated fear and threatened day-to-day coping strategies. AW project participants engaged in the active management of their sense of well-being by avoiding some topics of information in order to stay happy.	Authors highlight the complex and contradictory consequences of unwelcome health information and the welcome social interactions to combat isolation and loneliness in order to promote older people's sense of well-being and happiness.

He then presents a careful account of mechanisms whereby race, psychological sense of belonging and neighborhood economic deprivation interact to shape mental and emotional health and well-being of adolescents in an anonymous American city located in the North-east. This study addressed three questions: "(a) Do African American youth who live in self-reported unsafe neighborhoods show higher levels of depression? (b) Are there gender differences according to perception of calamity, social capital and depression? and (c) Do adolescents from supportive families and neighborhoods demonstrate healthier psychological outcomes compared to adolescents who have only one of these supports?" (p. 49). Stevenson's insightful analysis highlighted the need for interventions to recognize and bolster existing support systems available to adolescent boys and girls living in racially segregated socio-economically disadvantaged urban quarters. Stevenson observed gender differences in perceptions of potential calamity and expressions of fear. Adolescent girls were more likely to express fear of

TABLE 9.4. Studies with primary data linking social capital and mental health with reference to health care and service provision.

Author (year), location of study site(s)	Study design, sample size & unit(s) of analysis	Indicator of social capital & scale(s) used	Indicator of mental health & scale(s) used	Key findings	Policy/practice implications & remarks
Rosenheck et al. (2001) USA	Cross-sectional, one year follow-up observational study of 18 sites participating in the ACCESS (Access to Community Care and Effective Services and Supports) program for homeless seriously mentally ill patients (entered in the study in two cohorts) in the USA (9 States). N=2,668 (mean age 38.5 yrs; 64.4% male; 45.3% African American.	Number of club meetings attended in past 12 months; number of community projects worked on; number of participants in volunteer work; general belief that other people are honest; proportion of adults who voted in the 1994 and 1996 elections.	Clinical diagnoses of mental illness: psychiatric problems and substance abuse problems.	community social capital associated with greater system integration and greater access to assistance from a public housing agency and to a greater probability of exit from homelessness at 12 months. No associations between environmental factors, or systems integration and psychiatric problems.	Collaboration between service providers and service integration may improve outcomes for homeless mentally ill people. More data expected to become available at the end of the ACCESS demonstration period to guide policy and practice more specifically.
Campbell et al. (2004) UK	Qualitative study (indepth interviews, N=30; and two focus groups) with local community "stakeholders" from or working with the African-Caribbean community in an unnamed southern	Participation in local community networks, perception of trust, solidarity, community capacity for forming partnerships, and sense of agency.	Perception of quality of, and access to mental health services	Interviewees had high enthusiasm for participation in local mental health initiatives but were very skeptical of the possibility of effective partnership because of distrust, disillusionment, and disempowerment in the	Local & statutory partnerships are necessary to reduce health inequalities. Such partnerships require trust between voluntary and statutory sectors and require inclusion of the local community in mental health initiatives. It will

English town analyzed using a grid-coding method.		Not specified.	African-Caribbean community with respect to the statutory mental health service sector. … be important for these groups to have a common understanding of the meaning of a "partnership."
van der Linden *et al.* (2003) Maastricht, The Netherlands	Cross-sectional, case-control (mental health service users versus non-users). N=262 children (56 cases and 206 controls) living in Maastricht neighborhoods; Multi-level logistic regression models.	Neighborhood informal social control, social cohesion and trust; translated and adapted ISC and SC&T scales (with 5 site/culture-specific questions added).	More children from lower SES neighborhoods seen by mental health care services; Neighborhood social capital (social cohesion & trust) mitigate the effects of lower SES and children's coming into contact with mental health services. This study makes explicit justification for 'early intervention': parenting and family support strategies. Authors argue that prevention/programs for high-risk children should seek to alleviate neighborhood deprivation by creating safe areas for children to play and for their parents to meet and increase social cohesion.

calamity and benefit from access to neighborhood social capital than their fear-less counterparts. Girls were less likely to report depressive ideation including lethargy, instrumental helplessness, and cognitive difficulties even when they lived in high risk locations. Being fearful of violent calamity and articulating this fear is shown to be an emotionally adaptive strategy teen-age girls use to both generate and access social capital. Moreover, social isolation resulting from fear of violent calamity may promote resilience (p. 56). Stevenson couches his crime prevention and mental health promotion policy and practice recommendations in a comprehensive discussion in favor of building neighborhood social capital and healthy communities through adult supervision and care of adolescents (see also Stevenson, 1997).

Beyers et al.'s longitudinal study (2003) conducted in three southern cities of the USA (Nashville, TN, Knoxsville, TN, and Bloomington, IN) independently reinforces Stevenson's call for concerted efforts to build and strengthen struc-tural and cognitive social capital through prevention/intervention programs. This study addressed two questions: "i) do neighborhood structural disadvantage, concentrated affluence, and residential instability relate to initial levels of and/or growth in adolescence externalizing behavior after controlling for individual and family factors? and ii) do gender and parenting practices differentially affect the development of externalizing behaviors depending on the social structure of neighborhoods in which families reside?" (p. 36) Jennifer Beyers and her team use Coleman's definition of social capital as " . . . physical presence of adults in the family and the quality of relations among family members" (p. 46), and describe family-level collective efficacy as connectedness of social networks among resident adults and youths (after Sampson et al., 1997). They confine their investigation to externalizing behavior problems among youth, and conclude that while neighborhood structure does not directly impact externaliz-ing behavior, it contributes to the socialization of adolescents via the moderating effects of parental monitoring. The authors are careful to point out that their findings are not generalizable to African American youths and/or low SES densely populated urban American neighborhoods, as this category constituted only 17% of their study sample across three southern American cities. However, their findings resonate with "neighborhood-effect" studies of SES in relation to adolescent behavior and mental health, most notably Anneshensel & Sucoff's evidence (1996) from Los Angeles neighborhoods.

Weine, Ware, and Klebic (2004) conducted an ethnographic study among teen-age refugees from Bosnia-Herzegovina living in Chicago, Illinois. Participant obser-vations and in-depth interviews were conducted by an American and Bosnian pair of fieldworkers who focused on refugee adolescents and their families said to have been exposed to refugee trauma, defined as "senses of sadness, isolation, confusion, degradation, dissatisfaction, and anomie" (p. 926). The authors use Bourdieu's con-cept of "cultural capital" to analyze the ways in which Bosnian youth have been adapting to life in Chicago with the support of cohesive family and community struc-tures that affirm and build their ethnic identity, while they are absorbing certain aspects of their new (American) culture at the same time. The authors identify nine mechanisms whereby cultural capital is "converted" (presumably into social capital of the bonding type): using own language; obliging family; sticking together; returning to religion; going ghetto; building a future; taking pride in tradition; critiquing America; and seeking freedom. This study is ongoing, and may be expected to contribute to the wider discourse on positive psychology and promotion of resilience in the context of international humanitarian policy concerning psychosocial support.

Caughy et al. (2003) focus on African American mothers/carers of young - children in a racially-segregated American city (Baltimore, Maryland) and find that the mother/carer's "lack of attachment to community was a risk factor for behavior problems for children living in wealthy communities but, a protective factor for children living in highly impoverished neighborhoods." (p. 231). This study demonstrates a somewhat muddled view of social capital. Social capital (bonding and not bridging type) is investigated in this study in relation to neighborhood "context" with contradicting results. Margaret Caughy and her team use "census block" as a proxy for neighborhood, and do not attempt to examine the meaning of "community" in the context of their study site and sample of respondents. Their suggestion that weak neighborhood ties may be indicative of weak community ties and that African American mothers and/or pre-school children may be better off without their communities is questionable. "Contextual analysis" without enquiry into the meanings and boundaries of the community in question presents a serious limitation given what is already known about the issues of community, particularly in the context of health research.

It would be reasonable to suggest that social cohesion in the context of poverty and structural disadvantage poses mental health risks to women either because they tend to be giving more than receiving, or because they may be constrained by the norms and expectations of their social ties (Kawachi & Berkman, 2001), but Caughy et al.'s study does not consider such possibilities. Mindy Fullilove (1998), a social psychiatrist, analyzing the insights of insiders has demonstrated that building social cohesion and collective efficacy in four different American inner-city locations was beneficial for women, because "*women have major responsibility for raising children . . . The importance of social connections is not simply a matter of social intercourse, but more profoundly a matter of getting women's work done. Loss of social cohesion in the larger community will make women's work more onerous. Conversely, improvements in social organization create networks that allow women to share responsibilities and aid each other.*" (p. 76) Caughy et al.'s suggestion that "being alone might be better" thus runs counter to Fullilove's, Stevenson's, and Beyers et al.'s assertions. The latter highlight positive aspects of social capital with respect to the behavioral development and social adjustment of children and youth; while the former expressly set out to find non-salutary effects of communitarian social capital on individual well-being. Caughy et al.'s study is likely to fuel the ongoing politically-charged debate in epidemiology regarding social capital and public health in general and mental health in particular.

In sharp contrast, Drukker et al. (2003) define neighborhood in an "ecologically meaningful" way, and demonstrate care in fine-tuning their chosen measurement scale for specific components of social capital to suit their study participants.

These authors adopted Sampson et al.'s ISC and SC&T scale (1997) and translated it into Dutch, adding five new questions in order to make it specifically relevant to Maastricht (small city) neighborhoods. This study benefits from and reinforces a related case-control study of children's mental health services in Maastricht (van der Linden et al., 2003) which is discussed in section IV below. Drukker et al.'s longitudinal study was designed to investigate associations between SES and social capital; and how these influence behavior and quality of life of children on the brink of adolescence. The evidence pinpoints children's mental health and social behavior association with one particular aspect of social capital: informal social control. The study design is robustly eco-epidemiological, and the baseline evidence indicates that children living in "better" economic and social capital (low instability) neighborhoods enjoy better quality of life, better general and mental health and exhibit more pro-social behavior as they embark on adolescence. However, a more recent report from this study shows that those living in socio-economically deprived but stable neighborhoods make less use of mental health services (Drukker et al., 2004). The association between socioeconomy, informal social control (social capital) and rates of mental health service use could not be explained by individual differences. It is possible that residentially stable neighborhoods with high levels of informal social control may be more likely to foster and sustain resilience in the face of relative economic deprivation. Mental health care services may well have the effect of undermining resilience, or may be perceived as such. The lack of qualitative data to help interpret the statistical findings is a serious limitation of this study.

9.4. Social Capital and Adult Mental Health and Emotional Well-being

Papers summarized in Table 9.3 include two cross-cultural studies of social capital and emotional/mental health (Harpham et al., 2004; Rose, 2000a). Richard Rose's New Russia Barometer (NRB) study (2000a) sets out to find out whether it is human capital (education, subjective social status, and household income), or social capital (social integration, formal and informal links with others, someone to rely on if ill, etc.), or both human and social capital combined which primarily determine individual health. (p. 1423) Rose's NRB questionnaire was designed to measure "different forms of networking, some familiar in Russia and unfamiliar in the West, and some common to both types of societies" and "administered to a full-scale multi-stage randomly stratified sample covering the whole of the Russian Federation, urban and rural . . ." (p. 1425) This study presents purposely collected data on social capital in the Russian Federation; an improvement on previous studies such as for example, Kennedy et al., 1998 which involved secondary analysis of survey data, "retro-fitting" the concept of social capital on data collected for other purposes. However, it is worth noting that Rose's data on emotional health are subject to significant recall error. In anthropological and related areas of health research, 12-month recall is considered too long to produce reliable information. Nevertheless, Rose's multiple regression models showed that human capital could explain 12.3% of the variance in emotional health; while social capital explained 15.7%, and a composite model with human capital and social capital variables together explained 19.3% of variance in emotional health. Social capital significantly influenced involvement in or exclusion from formal and informal networks; friends to rely on when ill; control over one's own life; and "trust". Younger Russians (< 40 years of age) had greater sense of control of their lives compared to their middle-aged and older compatriots. Rose argued that social capital, a multifaceted construct, cannot be reduced to a single measure, and cautioned against using aggregate membership statistics as a proxy for social capital in aggregate analysis because, "The fullest understanding of the influence of social factors on health is best achieved by recognizing the independent influence of selective forms of both individual *and* social capital." (p. 1431) Rose concluded that public policy can only intervene in economic terms – to ensure sustained growth in household incomes and to promote resilience. It is worth noting here the prominence of "anti modern" society and culture in contemporary Russia contributes to the complexity of the picture partially presented in this study – see also Rose, 2000b, 2001).

Steptoe and Feldman (2001) investigated neighborhood-level effects of deprivation and deficit of social capital on self-rated health and psychological distress (measured using the GHQ-12). Neighborhood problems, including litter in the streets, air pollution, noise, vandalism and disturbance by neighbors or youngsters correlated with poor self-rated health, psychological distress and impaired physical function independent of age, gender, neighbourhood SES, individual deprivation, and social capital. The study participants represented a "stable residential population" with a very wide age range (18–94 years; M=52, SD, 18), and the authors posit and confirm that higher SES neighborhoods had higher levels of social capital. This could however be an artifact of postal questionnaire response – a response rate of 24% is low. Descriptive epidemiological studies such as this one tend to be limited, as that they confine themselves to quantitative methods of analysis, and do not adequately investigate underlying context and meaning.

Evidence presented by Terrie Moffitt and the "Environmental Risk team" (2002) serves to demonstrate how quantitative data from descriptive epidemiological studies may benefit from existing qualitative data to enhance the quality and applicability of evidence for policy and practice. This study is discussed within the sub-group of reviewed papers on social capital and mental health of adults and young people because the authors expressly focus on and prioritize mother-centered interventions. Moffitt and her team compared younger mothers of twins in England and Wales with older ones in order to examine a wide range of social and behavioral risk factors associated with poor child mental health outcomes. Environmental factors (including younger mothers' mental health history, biological father's mental health history, social support for parenting, neighborhood social cohesion, and twins' cognitive development and behavior at age 5) had negative prognoses for younger mothers and their twins compared to older mothers and their twins. This study's findings and recommendations merit discussion in the wider context of UK health policy and practice reform.

Reducing social exclusion and building social capital have been New Labour's explicit goals of health service modernization; and reducing (unwanted) teenage pregnancy and mental health promotion focusing on children and young people had been prioritized (see Social Exclusion Unit, 1999 a & b). The term "teenage" is not unambiguous, however. It needs careful defining. A qualitative study designed to assess health needs, attitudes and aspirations of young people in South London where teenage pregnancy rated highest in Europe, had revealed that "teenage pregnancy" was a heterogeneous category that embraced cases of under-age (unwanted) pregnancy occurring before girls reached the age of consent (sometimes as young as 12) as well as deliberate (wanted) pregnancy among 16 -19 year olds who often considered themselves "adults" (Health First, 1999). This latter group disapproved of "infantalizing" approaches to their needs on the part of practitioners in health and social services who summarily prob-lematized teenage childbearing. Parenthood in (late) teens was often a function of life aspirations, economic and social needs – a deliberate choice on the part of girls and young women, mainly in working class families following their own mothers'/role models' example concerning early parenting. Considering Moffitt et al.'s findings alongside the qualitative evidence summarized above would strengthen their policy recommendations. Practitioners involved in the allocation of resources to facilitate child care access for "teenage" mothers to enable them to build their human capital through education and employment would gain better understanding of their clients by integrating qualitative research evidence. Lack of communication and coordination between quantitative and qualitative researchers, and between researchers and practitioners has continued to hinder social inclusion and achievement of health improvement policy goals in the UK and other countries such as the USA. The problems are magnified when questions of race and/or immigration status limit the extent to which teenagers (or any other "target groups") may access and benefit from bridging social capital (see for example Almedom & Gosling, 2003; Geronimus, 2003).

Mulvaney and Kendrick (2005) investigated the risk of depression among mothers of young children living in deprived areas of Nottingham using a postal questionnaire survey of depressive symptoms as part of an ongoing randomized controlled trial designed to assess the effectiveness of safety advice given to mothers by health visitors. The results showed that mothers with three or more children under five years of age were at significantly higher risk of depression due to increased stress and/or lack of social support and socioeconomic deprivation as those receiving means-tested benefits reported more depressive symptoms. This study had considerable methodological limitations including response bias and confounding variables for which the analysis could not control.

By contrast, Maryah Fram's qualitative study (2005) assessed the types and levels of social capital developed by parents through participation in a Family Support Center (FSC) in a major city in the West Coast of the USA. Her findings showed that the diverse skills, experiences, and backgrounds of participants in the FSC allowed for helpful social networking. Most FSC relationships generated both bonding and bridging types of social capital. This was facilitated by tree aspects of the FSC: focus on commonalities in the parent/family developmental stage to bring diverse families together; its location in a diverse community; and activities built on diverse strengths and common concerns of parents and staff. Fram argued that efforts to generate social support in family services should aim to shape, rather than respond to the socioeconomic and demographic characteristics of the communities in which families with small children live. This study's focus on both structural and cognitive components of social capital – emphasis on service provision and promotion of family functioning makes useful for policy makers and planners responsible for resource allocation for family services and further research.

Mitchell and La Gory (2002) employ Putnam's Social Capital and Community Benchmark Survey and Mirowsky and Ross' psychological distress scale to examine how individual level social capital and individual sense of mastery may avert mental distress in an impoverished "ghetto" setting in Birmingham, Alabama. The authors report strong bonding ties within community and weak bridging ties to other groups: 71% of the study participants, pre-dominantly African American, trusted their neighbors, while 32% reported trust in people in general. Women and the unemployed experienced greater numbers of economic and environmental stressors. According to Mitchell and LaGory, bonding social capital significantly increased mental distress, and individual sense of mastery played a more important role than social capital: those with lower levels of mastery experienced more mental distress. It is likely that social cohesion would enhance mastery in individuals and thereby promote collective resilience in the face of socio economic adversity and absence of bridging social capital. However, the authors appear to "blame the victim" by implying that their study participants' cooperation with them could have been transferred to social action on the part of the study participants in order to solve social problems. It is possible that the researchers were viewed (by the respondents) as possible links between the community in distress and external structures of power. Other studies have shown that Birmingham, Alabama is among the cities where impoverished as well as better-off Black neighborhoods demonstrate high levels of political participation (see for example Portney & Berry, 1997).

Trudy Harpham and her team (2004) developed, tested and validated an adapted form of Sampson et al.'s social capital measurement scale (1997) prior to its application in a South American city. They conclude that in the presence of violence, social capital, namely, trust, is not as closely associated with mental health as is socioeconomic status, specifically, poverty and unemployment. The distinction between thin and thick trust helps to dissociate personal from structural stressors; however, it is not surprising that in a setting where crime and political violence are widespread, bonding social capital may accrue negative effect on mental health, and may even serve to perpetuate conflict in the absence of, or due to breakdown in bridging social capital. Nevertheless, Harpham et al. found that only 24 % of their study participants were "probable cases of mental ill health" and only "13% of the youth admitted considering suicide in the last month" (p. 2272). This may not be as "disturbing" as Harpham et al. suspect, given that a large majority (84%) did not report suicidal ideation, the exact meaning and significance of which is unknown for this sample. In Harpham, Snoxell, Grant, and Rodriguez's more recent report (2005), being mentally ill is referred to as "caseness" and although the prevalence of common mental disorders remains the same, in the absence of statistical associations between mental health and social capital, the authors recommend "more qualitative research to inform potential intervention" (p. 166). Their approach does not take into account their study populations' own views on the matter – only social capital was talked about in the focus group discussions, and mental health left unmentioned for "reasons of sensitivity" (p. 162). It is a matter of concern that this approach may inadvertently reinforce undue pathologization of youth behavior and undermine resilience. It is well accepted in mental health policy circles that the mentally ill resent interventions that (metaphorically) lock them up in the "case management" paradigm of health care provision – "I am not a case, and I can manage" is often the sentiment expressed (see Sayce, 2000).

Taken together, the evidence from Russia (Rose, 2000a) and London, England (Mulvaney & Kendrick, 2005; Steptoe & Feldman, 2001), England and Wales (Moffit et al., 2002), respectively West Coast and Alabama, USA (Fram, 2005; Mitchell & La Gory, 2002), Cali, Colombia (Harpham et al., 2004), confirm earlier research reports showing more reports of depression in women compared to men; implicating social support (giving and receiving differentials) and gender specific economic and social inequalities (see Aneshensel, Frerichs, & Clark, 1981; Aneshensel, Estrada, Hansell, & Clark, 1987;; Antonucci & Akiyama, 1987; Brown & Harris, 1978; Dohrenwend, Levav, & Shrout, 1992; Pevalin & Goldberg, 2003). Randomized controlled trials have also confirmed that social intervention aimed at treatment of depression may be more effective than medical intervention (Harris, Brown, & Robinson, 1999 a & b). Building and/or strengthening bonding as well as bridging social capital is therefore salutary for mental health; but it is worth noting that top-down models that inhibit bottom-up efforts may not be successful at preventing mental ill-health or promoting health and well-being.

9.5. Social Capital and Senior Citizens' Mental and Emotional Well-being

Cotterill and Taylor's evaluation of Plymouth Health Action Zone's "Ageing Well (AW)" project (2001) comprises a qualitative study of a portion of a complex inter-sectoral, multi-agency government supported initiative to build social capital. Health Action Zones (HAZ) are area-based British government-initiated interventions to tackle health inequalities and social exclusion, with explicit mandate to build social capital. Policy analysts and practitioners have expressed both support for and concern over the prospects of evaluating such complex initiatives with compound structural and functional opportunities and challenges (Higgins, 1998; Jacobson & Yen, 1998; Powell & Moon, 2001). In response, a national

HAZ evaluation commissioned to examine successes and failures of all 26 HAZ in England (plus one in northern Ireland) had proposed combined "Theories of Change" and "Realistic Evaluation" models of evaluation (see Judge, 2000). These did not incorporate specific measures of social capital. Moreover, one of the challenges to local evaluation design has been the absence of baseline data on pre-HAZ levels of social capital against which the success of targeted interventions can be measured. However, the health service modernization programme is said to be progressing steadily, and HAZs are currently in the process of relocating from local Health Authority to Primary Care Trust (PCT) settings in order to accomplish institutional "Whole Systems" change. It is worth noting here that HAZ funding timeframe of seven years may be too short to effect real change. As Putnam, Leonardi, and Nanetti (1993) observed from the Italian experiment, the development of effective democracy and meaningful civic engagement involves lengthy processes of public discussion, reasoning and decision-making for which government-led, time limited time and funding-bound initiatives hardly allow.

Cotterill and Taylor's qualitative assessment of effectiveness of a social capital building intervention (2001) exposes the contradictory effects of dissemination of health information intended to empower senior citizens (which threatens their emotional well-being by introducing fear about their health) and building bonding social capital to reduce isolation and thereby promote mental health. Enabling senior citizens to generate bonding and bridging social capital in order to "manage health information" thrown at them by health professionals with whom they have unequal power relationships may indicate positive overall outcome. This study brings to the fore inherent problems in social engineering, namely, the contradictions of "empowerment" and target-driven health promotion activities aimed at the production of statistically significant measurable results in time for local and/or general election campaigns. It is well known that social capital in terms of reciprocity, availability of social networks and access to social support involves delicate negotiations, time-intensive processes of social interaction and individually-crafted balances between dependence and autonomy (see Antonucci, Fuhrer, & Jackson, 1990; Krause, 1997; Liang et al., 2001). External agency interventions may thwart more rather than enhance these salutary processes. The UK social and health modernization policy has set in train processes of decentralization and devolution of public health (Evans, 2003) which may serve to empower health workers at the expense of excluded groups for whom prospects of social inclusion and civic participation may be a long way away (see for instance Almedom & Gosling, 2003). While advances in operational research (OR) herald promise of real integration of participatory and cross-cultural multimethod (Taket & White, 1994, 1998, 2000; White & Taket, 1994), translation of research into action may be pie in the sky. Real improvements in health and social development are likely to progress at a slow and arduous pace as and when the poor and marginalized gain control over their own health and social welfare.

9.6. Social Capital and Mental Health Service and Care Provision

The former WHO Mental Health Division head Norman Sartorius' valedictory appeal for social capital highlights a two-way process whereby efficient and effective mental health services help to build and/or strengthen social capital in the communities they serve, and are in turn built and strengthened by the social capital of service users (2002, 2003). Rosenheck et al. (2001) and van der Linden et al. (2003) independently reinforce Sartorius' views.

Rosenheck et al. (2001) demonstrate effectively that structural bonding and bridging social capital in mental health and housing service integration "reflect the state of civic culture in the community at large." (p. 701). This supports Sartorius' argument (2002) and is borne out by the findings of other studies (see Ahern & Hendryx, 2003; Hendryx & Ahern, 2001; Hendryx, Ahern, Loverich, & McCurdy, 2002). Similarly, van der Linden et al.'s report of children's use of mental health services substantiates the view that deficit in social capital in the shared social environment contributes to increased exposure of children to mental health services. The Rosenheck team's interest in studying the links between communitarian social capital and mental health care services has extended to investigating the quality of mental health care service in department of Veterans Affairs (VA) hospitals across the United States. According to Desai, Dausey, and Rosenheck (2005) who conducted a prospective mortality study of psychiatric inpatients of 128 VA hospitals around the country (a total sample of 121,933 patients discharged with a diagnosis of major affective disorder, bipolar affective disorder, posttraumatic stress disorder (PTSD), or schizophrenia between 1994 and 1998), only 2.9 per cent died within a year of discharge; and of those only 481 (0.4 per cent of the sample) committed suicide, mostly during the first 6 months following discharge from hospital. Desai et al.'s presentation appears to be overkill (no pun intended!) as the proportion of suicides is so small. Moreover, given the levels of variation in individual diagnosis, length of hospitalization, and (unknown) post-discharge circumstances, it seems that this study started out with an overstretched hypothesis in trying to test whether or not suicide risk could be an indicator of quality of care in mental health hospitals. The study may have benefited from investigating individual level access to social capital, but as it stands, it is an example of the way in which "social capital and mental health" research can sometimes fail to see the wood for the trees.

In contrast, Campbell, Cornish, and McLean (2004) shed light on both the structural and cognitive obstacles to mental health care improvement in England. Using robust qualitative methods of investigation and analysis, Catherine Campbell and her team unveil the depth of distrust between African-Caribbean community and statutory sectors that inhibit meaningful partnerships. Three factors, social capital (considered to have complementary explanatory power to income and health inequalities), social identity ((based on content of social representations of group membership), and social representation (systems of shared social knowledge that help people make sense of their world and communicate it to others) comprise the "social psychology of participation" applied in their analysis of the processes involved in the functioning of community participation. As would be expected, Campbell and her team's data revealed multiple meanings of "community participation" among those represented in their sample often hampered by the lack of resources and capacity to engage in meaningful partnerships with the statutory sector, over and above the deeply entrenched perceptions of institutional racism.

In summary, this evaluative review serves to derive from the findings a set of guidelines for interdisciplinary research aimed at unraveling the complex associations between social capital and mental health. What is known so far about the associations between social capital and mental health is outlined herewith. Neighborhood safety is a function of informal social control, social cohesion and trust whereby prevention of vandalism and violent crime, parental active involvement in children's and adolescents' activity generates collective efficacy. Residents' sense of physical and mental or emotional well-being cannot be disaggregated into separate categories or promoted by means of social in the absence of economic and capacity building interventions. Furthermore, the value of qualitative studies in illuminating the areas that are often overshadowed by quantitative data that are, on their own, difficult to interpret and use has been demonstrated. The challenge remains to combine both qualitative and quantitative analyses in the quest for a better understanding of the ways in which social capital and mental health are inter-connected.

References

Adger, W. N, Hughes, T. P., Folke, C., Carpenter, S. R., Rockstiön, J., (2005). Social-ecological resilience to coastal disasters. *Science, 309*, 1036–1039.

Ahern, M., & Hendryx, M. S. (2003). Social capital and trust in providers. *Social Science & Medicine, 57*, 1195–1203.

Almedom, A. M. (2005). Social capital and mental health: An interdisciplinary review of primary evidence. *Social Science & Medicine, 61*, 943–964.

Almedom, A. M., & Gosling, R. (2003). The health of young asylum seekers and refugees in The United Kingdom: Reflection from research. In Allotey, P. (Ed.), *The health of refugees: Public health perspectives from crisis to settlement* (pp. 169–184). Melbourne: Oxford University Press.

Aneshensel, C. S., Estrada, A. L., Hansell, M. J., & Clark, V. A. (1987). Social psychological aspects of reporting behavior: Lifetime depressive episode reports. *Journal of Health and Social Behavior, 28*, 232–246.

Aneshensel, C. S., Frerichs, R. R., & Clark, V. A. (1981). Family roles and sex differences in depression. *Journal of Health and Social Behavior, 22*, 379–393.

Aneshensel, C. S., & Sucoff, C. A. (1996). Jue neighborhood context of adolesceut meutal health. *Journal of Health and Social Behavior, 37*(4), 293–310.

Antonucci, T. C., & Akiyama, H. (1987). An examination of sex differences in social support among older men and women. *Sex Roles, 17*, 737–749.

Antonucci, T. C., Fuhrer, R., & Jackson, J. S. (1990). Social support and reciprocity: A cross-ethnic and cross-national perspective. *Journal of Social and Personal Relationships, 7*, 519–530.

Beyers, J. M., Bates, J. E., & Pettit, G. S. & Dodge, K. A. (2003). Neighborhood structure, parenting processes, and the development of youths' externalizing behaviors: A multilevel analysis. *American Journal of Community Psychology, 31*, 35–53.

Brown, G. W., & Harris, T. (1978). *Social origins of depression: A study of psychiatric disorder in women*. New York: Free Press.

Caughy, M. O., O'Campo, P. J., & Muntaner, C. (2003). When being alone might be better: neighborhood poverty, social capital, and child mental health. *Social Science & Medicine, 57*, 227–237.

Campbell, C., Cornish, F., & McLean, C. (2004). Social capital, participation and the perpetuation of health inequalities: Obstacles to African-Caribbean participation in 'Patrtnerships' to improve mental health. *Ethnicity & Health, 9*, 313–335.

Cotterill, L., & Taylor, D. (2001). Promoting mental health and wellbeing amongst housebound older people. *Quality in Ageing, 2*, 32–46.

Davis, M. (1998). *Ecology of fear*. New York: Vintage.

Desai, R. A., Dausey, D. J., & Rosenheck, R. A., (2005). Mental health delivery and suicide risk: The role of individual patient and facility factors. *American Journal of Psychiatry, 162*, 311–318.

Dohrenwend, B. P., Levav, I., Shrout, P. E. Schwartz, S., Naveh, G., Link, B. G., Skodol, A. E., & Stueve, A. (1992). Socioeconomic status and psychiatric disorders: The causation-selection issue. *Science, 255*, 946–952.

Drukker, M., Driessen, G., Krabbendam, L., & van Os J.(2004). The wider social environment and mental health service use. *Acta Psychiatrica Scandinavica, 110*, 119–129.

Drukker, M., Kaplan, C., & Feron, F. & van Os J. (2003). Children's health-related quality of life, neighbourhood socio-economic deprivation and social capital: A contextual analysis. *Social Science & Medicine, 57*, 825–841.

Evans, D. (2003). 'Taking public health out of the ghetto': The policy and practice of multi-disciplinary public health in the United Kingdom. *Social Science & Medicine, 57*, 959–967.

Fram, M. S. (2005). "It's just not all teenage moms": Diversity, support, and relationship family services. *American Journal of Orthopsychiatry, 75*, 507–517.

Fullilove, M. T. (1998). Promoting social cohesion to improve health. *Journal of American Medical Women's Association, 52*, 72–76.

Geronimus, A. T. (2003). Damned if you do: culture, identity, privilege, and teenage childbearing in the United States. *Social Science & Medicine, 57*, 881–893.

Hardin, G. (1968). The tragedy of the commons. *Science, 162*, 1243–1248.

Harpham, T., Snoxell, S., Grant, E., & Rodriguez, C. (2005). Common mental disorders in a young urban population in Colombia. *British Journal of Psychiatry, 187*, 161–167.

Harpham, T., Grant, E., & Rodriguez, C. (2004). Mental health and social capital in Cali, Colombia. *Social Science & Medicine, 58*, 2267–2277.

Harris, T., Brown, G. W., & Robinson, R. (1999a). Befriending as an intervention for chronic depression among women in an inner city. 1: Randomized controlled trial. *British Journal of Psychiatry, 174*, 219–224.

Harris, T., Brown, G. W., & Robinson, R. (1999b). Befriending as an intervention for chronic depression among women in an inner city. 2: Role of fresh-start experiences and baseline psychosocial factors in remission from depression. *British Journal of Psychiatry, 174*, 225–232.

Health First (Community Health South London). (1999). *Health needs and perceptions of young people in Lambeth*. Report prepared by Carrick James market Research, June 1999, London.

Hendryx, M. S., & Ahern, M. M. (2001). Access to mental health services and health sector social capital. *Administration and Policy in Mental Health, 28*, 205–218.

Hendryx, M. S., Ahern, M. M., Loverich, N. P., & McCurdy, A. R. (2002). Access to health care and community social capital. *Health Services Research, 31*, 85–101.

Higgins, J. (1998). HAZs warning. *Health Service Journal*, 24–25.

Jacobson, B., & Yen, L. (1998). Health action zones offer the possibility of radical ideas which need rigorous evaluation. *British Medical Journal, 316*, 164.

Judge, K. (2000). Testing evaluation to the limits: the case of English Health Action Zones. *Journal of Health Service Research Policy, 5*, 3–5.

Kawachi, I., & Berkman, L. F. (2001). Social ties and mental health. *Journal of Urban Health-Bulletin of the New York Academy of Medicine, 78*, 458–467.

Kennedy, B., Kawachi, I., & Brainerd, E. (1998). The role of social capital in the Russian morality crisis. *World Development, 26*(11), 2029-2043.

Klinenberg, E. (2002). *Heat wave: A social autopsy of disaster in Chicago*. Chicago: University of Chicago Press.

Krause, N. (1997). Anticipated support, received support, and economic stress among older adults. *Journal of Gerontology: Psychological Sciences, 52B*, 284–293.

Liang, J., Krause, N. M., & Bennett, J. M. (2001). Social exchange and well-being: Is giving better than receiving? *Psychology & Aging, 16*, 511–523.

Lindström, M., Merlo, J., & Östergren, P-O. (2003). Social capital and sense of insecurity in the neighborhood: a population-based multilevel analysis in Malmö, Sweden. *Social Science & Medicine, 56*, 1111–1120.

Mitchell, C. U., & LaGory, M. (2002). Social capital and mental distress in an impoverished community. *City & Community, 1*, 195–215.

Moffitt, T. E., the E-Risk Study Team. (2002). Teen-aged mothers in contemporary Britain. *Journal of Child Psychology and Psychiatry, 43*, 727–742.

Mulvaney, C., & Kendrick, D. (2005). Depressive symptoms in mothers of pre-school children: Effects of deprivation, social support, stress and neighbourhood social capital. *Social Psychiatry and Psychiatric Epidemiology, 40*, 2002–2008.

Pevalin, D. J., & Goldberg, D. P. (2003). Social precursors to onset and recovery from episodes of common mental illness. *Psychological Medicine, 33*, 299–306.

Portney, K. E., & Berry, J. M. (1997). Mobilizing minority communities: Social capital and participation in urban neighborhoods. *American Behavioral Scientist, 40*, 632–644.

Powell, M., & Moon, G. (2001). Health action zones: the 'third way' of a new area-based policy? *Health and Social care in the Community, 9*, 43–50.

Pretty, J. (2003). Social capital and the collective management of resources. *Science, 302*, 1912–1914.

Putnam, R. D., Leonardi, R., & Nanetti, R. Y. (1993). *Making democracy work, civic traditions in modern Italy*. New Jersey: Princeton University Press.

Rose, R. (2001). When government fails: Social capital in an antimodern Russia. In B. Edwards, M. W. Foley, M. Diani (Eds.), *Beyond tocqueville* (pp. 56–69)., Hanover and London: Tufts University, University Press of New England..

Rose, R. (2000a). How much does social capital add to individual health? A survey study of Russians. *Social Science & Medicine, 51*, 1421–1435.

Rose, R. (2000b). Uses of social capital in Russia: Modern, pre-modern, and anti-modern. *Post-Soviet Affairs, 16*, 33–57.

Rosenheck, R., Morrissey, J., Lam, J., Calloway, M., Stolar, M., Johnsen, M., Randolph, F., Blasinsky, M., & Goldman, H. (2001). Service delivery and community: Social capital, service systems integration, and outcomes among homeless persons with severe mental illness. *Health Services Research, 36*, 691–710.

Ross, C. E., Reynolds, J. R., & Geis, K. J. (2000). The contingent meaning of neighborhood stability for residents' psychological well-being. *American Journal of Social Review, 65*, 581–597.

Sampson, R. J., Stephen, W. R., & Earls, F. (1997). Neighborhoods and violent crime: A multilevel study of collective efficacy. *Science, 277*, 918–924.

Sartorius, N. (2003). Social capital and mental health. *Current Opinion in Psychiatry, 16*, S101–S105.

Sartorius, N. (2002). *Fighting for mental health.* Cambridge: Cambridge University Press.

Sayce, L. (2000). *From psychiatric patient to citizen: Overcoming discrimination and social exclusion.* London and New York: Macmillan and St. Martin's Press.

Social Exclusion Unit, 1999a. *Teenage Pregnancy* Report presented to Parliament by the Prime Minister by Command of Her majesty (June 1999), London.

Social Exclusion Unit, 1999b. Bridging the Gap: *New opportunities for 16–18 year olds not in education, employment or training* London.

Steptoe, A., & Feldman, P. J. (2001). Neighborhood problems as sources of chronic stress: Development of a measure of neighborhood problems, and associations with socioeconomic status and health. *Annals of Behavioral Medicine, 23*, 177–185.

Stevenson, H. C. (1998). Raising safe villages: Cultural-ecological factors that influence the emotional adjustment of adolescents. *Journal of Black Psychology, 24*, 44–59.

Stevenson, H. C. Jr. (1997). "Missed, dissed, and pissed": Making meaning of neighborhood risk, fear and anger management in urban black youth. *Cultural Diversity and Mental Health, 3*, 37–52.

Taket, A., White, L. (2000). *Partnership & participation.* Chichester: John Wiley & Sons.

Taket, A., & White, L. (1998). Experience in the practice of one tradition of multimethodology. *Systemic Practice and Action Research, 11*, 153–168.

Taket, A., & White, L. (1994). Doing community operational research with multicultural groups. *Omega, International Journal of Management Science, 22*, 579–588.

van der Linden, J., Drukker, M., Gunther, N., Feron, F., & van Os, J. (2003). Children's mental health service use, neighbourhood socioeconomic deprivation, and social capital. *Social Psychiatry & Pshychiatric Epidemiology, 38.* 507–514.

Weine, S. M., Ware, N., & Klebic, A. (2004). Converting cultural capital among teen refugees and their families from Bosnia-Herzegovina. *Psychiatric Services, 55*, 923–927.

Weine, S. M., Ware, N., & Klebic, A. (2004). A family approach to severe mental illness in post-war Kosoro. *Psychiatry, 68*(1), 17–27

White, L., & Taket, A. (1994). The death of the expert. *Journal of Operational Research Society, 45*, 733–748.

10
Social Capital and Health-Related Behaviors

MARTIN LINDSTRÖM

10.1. Health-Related Behaviors in a Social Context

10.1.1. Environmental Conditions and Health-Related Behaviors

Behaviors such as tobacco smoking, alcohol consumption, physical activity (or a sedentary lifestyle) and diet are major determinants of health because of their causal effects on cardiovascular diseases, cancers, and many other chronic diseases (The World Health Report, 2002). Some other health-related behaviors such as the abuse of narcotic drugs (which lead to premature death for a variety of reasons) and sexual behaviors (which lead to sexually transmitted diseases/infections) are mainly causally linked to health for other reasons.

Causal linkages between environmental factors and health-related behaviors have been recognized for decades in social and behavioral science theories (Bandura, 1986; McLeroy, Bibeau, Steckler, & Glantz, 1988) and are supported by empirical findings. Factors in the physical environment have been thoroughly investigated (MacIntyre, MacIver, & Sooman, 1993). The social environment also affects health. Cassel hypothesized in 1976 that aspects of the social environment may have an effect on health (Cassel, 1976), and the association between social circumstances and health-related behaviors is now widely accepted as a major health determinant (Emmons, 2000). The social environment affects individual health-related behavior through a number of causal mechanisms by shaping norms, enforcing social control, enabling or not enabling people to participate in particular behaviours, reducing or producing stress, and constraining individual choice (Institute of Medicine, 2003). A comprehensive list of social environmental factors which influence behavior has recently been given by McNeill, Kreuter, and Subramanian (2006), and this list is shown in Table 10.1. Social support and social networks, listed at the top of Table 10.1, may enable or constrain the adoption of health-promoting behaviors, provide access to resources and material goods, provide individual and community-coping resources, buffer negative health outcomes, and restrict contact to infectious diseases. Low socioeconomic position (as typically measured by education, income and/or occupation) may increase biological

Table 10.1. Social environment dimensions, descriptions and key elements, and mechanisms by which they influence behavior.

Dimension	Description/key elements	Mechanism
Social support and social networks	The presence and nature of interpersonal relationships and interactions; extent to which one is interconnected and embedded in a community; interpersonal level characteristic	Enables or constrains the adoption of health-promoting behaviors; provides access to resources and material goods; provides individual and community coping responses; buffers negative health outcomes; and restricts contact to infectious diseases
Socioeconomic position (SEP) and Income Inequality (II)	SEP: Reflects one's social standing in society; commonly measured using educational attainment, occupation, and individual income II: Reflects the unequal distribution of income; signifies the gap between the rich and poor	SEP: Increases biological stress and thereby adversely affects health; reduces accumulation of and access to material resources that can protect against stress. II: Creates less socially cohesive communities through disinvestments in social capital; reduces social spending on programs and services; and increases psychosocial conditions (e.g., frustration, social comparison)
Racial discrimination	Interpersonal or institutional bias that results in psychological harm; limits opportunities for advancement	Produces economic and social deprivation; increases exposure to harmful substances; and creates psychological trauma. Inadequate health care and targeting of harmful substances to marginalized groups is also a byproduct of racial discrimination
Neighborhood factors	Also described as neighborhood deprivation; represents independent environmental factors of "place" rather than the aggregation of individuals living in an area	Exposure to harmful elements of the physical environment (e.g., water quality), availability of health, social and community support services, community reputaton and other historical and cultural features
Social cohesion and social capital	Extent of connectedness and solidarity among groups; shared resources that allow people to act together; area or community-level characteristic	Ability to enforce and/or reinforce group or social norms for positive health behaviors; provision of tangible support (e.g., transportation)

L.H. McNeill et al. 2006, Social Science and Medicine

stress and reduce access to material resources. Income inequality may create less cohesive communities through disinvestments in social capital, reduced social spending on programs and services, and increased frustration originating in social comparisons. Racial discrimination produces economic and social deprivation, increases exposure to harmful substances, and creates psychological trauma. Neighborhood factors such as neighborhood deprivation may result in exposure to harmful elements of the physical environment (e.g., water quality, air pollution, housing), or may be related to the availability of health, social, and community support services, and a community's reputation. Social cohesion and social capital may increase the ability to enforce/reinforce social norms for positive health behaviors. This list gives a picture of the variety of plausible social influences on health behaviors, although it is not complete. For instance, social capital may also affect health-related behaviours by a direct psychosocial stress mechanism (Kawachi, Kennedy, & Glass, 1999). Social capital is the most recently conceptualised and investigated of the social items listed in Table 10.1 which influences health-related behaviors.

10.1.2. Social Capital and Health-Related Behaviors

Social capital is a very recent concept in the public health literature. The progress in public health studies analyzing social capital as a health determinant has been exponential in recent years. Whereas Macinko and Starfield (2001) only found 10 articles on social capital within the public health literature in 2001, Kawachi, Kim, Coutts, and Subramanian (2004) found 50 papers published on this subject in 2002, just a year later. Social capital is defined as those features of social structures - such as levels of interpersonal trust and norms of reciprocity and mutual aid - which constitute resources for individuals and facilitate collective action (Coleman, 1990; Kawachi & Berkman, 2000; Putnam, 1993, 2000). Social capital forms a subset of the notion of social cohesion. Social cohesion refers to two broader, intertwined features of society, which may be described as the absence of latent social conflict (in the form of income inequality, racial/ethnic conflict dimensions, disparities in political participation or other forms of polarization), and the presence of strong social bonds (as measured by levels of trust and norms of reciprocity, i.e., social capital, the abundance of associations that bridge social divisions and create "civil society", and the presence of institutions of conflict management, e.g., a responsive democracy, an independent judiciary, and so forth) (Kawachi & Berkman, 2000). Social capital is always a contextual phenomenon in the sense that it is a characteristic of the relations and interactions *between* individuals, groups of individuals, organizations and institutions rather than a characteristic of the individuals, groups, organizations and institutions *themselves*. The concept of social capital can thus be clearly distinguished from the concept of human capital, which denotes the formal education and experience of the individual person (Coleman, 1990). The concept of social capital should also be distinguished from the concept of social support in the narrow sense of the social embeddedness in the closest social network of the individual

(Lochner, Kawachi, & Kennedy, 1999). This distinction is also important because the social support and also the social network (in connection with social support) concepts are derived from the psychosocial stress theory and have been analyzed within the public health literature for decades (see for e.g., Berkman & Syme, 1979; House, Landis, & Umberson, 1988), although the line between social support and social capital may not always be easy to draw. The three concepts of bonding, bridging, and linking social capital have also been introduced. Bonding social capital refers to "trusting and cooperative relations between members who see themselves as being similar in terms of their shared social identity", bridging social capital to "relations of respect and mutuality between people who know they are not alike in some sociodemographic (or social identity) sense (differing by age, ethnic group, social class, etc.)", and linking social capital to "norms of respect and networks of trusting relationships between people who are interacting across explicit, formal or institutionalised power or authority gradients in society" (Szreter & Woolcock 2004). It seems possible that the "bonding" social capital concept would also border the social network and social support concepts derived from the psychosocial stress theory.

Social capital has been suggested to have beneficial effects on health by several different causal mechanisms which include: 1) the norms and attitudes which affect health-related behaviors; 2) psychosocial mechanisms which both serve to enhance self-esteem, confidence, and control, and may have biological effects (for instance, by activating the hypothalamic-pituitary-adrenocortical axis); 3) social networks, which tend to increase access to health care and amenities; and 4) by having a lowering effect on crime rates (Kawachi, Kennedy & Glass, 1999; Kawachi & Berkman, 2000).

Although social capital is a clearly contextual concept, both the nature (definition/operationalization) and level of analysis differ in the literature concerning social capital and health. First, social capital has been defined and analyzed as civic engagement, social networks/social participation, generalized trust in other people (horizontal trust), trust in the institutions of society (vertical trust), and reciprocity (expectation of helpfulness from other people) (Putnam 1993, 2000). While some theorists construe social capital as "ties" and norms binding individuals within constituent elements of large organizations or linking them across a variety of institutional and formal and informal associational realms (Granovetter, 1973), others regard social capital as a "moral resource" such as trust (Fukuyama, 1995, 1999). The debate concerning the "essence of social capital", i.e., norms and values in social participation/networks or trust, is still unresolved. As Woolcock has noted, "This leaves unresolved whether social capital is the infrastructure or the content of social relations, the 'medium' as it were, or the 'message'" (Woolcock, 1998). Second, Macinko and Starfield (2001) have defined and identified at least four different levels at which the analysis of social capital and health have been conducted. These include the macro (countries, regions, municipalities), meso (neighbourhoods, city quarters), micro (social networks and social participation of individuals), and individual psychological (trust) levels. Some authors study social capital at the macro and meso levels (Putnam, 2000;

Woolcock, 2001). In contrast, others study how relations between individuals and social networks are organized in local environments (Coleman, 1990). These differing definitions and levels of analysis must be taken into consideration in the following sections on social capital and health-related behaviors of this chapter. The contextual characteristic of social capital must also be related to the growing literature on individual and community interventions targeting health-related behaviors.

10.1.3. Individual and Community Interventions Targeting Health-Related Behaviors

In recent decades a large volume of intervention research has been conducted targeting health-related behaviors. Individual-targeted interventions, e.g., in the primary health care setting, have been most commonly used. These interventions, although being intensive in impact at the individual level, mostly run the risk of reaching only an extremely limited proportion of the population. Individual-level interventions have also used tailored telephone counselling or tailored print communications. However, such individual-level interventions do not take into account the fact that socially and economically deprived groups with a concentration of risk behaviors to a lesser extent have access to a telephone (Resnicow et al., 1996) and to a considerably higher extent have low literacy skills (Williams et al., 1995). The population-based intervention approach is considered by many as superior to those interventions only targeting the individual level, because a much larger population is targeted. Some community-based studies have found no intervention effects on risk factors (Glasgow, Terborg, Hollis, Severson, & Boles, 1995), while others have found intervention effects only on some risk factors (Sorensen, Emmons, Hunt, & Johnston, 1998). Intervention studies on health-related behaviors thus entail a paradox. Intervention studies targeted at individuals are often effective in achieving health behavior change at the individual participant level, but are less effective in achieving measurable health behavior change at the population level. In contrast, intervention studies targeted at the population level often include a large proportion of the population, but are less effective at the individual level compared to individual level interventions. However, small changes in health-related behaviors at the population level can lead to large overall effects on disease burden (Rose, 1992). Evaluations of health behavior interventions must thus be conducted both in terms of their benefits in producing individual changes, and in terms of their reach or penetration within the population (Abrams et al., 1996). Although there is a tendency towards recommending community interventions, very little work has so far been conducted directly using social capital to improve health-related behaviors.

Studies on the association between social capital and health in general as well as between social capital and health-related behaviors in particular have mostly been conducted in industrialised countries. Hence, the relations between socioeconomic gradients, social capital, health behaviours and health are mainly discussed in relation to these social and economic contexts.

10.2. The Influence of Social Capital on Specific Health-Related Behaviors

10.2.1. Alcohol and Narcotic Drugs

The links between social deprivation and health behaviors are very strong in the case of both legal and illegal drug use. In a significant number of cases, the latter result in suicide, homicide, violent crime, and accidents. Alcohol is associated as a misk factor with more than 60 diagnoses, but there is also an inverse association between alcohol and adverse health effects in the case of ischemic heart disease, stroke, and type II diabetes (Murray & Lopez, 1996). Alcohol abuse has an important impact on death rates. Alcohol has recently been estimated to contribute to 3.2% of the total mortality in the world and to 4.0% of the total disease burden, and these proportions reach above 10% in western countries (Rehm, Room, & Moneiro, 2004). There are also many illegal drugs (in most countries), cannabis being the most important in many countries in terms of prevalence, primarily among young people (Gilvarry, 2000; Smart & Ogborne, 2000). Drug users are mostly recruited from groups with disturbed family backgrounds, low self-esteem, and impaired psychological functioning. Apart from its own health-detrimental effects, cannabis use is an important precursor to the use of other drugs (Dupre, Miller, Gold, & Rospenda, 1995).

Adolescence and early adulthood are the periods when in most persons health-related behaviors such as alcohol consumption, other drug use, and smoking are founded. Low levels of parental monitoring have been shown to be associated with children's initiation of substance use (alcohol, smoking and other drugs) at earlier ages (Chilcoat & Anthony, 1996). The social context in peer groups as well as in schools has also been shown to be important for the risk of initiating drug abuse (Dupre, Miller, Gold and Rospenda, 1995). The extent to which school is a functional community with supportive social relationships, social participation in school activities, and shared norms, goals, and values, may also moderate individual risk of initiating adverse health behaviors such as high alcohol consumption and drug use (McMillan & Chavis, 1986). Multilevel analyses, which take both individual-level composition of individuals and contextual-level characteristics into account, have shown some contextual effects of the family (adolescents living with both parents or not) (Bjarnason et al., 2003), school (Maes & Lievens, 2003), and university (Kairouz, Gliksman, Demers, & Adlaf, 2002) in different Western countries. However, only a few theoretical models of contextual effects of alcohol and narcotic drugs have been suggested. Coleman has proposed that the socialization of children is facilitated by normative consensus among community members, plausibly through both increased clarity concerning appropriate and inappropriate behaviors and increased monitoring and enforcement of community norms (Coleman & Hoffer, 1987; Coleman, 1988). The results of a few multilevel studies in the

US have indicated that low social cohesion in neighborhoods is significantly associated with neighborhood youth and alcohol arrests (Duncan, Duncan, & Strycker, 2002), that college social capital (measured as college mean aggregate reports of student voluntarism) is significantly associated with alcohol abuse and harm (Weitzman & Chen, 2005), and that college social capital (measured as the individual's daily time volunteering in the past 30 days, aggregated to the college campus-level) has protective effects on binge drinking, i.e., the consumption of large amounts of alcohol on one occasion (Weitzman & Kawachi, 2000). In southern Sweden one individual- level social capital study has shown that social capital, indicated by measures of social participation and trust, was inversely correlated with the probability of tobacco smoking and illicit drug use, but that social capital showed no statistically significant correlation with the probability of binge drinking among adolescents aged 12–18 years (Lundborg, 2005). Another multi-level analysis conducted across 34 different countries demonstrated a significant positive association between income inequality and alcohol use and the frequency of drunkenness among adolescents (aged 11, 13 and 15 years) (Elgar, Roberts, Parry-Langdon, & Boyce, 2005).

In adult populations, high (in terms of health-threatening) alcohol consumption, currently defined as 168 grams/week or more for men and 108 grams/week or more for women (British Medical Association, 1995), mostly has a positive association with high socioeconomic status (Blaxter, 1990; Lindström, 2005a; Pollack, Cubbin, Ahn, & Winkleby, 2005). This pattern clearly differs from other health behaviors such as smoking, physical activity, and diet, for which the adverse health effects are concentrated in lower socioeconomic strata. The socioeconomic patterns for high alcohol consumption also seem to be reflected in the association between aspects of social capital and alcohol consumption. Individual-level cross-sectional studies in southern Sweden have indicated a significant association between social capital and high alcohol consumption (see above) among adults 18–80 years (Lindström, 2005a), consumption of illegal alcohol (home made and smuggled) among adults 18–80 years (Lindström, 2005b), and experience of cannabis use among young adults aged 18–34 years (Lindström, 2004), respectively. However, the patterns differ for social participation (measured as participation in 13 different social activities at some occasion during the past year) compared to generalized trust in other people. Social participation was only associated with consumption of illegal alcohol during the past year, i.e., high social participation was significantly associated with higher odds of consumption of illegal alcohol. There were no significant associations between social participation and high alcohol consumption and experience of cannabis use. In contrast, low generalized trust in other people was significantly associated with all three behavioral outcomes. The associations between the combination of high social participation and low trust, and all three behavioural outcomes were also significant. First, these findings imply that the psychological aspect of social capital (trust in other people) may be important in connection with drug (both alcohol and cannabis) use/abuse, a finding which supports the notion that psychological factors and the psychosocial conditions during childhood and adolescence are crucial as predictors of drug use/abuse (see above). Second, the findings also imply that the "miniaturization of community", i.e., high or average levels of social participation combined with low levels of trust (Fukuyama, 1999), may be associated with drug use/abuse. It seems that people in high or average socioeconomic positions with high or average social participation but consistently low trust have the highest odds of high alcohol consumption, consumption of illegal alcohol, and previous experience of cannabis use. In contrast, a recent American study found no significant individual-level association between trust in one's community, social participation, and binge drinking (Greiner, Chaoyang, Kawachi, Hunt, & Ahluwalia, 2004).

Many multilevel analyses which include effects of both individual-level and contextual-level characteristics on alcohol consumption or binge drinking in the general adult population in different countries have been conducted at contextual levels such as the state level in India concerning effects of prohibition policy (Subramanian, Nandy, Irving, Gordon, & Smith, 2005), regional-level effects of per capita income in Japan (Fukuda, Nakamura, & Takamo, 2005), neighbourhood-level effects of deprivation in the US (Pollack, Cubbin, Ahn & Winkleby 2005), regional-level effects of the proportion of manual workers, unemployment, median household income, the Gini coefficient (income distribution), family cohesion, voting turnout, level of urbanisation, and proportion of Swedish-speaking persons in Finland (Blomgren, Martikainen, Makela, & Valkonen, 2004), and household-level effects in England (Rice, Carr-Hill, Dixon, & Sutton, 1998), mostly finding significant contextual-level associations with harmful levels of alcohol consumption or alcohol-related mortality. However, it seems that specific multilevel analyses on the effects of contextual-level social capital on alcohol consumption in adult populations are yet to come.

In conclusion, the main finding so far seems to be that some studies indicate an influence of social capital on alcohol and other drug use during childhood and adolescence as well as during adulthood. Both the theoretical social capital literature and empirical evidence suggest that norms, values, and beliefs (such as generalized trust in other people) are founded and formed by psychosocial conditions (intact families, parental monitoring, conditions in school, etc.) during childhood and adolescence, and that they affect alcohol and other drug use both during adolescence and adulthood. Results in adult populations suggest that trust, i.e., the psychological aspect of social capital, which has been suggested to be created during childhood and adolescence and to remain rather stable during the life course (Putnam, 2000), is protective against alcohol consumption above recommended levels, the consumption of illegal alcohol, and cannabis use.

10.2.2. Cigarette Smoking

Unlike alcohol consumption and narcotic drug use, cigarette smoking is not a behavior with potentially acute effects in terms of accidents, crime and suicide, but it still imposes the greatest costs of all health-related behaviors in terms of premature death globally. Cigarette smoking is an individual behavior, but the underlying causal determinants of cigarette smoking are predominantly social. Socially- and economically-deprived people in lower socioeconomic positions are heavily overrepresented among daily smokers. In many western countries the prevalence of smoking has been declining for decades, which has somewhat paradoxically led to increasing socioeconomic differences in smoking (Jarvis & Wardle, 2006).

Most smokers become smokers during adolescence, some during early adulthood and very few later than that. Smoking prevention is thus a matter of two principally different strategies: to stop young people (adolescents and young adults) from initiating tobacco smoking, and to make adults of all ages stop smoking. Both smoking initiation and smoking cessation depend on social and psychosocial factors. Smoking initiation during adolescence has been shown to be a phenomenon with a clear socioeconomic gradient with higher risk of initiation in socially- and economically-deprived socioeconomic groups and neighborhoods. Children who grow up in social environments with many adult smokers are more likely to become smokers themselves due to parental, family, and social behavioral role modelling. In addition, there is evidence that smoking is a measure of smoking trajectory, with prevalence being even more closely related to people's social destination than their original social circumstances during childhood (Glendinning, Shucksmith, & Hendry, 1994). Smoking cessation is a dynamic process which begins with a decision to stop smoking and ends with abstinence maintained over a long period of time. Smoking cessation is thus not a single event, but rather a process influenced by social, psychosocial, psychological, and biological factors (Gulliver, Hughes, Solomon, & Dey, 1995; Hajek, West, & Wilson, 1995; Pomerleau & Pomerleau, 1991). Occasions with negative events and perceived stress are associated with smoking and urges to smoke (Todd, 2004).

The results of two studies in Malmö in southern Sweden suggest that social participation in formal and informal associations but also participation in cultural activities are important determinants of smoking cessation. In contrast, social anchorage in the closer proximity of the individual, i.e., the feeling of "social embeddedness" with friends and neighbors, as well as the two other psychosocial factors of emotional and instrumental support, were not significantly associated with smoking cessation (Lindström & Isacsson, 2002; Lindström, Isacsson, & Elmståhl, 2003). Social participation can be interpreted either as a distinct social science concept measuring the diffusion of innovations (Rogers, 1983) and measuring the norms, rules, values, and control within formal and informal social networks and organisations (Putnam, 1993), or as a protective buffer against psychosocial stress. The lack of significant associations with all of the other three psychosocial variables seems to support the social context/social capital interpretation. Another individual-level study from southern Sweden showed that both low social participation and lack of generalised trust in other people were significantly associated with daily smoking, a result which seems to further support the norms and values interpretation of the relationship between social participation and smoking cessation (Lindström, 2003).

Studies at the contextual, mainly school or area, level often demonstrate that smoking prevalence varies with social contexts and may be affected by social, economic and psychosocial traits of these varying administrative or geographic contexts. A group randomised controlled trial in 26 Dutch schools which provided junior secondary education demonstrated that promotion of certain norms and peer pressure could be a promising strategy in terms of preventing smoking among adolescents (Crone et al., 2003). A cross-sectional multilevel study of 55 secondary schools in the United Kingdom which also analysed school-level and pupil-level data also demonstrated an association between policy strength, policy enforcement, and the prevalence of smoking among pupils, after adjustments for pupil-level characteristics (Moore, Roberts, & Tudor-Smith, 2001). A multilevel discrete-choice models study concerning young adolescents attending 30 secondary schools in Spain demonstrated that a substantial part of individual differences in smoking may be explained by factors at the school level (Pinilla, Gonzalez, Barber, & Santana, 2002). Multilevel studies on adult populations show that tobacco smoking is associated with local neighborhood characteristics such as deprivation in the United Kingdom (Duncan, Jones, & Moon, 1999), level of neighborhood unemployment in Sweden (Öhlander, Vikström, Lindström, & Sundquist, 2006), Gross Domestic Product (GDP) at the area level in France (Chaix, Guilbert, & Chauvin, 2004), and state-level income inequality in the US (Kaplan, Pamuk, Lynch, Cohen, & Balfour, 1996). However, contextual and area differences or variance do not always remain after adjustment for relevant individual factors in multilevel models. Some multilevel studies have reported no remaining district variation in adult smoking in the United Kingdom (Hart, Ecob, & Smith, 1997), no remaining differences in smoking in deprived compared to affluent urban areas in Amsterdam (22 areas) and the Netherlands (Reijneveld, 1998), and no remaining neighbourhood variance in daily smoking in Malmö (74 neighbourhoods) in southern Sweden (Lindström, Moghaddassi, Bolin, Lindgren, & Merlo, 2003) after adjustments for individual compositional factors. In the latter study, the lack of neighborhood variance after adjustment for individual characteristics meant that there was no point in including neighbourhood-level social capital in the analyses. Compared to the rather high number of multilevel studies on the influence of area-level economic conditions on smoking, only a few multilevel studies have investigated the relationship between community-level social capital and smoking. These few studies mostly concern adolescents in school settings (see above). A contextual econometric analysis on 39,369 adults in the US modeling community-level fixed effects, tobacco price (including excise taxes), family income, a tobacco smuggling indicator, non-smoking regulations, education, marital status, sex, age, and race/ethnicity indicated that the proportion of community social capital attributable to religious groups was inversely and strongly related to the number of cigarettes that smokers consumed, but it was not, in contrast, attributable to the overall prevalence of smoking (Brown, Scheffler, Seo, & Reed, 2006).

Although much more research is needed, the results still imply that preventive measures against tobacco smoking should be designed to improve aspects of social capital and social cohesion (Lomas, 1998).

10.2.3. Leisure-Time Physical Activity

Physical activity is an important determinant of health and benefits many aspects of health. It has for a long time been recommended that physical activity should be performed regularly for at least 30 minutes on five or more days of the week. The intensity of this physical activity should be moderate such as brisk walking (US Department of Health and Human Services, 1990). The major part of the health benefits occur when adults with a sedentary lifestyle become moderately active (Haapanen, Miilunpalo, Vuori, Oja, & Pasanen, 1996).

Changing work contexts (i.e., a much lower proportion of the population in developed countries performing physically strenuous work tasks, and an increasing proportion of many adult western populations being unemployed for various reasons) have made leisure-time physical activity the crucial component of physical activity. Leisure-time physical activity is a socially patterned health-related behavior with a socioeconomic gradient according to occupation, education, or income with a higher risk of sedentary physical activity status among groups with lower socioeconomic position such as blue collar workers and those unemployed in many developed countries (see e.g., Blaxter, 1990; Burton, Turrell, & Oldenburg, 2003; Lindström, 2000). One individual-level causal mechanism explaining this socioeconomic gradient may be a corresponding socioeconomic gradient in access to transportation to facilities for physical activity and access to material resources to be able to afford to pay for leisure-time activities and sports (Chinn, White, Harland, Drinkwater, & Raybould, 1999). Another causal mechanism may be that low socioeconomic position increases psychosocial stress, which leads to less physical activity and subsequently adverse health effects (McNeill et al., 2006). Individual-level studies in southern Sweden have consistently shown a strong positive association between social capital measured as participation in different social activities and leisure-time physical activity (Ali & Lindström, 2006; Lindström, Hanson, & Östergren, 2001; Lindström, Moghaddassi, & Merlo, 2003). These findings may be interpreted as either a consequence of the "healthy" norms and values in Swedish society being transmitted through formal and informal organizations and social networks, or as a result of the lower levels of psychosocial stress among participants in social networks resulting in higher levels of physical activity.

Contextual factors are also important for both the motivation and possibility to perform physical activity. Physical environment factors such as beautiful scenery, access to pavements, access to trails, and green surroundings have consistently been shown to be positively associated with physical activity (Humpel,

Owen, & Leslie, 2002; Leyden, 2003; van Lenthe, Brug, & Mackenbach, 2005; Wilson, Kirtland, Ainsworth, & Addy, 2004). A Dutch study has also demonstrated that the higher risk of almost never participating in sports activities in the most disadvantaged neighbourhoods of Eindhoven was partly mediated by larger amounts of required police attention (van Lenthe, Brug & Mackenbach 2005). This finding suggests an indirect effect of crime rates in the neighborhood on physical activity, the crime rates in the previous step in a chain of causality plausibly being an effect of low social capital (Sampson, Raudenbush, & Earls, 1997). Neighborhood-level social capital may also affect physical activity through mechanisms which include the norms and values, trust, and generalised reciprocity, or the social cohesion prevailing in the neighborhood. A multilevel analysis concerning self-reported physical activity among older adults in 56 neighbourhoods in Portland in the US found that social cohesion was associated with higher levels of physical activity, with a significant second-level variance with an intra-class correlation (ICC) of 4% remaining after adjustments for individual-level factors in the model (Fisher, Li, Michael, & Cleveland, 2004). Another American hierarchical study, analyzing urban-rural communities/the geographic areas of Kansas, found significant individual-level associations between trust in one's community, social participation, and physical activity (Greiner et al., 2004). A likely mechanism by which generalized trust in other people could affect physical activity is through feelings of security or lack of security in the community connected with trust. A third multilevel study in the US with a second county level and a third state level of analysis demonstrated significant inverse contextual-level associations between social capital indices, including indicators of trust, different aspects of social participation, mean number of non-profit organizations per 1,000 inhabitants, mean number of civic and social organizations per 1,000 inhabitants, times worked on community project and percentage turnout in presidential elections, and physical inactivity (Kim, Subramanian, Gortmaker, & Kawachi, 2006). In contrast, a multilevel analysis of the adult population in the city of Malmö, southern Sweden, residing in 77 neighbourhoods, showed no remaining variance (intra-class correlation, ICC = 0%) after adjustments for individual factors. In contrast, individual-level social participation was significantly associated with leisure-time physical activity (Lindström, Moghaddassi & Merlo   2003). The different results of the American studies as opposed to the Swedish study may reflect differences between the US and Sweden in neighborhood social capital and other neighborhood characteristics, and their effects on physical activity.

In conclusion, the literature presents strong evidence for contextual effects on physical activity through several different and distinct causal mechanisms. The social capital approach to contextual-level differences in physical activity find strong support in the US but not to the same extent in Europe. The single study in Europe shows absence of significant contextual-level associations. There are significant micro-level (social participation/social network of the individual) associations between social capital and physical activity in Europe, but more studies are required, especially in Europe.

10.2.4. Diet

A large proportion (41%) of total disability-adjusted life-years (DALYs) lost in Europe result from cardiovascular diseases (CVD), type II diabetes, and cancers. These three groups of diseases all have nutrition as a major determinant. An additional 38% of DALYs lost is explained by lowered resistance to infection, oral diseases, and congenital abnormalities for which nutrition plays an important role. Of the seven major risk factors for CVD, six are related to diet and physical activity: 1) high blood pressure is directly related to salt intake and obesity, 2) serum cholesterol is directly linked to high intakes of saturated fats, 3) tobacco (the only CVD risk factor not directly related to diet), 4) overweight and obesity are strongly linked to CVD, type II diabetes, and some cancers, 5) low fruit and vegetable intakes are closely related to CVD and some cancers, 6) low physical activity, and 7) high intakes of alcohol (Robertson, Brunner, & Sheiham, 2006). In most European countries and some other industrialised countries, low-income families tend to spend less on food such as fruit and vegetables which are rich in micro-nutrients but comparatively low in energy, and more on foods rich in sugar and fat which are high in energy but low in micro-nutrients (De Irala-Estevez et al., 2000). The nutritional security of individuals and family members depends on a variety of factors such as macroeconomics, local accessibility and affordability, social and cultural influences on food choice, and individual preferences. Although initiatives to help low-income groups by religious, voluntary, and neighborhood organizations may be useful at the local level in some settings, comprehensive national food and nutrition policies must be developed (Robertson et al., 2006; World Health Organization, 2000).

We have already noted that more research is needed on the relationship between social capital and health behaviors such as tobacco smoking, alcohol consumption, drug abuse, and physical activity. The need for studies on the association between social capital and nutrition seems to be even more urgent. An individual-level study in southern Sweden found a statistically significant association between social participation, measured as participation in 13 different social activities outside of the family, and low vegetable consumption among both men and women (Lindström, Hanson, Wirfält, & Östergren, 2001). Area-level factors mediating the association between socioeconomic deprivation and poor nutrition include lower prevalences of supermarkets, higher prevalences of fast-food restaurants (Morland, Wing, & Diez Roux, 2002), and higher relative costs of healthy compared to unhealthy food in deprived neighbourhoods (Sooman, MacIntyre, & Anderson, 1993). The extent to which social capital may mediate the association between neighbourhood deprivation and diet largely remains to be investigated and empirically tested. Locher et al. (2005) have suggested a number of causal mechanisms by which social capital/lack of social capital may influence dietary behaviors and nutrition. First, socially-cohesive neighbourhoods may be an important source of social capital for many older adults. A major part of the care that community-dwelling older adults receive is provided for by relatives, friends, and neighbors (Rabin & Barry, 1995). However, this mechanism may not hold for all, because neighborhood stability seems to be associated with reduced distress in affluent communities, but not in those that are poor (Ross, Reynolds, & Geis, 2000). Second, various forms of religion, which may be seen as both a source of norms and values and as a source of network/social participation, have been shown to have significant positive effects on health. Religious commitment has been reported to be associated with better dietary behavior and dietary adequacy (McIntosh & Schifflett, 1984). Third, the generalised trust in other people of the individual as well as neighborhood-level trust in other people may affect the inclination to perform leisure-time physical activity (Madriz, 1997; see also Sampson et al., 1997), which may affect the balance between energy intake and energy expenditure. This may, in the next step, lead to increased body mass index. The lack of generalised trust in other people in the neighborhood my also result in the reluctance of older people to even go to the store to buy food.

10.2.5. Sexual Behavior

The study of sexual health has increased dramatically in recent decades following the HIV/AIDS epidemic. The risk of acquiring sexually transmitted diseases (STDs) is related to a number of factors such as the number of partners and sexual orientation, with people with higher numbers of partners and homosexual individuals being at higher risk. The highest rates of partner change are seen among the young and unmarried (Johnson, Wadsworth, & Wellings Field, 1994). The rates of partner change do not vary greatly by social class but tend to be higher in higher social classes (Johnson, Mercer, & Cassell, 2006). Recent evidence from the UK suggests variation by ethnicity, with less risk behaviors among those from the Indian sub-continent and more risk behaviors and poorer sexual outcomes among African and Afro-Caribbean communities (Fenton et al., 2005).

Some cross-sectional studies using social capital indicators such as community organizational life, civic engagement, informal sociability and trust (comprising one social capital index) to analyse the impact of social capital on adolescent sexual risk and protective behaviors in 28 US states (Crosby, Holtgrave, DiClemente, Wingood, & Gayle, 2003) and case rates of gonorrhoea, syphilis, Chlamydia and AIDS in 48 US states (Holtgrave & Crosby, 2003), show the social capital index to be inversely associated with sexual risk behaviors, positively associated with protective sexual behaviours, and inversely associated with gonorrhoea, syphilis, Chlamydia and AIDS case rates. In the southeastern US the black community has 30 times higher rates of sexually transmitted bacterial infections such as syphilis and gonorrhoea compared to other racial groups, and most of these higher rates cannot be explained by traditional measures of socioeconomic differences. Key factors explaining these differences include chronic joblessness, drug and alcohol marketing, social disorganization (or lack of social capital), and male incarceration (Farley, 2006). Another US study concludes that these racial disparities in the US can still only be explained by the underlying social context, which means that prevention targeted at certain individuals and groups according to race but ignoring underlying social and economic conditions are fruitless (Adimora & Schoenbach, 2005). However, as already mentioned, the impact of some aspects of social capital are not always protective against sexually transmitted diseases. High social participation within adolescent and young adult peer groups with norms and values that increase the risk of acquiring a sexually transmitted infection is a substantial public health problem. A qualitative study of heterosexual Asian Indian immigrant men residing in New York City demonstrated that not only lack of knowledge concerning sexually transmitted infection and HIV transmission but also peer solidarity and adherence to negative peer norms (e.g., alcohol use with sex) was significantly associated with elevated risks for HIV (Bhattacharya, 2005).

10.3. Conclusions and Implications for Prevention and Research

Social capital affects health-related behaviors according to the results of a great number of studies. The causal mechanisms by which social capital may influence health-related behaviors plausibly include both norms and values, channels of communication and information, and psychosocial stress mechanisms. However, the academic debate concerning social capital still revolves around basic issues such as its definition and the most adequate level of analysis. Social capital is basically a contextual concept. At the contextual area level previous studies also confirm that the influence of geographic area on health-related behaviors varies according to the behavior and the way it is measured, and that the influence of area deprivation, which is the measure of contextual characteristics mostly studied, can vary by age and household deprivation (Ecob & MacIntyre, 2000). The influence of social capital on health-related behaviors also seems to vary by not only demographic and social factors such as age group and household deprivation, but also by social, cultural, and historical setting, as illustrated by for instance the presence of significant contextual effects of social capital on physical activity in several US studies, but not in the Swedish study (see above).

The social capital debate not only concerns the definition and level of analysis of social capital. It also has policy implications which some perceive as an ideological dimension. The so-called neo-materialists have suggested that the research on social capital and public health only obscures the underlying ideological, political, administrative, and economic determinants of health inequalities and other public health issues. The neo-materialists emphasize politics, governments, welfare programs, and good material conditions as crucially important for public health instead of social capital and civil society. They also claim that the social capital authors within the public health literature are "blaming the victim", which would imply that the source of many health problems in deprived socioeconomic groups and among people in deprived neighbourhoods is the lack of initiative in forming and participating in social networks, or building other forms of social capital (Navarro & Shi, 2001; Pearce & Davey Smith, 2003). The social capital position is also questioned for creating an artificial dichotomy between civil society and the political system (Navarro, 2004), for introducing a dichotomy between material and psychosocial factors, which by the neo-materialists are suggested to be determined by the same underlying socioeconomic conditions, for reintroducing the psychosocial stress theory which has already proven to accumulate scientific knowledge poorly, and for ignoring the importance of politics in general and welfare politics in particular for health (Muntaner, 2004). Although the impact of welfare policies on health-related behaviors may be hard to discern and the expected outcomes not obvious, dependent on factors such as culture (norms and values), religion, and level of economic development, other political decisions and public policies may have direct impacts on health-related behaviors. Since the 1998 Master settlement (MSA) between states and the tobacco industry in the US, states have unprecedented resources for programs to reduce tobacco use. Econometric analyses of the impact of tobacco control expenditures on aggregate tobacco use in all states and in selected states with comprehensive programs for the period from 1981 through 2000 have suggested that increases in funding for state tobacco control programs have reduced cigarette sales (Farrelly, Pechacek, & Chaloupka, 2003). The experience from Denmark during the inter-war and early post-war periods suggest that heavy price restrictions on alcohol severely limit availability and, thus, per capita consumption levels. During the 1920–1960 period when such heavy price restrictions were imposed in Denmark, alcohol consumption was only half to two-thirds compared to the consumption levels in Sweden, despite the fact that the amount of alcohol each Swedish citizen had access to was limited to a very restricted amount. In contrast, during both the pre-1920 and 1975–1995 periods, when there were no price restrictions imposed by the Danish state, alcohol consumption per capita was almost twice as high as in Sweden (Lindström, 2005c). A fruitful strategy to resolve the debate concerning social capital as opposed to material (neo-materialist) factors would be to analyse social capital and material contextual factors in the same empirical analyses, not only concerning access to health care and amenities (Lindström et al., 2006) but also concerning health-related behaviors.

Very little is known about how to build social capital in a society, although we know that high levels of social capital require social stability. The current basis for prevention must consequently be to use the social capital already available. This could be done both from a top-down and a bottom-up perspective. From a top-down perspective, government as well as the private sector may financially support local associations which foster social capital. From a bottom-up perspective, existing associations could encourage voluntarism and other acts entailing social capital (Kawachi & Berkman, 2000). The social capital approach, thus, does not exclude the possibility of state interference.

One strategy may also be the utilization of other channels of communication than traditional channels. In many western countries, membership in labor unions, political parties, and other traditional organisations is declining. In contrast, other new forms of social networks and trust creating social structures are evolving rapidly. One example is the internet, which may foster new identities and extend social networks, and thus create new social capital. The internet is a low-cost way to reach and educate large numbers of people (Putnam, 2000). An e-mail intervention for the promotion of physical activity and nutrition behaviour in the workplace context in Alberta, Canada, has recently demonstrated that e-mail is a promising mode of delivery for promoting physical activity and nutrition in the workplace (Plotnikoff, McCargar, Wilson, & Loucaides, 2005). The knowledge concerning the effects of the internet on health behaviors is very rudimentary and a challenge for future research.

The idea that all social networks and all forms of social participation do not enhance and strengthen trust in other people and/or trust in the institutions of society has already been referred to as "the miniaturization of community" following Fukuyama (1999). Several examples of the effects of this decreased radius of trust in some social contexts have been given in this chapter. A cross-sectional multilevel study on preschool children's behavioral problems in African-American families living in 39 neighbourhoods in Baltimore city with social capital conceptualised as the attachment to community also demonstrated that in wealthy neighbourhoods, low community attachment was associated with higher levels of behavioral and mental problems. In contrast, in poor neighborhoods, low community attachment was associated with lower rates of such problems (Caughy, O'Campo, & Muntaner, 2003). The "miniaturization of community" notion can be applied to yet other behaviors, and it highlights the fact that phenomena such as social networks, participation, attachment, and trust do not always enhance healthy behaviors.

Much more research is needed on how institutional (vertical) trust in institutions, for example, trust in physicians, primary health care, and the health care system in general, affects the effectiveness of information concerning health-related behaviors. A recent study from New Zealand found that the most trusted source of physical activity information was the general practitioner (Schofield, Croteau, & McLean, 2005). Another study showed that one third of the students at Lund University in southern Sweden lacked trust in the HIV health authorities and the mass media, and that an equal proportion felt that national campaigns lacked personal relevance (Svenson & Hanson, 1996). Much more research on institutional trust and its effects on health-related behaviors is needed. More research is also needed concerning the relationship between social capital and behaviors such as compliance with prescribed medications (Johnell, Lindström, Sundquist, Eriksson, & Merlo, 2006).

References

Abrams, D. B., Orleans, C. T., Niaura, R., Goldstein, M., Prochaska, J., & Velicer, W. (1996). Integrating individual and public health perspectives for treatment of tobacco dependence under managed health care: a combined stepped-care and matching model. *Annals of Behavioral Medicine, 18*, 290–304.

Adimora, A. A., & Schoenbach, V. J. (2005). Social context, sexual networks, and racial disparities in rates of sexually transmitted infections. *The Journal of Infectious Diseases, 191*, S115–S122.

Ali, S. M., & Lindström, M. (2006). Psychosocial work conditions and leisure time physical activity: A population-based study. *Scandinavian Journal of Public Health, 34*(2), 209–216.

Bandura, A. (1986). *Social foundations of thought and action.* Englewood Cliffs, NJ: Prentice-Hall.

Berkman, L. F., & Syme, S. L. (1979). Social networks, host resistance and mortality: A nine-year follow-up study of Alameda county residents. *American Journal of Epidemiology, 109*, 186–204.

Bhattacharya, G. (2005). Social capital and HIV risks among acculturating Asian Indian men in New York City. *AIDS Education and Prevention, 17*(6), 555–567.

Bjarnason, T., Andersson, B., Choquet, M., Elekes, Z., Morgan, M., & Rapinett, G. (2003). Alcohol culture, family structure and adolescent alcohol use: multilevel modeling of frequency of heavy drinking among 15–16 year old students in 11 European countries. *Journal of Studies on Alcohol, 64*(2), 200–208.

Blaxter, M. (1990). *Health and lifestyles.* London, New York: Tavistock and Routledge.

Blomgren, J., Martikainen, P., Makela, P., & Valkonen, T. (2004). The effects of regional characteristics on alcohol-related mortality– a register-based multilevel analysis of 1.1 million men. *Social Science and Medicine, 58*(12), 2523–2535.

British Medical Association. (1995). *Alcohol: Guidelines on sensible drinking.* London: National Institute on Alcohol Abuse and Alcoholism. Alcohol alert No. 16 PH 315.

Brown, T. T., Scheffler, R. M., Seo, S., & Reed, M. (2006). The empirical relationship between community social capital and the demand for cigarettes. *Health Economics, 15* (11), 159–72.

Burton, N. W., Turrell, G., Oldenburg. (2003). Participation in recreational: why do socioeconomic groups differ? *Health Education and Behavior, 30*(2), 225–244.

Cassel, J. (1976). The contribution of the social environment to host resistance: The Fourth Wade Hampton Frost Lecture. *American Journal of Epidemiology, 104*(2), 107–123.

Caughy, M. O., O'Campo, P. J., & Muntaner, C. (2003). When being alone might be better: neighbourhood poverty social capital and child mental health. *Social Science and Medicine, 57*, 227–237.

Chaix, B., Guilbert, P., & Chauvin, P. (2004). A multilevel analysis of tobacco use and tobacco consumption levels in France: are there any combination risk groups? *European Journal of Public Health, 14*(2), 186–190.

Chilcoat, H. D., & Anthony, J. C. (1996). Impact of parent monitoring on initiation of drug use through late adulthood. *Journal of the American Academy of Child and Adolescent Psychiatry, 35*(1), 91–100.

Chinn, D. J., White, M., Harland, J., Drinkwater, C., & Raybould, S. (1999). Barriers to physical activity and socioeconomic position: Implications for health promotion. *Journal of Epidemiology and Community Health, 53*, 191–192.

Coleman, J. (1988). Social capital in the creation of human capital. *American Journal of Sociology, 94*, 95–120.

Coleman, J. (1990). *Foundations of social theory.* Princeton: Harvard University Press.

Coleman, J., & Hoffer, T. (1987). *Public and private high schools: The impact of communities.* New York: Basic Books.

Crone, M. R., Reijneveld, S. A., Wilhelmsen, M. C., van Leerdam, F. J., Spruijt, R.D., & Sing, R. A. (2003). Prevention of smoking in adolescents with lower education: A school based intervention study. *Journal of Epidemiology and Community Health, 57*(9), 675–680.

Crosby, R. A., Holtgrave, D. R., DiClemente, R. J., Wingood, G. M., & Gayle, J. A. (2003). Social capital as a predictor of adolescent's sexual risk behaviour: A state level exploratory. *AIDS Behavior, 7*, 245–252.

De Irala-Estevez, J., Groth, M., Johansson, L., Oltersdorf, U., Prattala, R., & Martinez-Gonzalez, M. A. (2000). A systematic review of socio-economic differences in food habits in Europe: Consumption of fruit and vegetables. *European Journal of Clinical Nutrition, 54*, 706–714.

Droomers, M., Schrijvers, C. T., van de Mheen, H., & Machenbach, J. P. (1998). Educational differences in leisure-time physical activity: A descriptive and explanatory study. *Social Medicine and Science, 47*, 1665–1676.

Duncan, S. C., Duncan, T. E., & Strycker, L. A. (2002). A multilevel analysis of neighborhood context and youth alcohol and drug problems. *Prevention Science, 3*(2), 125–133.

Duncan, C., Jones, K., & Moon, G. (1999). Smoking and deprivation: Are there neighbourhood effects? *Social Science and Medicine, 48*(4), 497–505.

Dupre, D., Miller, N., Gold, M., & Rospenda, K. (1995). Initiation and progression of alcohol, marijuana and cocaine use among adolescent abusers. *American Journal of Addiction, 4*, 43–48.

Ecob, R., & MacIntyre, S. (2000). Small area variations in health related behaviours: Do these depend on the behaviour itself, its measurement, or on personal characteristics? *Social Science and Medicine, 6*(4), 261–274.

Elgar, F. J., Roberts, C., Parry-Langdon, N., & Boyce, W. (2005). Income inequality and alcohol use: a multilevel analysis of drinking and drunkenness in 34 countries. *Journal of Epidemiology and Community Health, 15*(3), 245–250.

Emmons, K. M. (2000). Health behaviors in a social context. In L. F. Berkman & I. Kawachi (Eds.), *Social epidemiology* (pp. 242–266). Oxford: Oxford University Press.

Farley, T. A. (2006). Sexually transmitted dieases in the southeastern United States: Location, race, and social context. *Sexually Transmitted Diseases, 33*(7 Suppl), S58–64.

Farrelly, M. C., Pechacek, T. F., & Chaloupka, F. J. (2003). The impact of tobacco control program expenditures on aggregate cigarette sales 1981–2000. *Journal of Health Economics, 22*(5), 843–859.

Fenton, K. A., Mercer, C. H., McManus, S., Erens, B., Macdowall, W., & Wellings, K. et al. (2005). Sexual behaviour in Britain: ethnic variations in high-risk sexual behaviour and STI acquisition risk. *Lancet, 365*, 1246–1255.

Fisher, K. J., Li, F., Michael, Y., & Cleveland, M. (2004). Neighborhood influences on physical activity among older adults: A multilevel analysis. *Journal of Aging and Physical Activity, 11*, 45–63.

Fukuda, Y., Nakamura, K., & Takamo, T. (2005). Accumulation of health risk behaviours is associated with lower socioeconomic status and women's urban residence: A multilevel analysis in Japan. *BMC Public Health, 5*(1), 53.

Fukuyama, F. (1995). *Trust. The social virtues and the creation of prosperity.* New York, London, Toronto, Sydney, Tokyo, Singapore: The Free Press.

Fukuyama, F. (1999). *The great disruption. Human nature and the reconstitution of social order.* London: Profile Books.

Gilvarry, E. (2000). Substance abuse in young people. *Journal of Child Psychology and Psychiatry, 41*, 55–80.

Glasgow, R. E., Terborg, J. R., Hollis, J. F., Severson, H. H., & Boles, S. M. (1995). Take heart: Results from the initial phase of a worksite wellness program. *American Journal of Public Health, 85*, 209–216.

Glendinning, A., Shucksmith, J., & Hendry, L. (1994). Social class and adolescent smoking behaviour. *Social Science and Medicine, 38*, 1449–1460.

Granovetter, M. (1973). The strength of weak of ties. *American Journal of Sociology, 78*, 1360–1380.

Greiner, K. A., Chaoyang, L., Kawachi, I., Hunt, D. C., & Ahluwalia, J. S. (2004). The relationships of social participation and community ratings to health behaviors in areas with high and low population density. *Social Science and Medicine, 59*, 2303–2312.

Gulliver, S. B., Hughes, J. R., Solomon, L. J., & Dey, A. N. (1995). An investigation of self-efficacy, partner supportand daily stresses as predictors of relapse to smoking in self-quitters. *Addiction, 90*, 767–772.

Haapanen, N., Miilunpalo, S., Vuori, I., Oja, P., & Pasanen, M. (1996). Characteristics of leisure time physical activity associated with decreased risk of premature all-cause and cardiovascular disease mortality in middle-aged men. *American Journal of Epidemiology, 143*, 870–880.

Hajek, P., West, R., & Wilson, J. (1995). Regular smokers, lifetime very light smokers and reduced smokers. Comparison of psychosocial and smoking characteristics in women. *Health Psychology, 14*, 195–201.

Hart, C., Ecob, R., & Smith, G. D. (1997). People, places and coronary heart disease risk factors: a multilevel analysis of the Scottish Heart Health Study Archive. *Social Science and Medicine, 45*(6), 893–902.

Holtgrave, D. R., & Crosby, R. A. (2003). Social capital, poverty, and income inequality as predictors of gonorrea, syphilis, Chlamydia and AIDS in the United States. *Sexually Transmitted Infections, 79*, 62–64.

House, J. S., Landis, K. R., & Umberson, D. (1988). Social relationships and health. *Science, 214*, 540–545.

Humpel, N., Owen, N., & Leslie, E. (2002). Environmental factors associated with adults' participation in physical: A review. *American Journal of Preventive Medicine, 22*(3), 188–199.

Institute of Medicine. (2003). *The future of the public's health in the 21st century*. Washington, DC: National Academies of Press.

Jarvis, M. J., & Wardle, J. (2006). Social patterning of individual health: the case of cigarette smoking. In M. Marmot & R. G. Wilkinson (Eds.), *Social determinants of health* (2nd edition, pp. 224–237). Oxford: Oxford University Press.

Johnell, K., Lindström, M., Sundquist, J., Eriksson, C., & Merlo, J. (2006). Individual characteristics, area social participation, and primary non-concordance with medication: A multilevel analysis. *BioMedCentral- Public Health, 6*, 52.

Johnson, A. M., Wadsworth, J., & Wellings Field, J. (1994). *Sexual attitudes and lifestyles*. Oxford: Bradford Academic Press.

Johnson, A. M., Mercer, C. H., & Cassell, J. A. (2006). Social determinants, sexual behaviour, and sexual health. In M. Marmot & R. G. Wilkinson (Eds.), *Social determinants of health* (2nd edition, pp. 318–340). Oxford: Oxford University Press.

Kairouz, S., Gliksman, L., Demers, A., & Adlaf, E. M. (2002). For all these reasons, I do . . .drink: a multilevel analysis of contextual reasons for drinking among Canadian undergraduates. *Journal of Studies on Alcohol, 63*(5), 600–608.

Kaplan, G. A., Pamuk, E. R., Lynch, J. W., Cohen, R. D., & Balfour, J. L. (1996). Inequality in income and mortality in the United States: Analysis of mortality and potential pathways. *British Medical Journal, 312*(7037): 999–1003.

Kawachi, I., & Berkman, L. F. (2000). Social cohesion, social capital, and health. In L. F. Berkman & I Kawachi (Eds.), *Social epidemiology* (pp. 174–190). Oxford: Oxford University Press.

Kawachi, I., Kennedy, B. P., & Glass, R. (1999). Social capital and self-rated health: a contextual analysis. *American Journal of Public Health, 89*(8), 1187–1193.

Kawachi, I., Kim, D., Coutts, A., & Subramanian, S. V. (2004). Commentary: Reconciling the three accounts of social capital. *International Journal of Epidemiology, 33*(4), 682–690.

Kim, D., Subramanian, S. V., Gortmaker, S. L., & Kawachi, I. (2006). US-state- and county-level social capital in relation to obesity and physical inactivity: A multilevel, multivariable analysis. *Social Science and Medicine, 63*, 1045–1059.

Leyden, K. M. (2003). Social capital and the built environment: The importance of walkable neighborhoods. *Social Science and Medicine, 93*(9), 1546–1551.

Lindström, M. (2000). *Social participation, social capital, and socioeconomic differences in health related behaviors.* Malmö: Lund University. (Doctoral dissertation).

Lindström, M., Hanson, B. S., & Östergren, P. O. (2001). Socioeconomic differences in leisure-time physical activity: the role of social participation and social capital in shaping health related behaviour. *Social Science and Medicine, 52*(3), 441–451.

Lindström, M., Hanson, B. S., Wirfält, E., & Östergren, P. O. (2001). Socioeconomic differences in the consumption of vegetables, fruit and fruit juices: The influence of psychosocial factors. *European Journal of Public Health, 11*, 51–59.

Lindström, M., Isacsson, S. O. (2002). Smoking cessation among daily smokers, aged 45–69 years: A longitudinal study in Malmö, Sweden. *Addiction, 97*, 205–215.

Lindström, M. (2003). Social capital and the miniaturization of community among daily and intermittent smokers: a population-based study. *Preventive Medicine, 36*, 177–184.

Lindström, M., Isacsson, S. O., & Elmståhl, S. (2003). Impact of different aspects of social participation and social capital on smoking cessation among daily smokers: A longitudinal study. *Tobacco Control, 12*(3), 274–281.

Lindström, M., Moghaddassi, M., Bolin, K., Lindgren, B., & Merlo, J. (2003). Social participation, social capital and daily tobacco smoking: A population-based multilevel analysis in Malmö, Sweden. *Scandinavian Journal of Public Health, 31*(6), 444–450.

Lindström, M., Moghaddassi, M., & Merlo, J. (2003). Social capital and leisure-time physical activity: A population-based multilevel analysis of individual- and neighbourhood level data in Malmö, Sweden. *Journal of Epidemiology and Community Health, 57*, 23–28.

Lindström, M. (2004). Social capital, the miniaturization of community and cannabis smoking among young adults: A population-based study. *European Journal of Public Health, 14*(2), 204–208.

Lindström, M. (2005a). Social capital, the miniaturization of community and high alcohol consumption: A population-based study. *Alcohol and Alcoholism, 40*(6), 556–562.

Lindström, M. (2005b). Social capital, the miniaturization of community and and consumption of home made and smuggled liquor during the past year: A population-based study. *European Journal of Public Health, 15*(6), 593–600.

Lindström, M. (2005c). Price restrictions and other restrictions on alcohol availability in Denmark and Sweden: A historical perspective with implications for the current debate. *Scandinavian Journal of Public Health, 33*, 156–158.

Lindström, M., Axén, E., Lindström, C., Beckman, A., Moghaddassi, M., & Merlo, J. (2006). Social capital and neo-materialist contextual determinants of lack of access to a regular doctor: A multilevel analysis in southern Sweden. *Health Policy, 79*, 153–164

Locher, J. L., Ritchie, C. S., Roth, D. L., Sawyer Baker, P., Bodner, E. V., Allman, R. M. (2005). Social isolation, support and capital and nutritional risk in an older sample: Ethnic and gender differences. *Social Science and Medicine, 60*, 747–761.

Lochner, K., Kawachi, I., & Kennedy, B. P. (1999). Social capital: a guide to its measurement. *Health and Place, 5*(4), 259–270.

Lomas, J. (1998). Social capital and health: Implications for health policy and epidemiology. *Social Science and Medicine, 47*, 1181–1188.

Lundborg, P. (2005). Social capital and substance use among Swedish adolescents- an explorative study. *Social Science and Medicine*, 1151–1158.

Macinko, J., & Starfield, B. (2001). The utility of social capital in research on health determinants. *The Milbank Quarterly, 79*(3), 387–427.

MacIntyre, S., MacIver, S., & Sooman, A. (1993). Area, social class and health: Should we be focusing on places or people. *Journal of Social Policy, 22*(2), 213–234.

Maes, L., & Lievens, J. (2003). Can the school make a difference? A multilevel analysis of adolescent risk and health behaviour. *Social Science and Medicine, 56*(3), 517–529.

Madriz, E. (1997). *Nothing bad happens to good girls: fear of crime in women's lives.* Berkeley, CA: University of California Press.

McIntosh, W. A., & Schifflett, P. A. (1984). Influence of social support systems on dietary intake of the elderly. *Journal of Nutrition for the Elderly, 4*(1), 5–18.

McMillan, D. W., & Chavis, D. M. (1986). Sense of community: a definition and theory. *Journal of Community Psychology, 14*, 6–23.

McNeill, L. H., Kreuter, M. W., & Subramanian, S. V. (2006). Social environment and physical activity: a review of concepts and evidence. *Social Science and Medicine, 63*(4), 1011–1022.

McLeroy, K. R., Bibeau, D., Steckler, A., & Glantz, K. (1988). An ecological perspective on health promotion programs. *Health Education Quarterly, 15*(4), 351–377.

Moore, L., Roberts, C., & Tudor-Smith, C. (2001). School smoking policies and smoking prevalence among adolescents: Multilevel analysis of cross-sectional data from Wales. *Tobacco Control, 10*(2), 117–123.

Morland, K., Wing, S., & Diez Roux, A. (2002). The contextual effect of the local food environment on resident's diets: The Atheroschlerosis risk in communities study. *American Journal of Public Health, 92*, 1761–1767.

Muntaner, C. (2004). Commentary: Social capital, social class, and the slow progress of psychosocial epidemiology. *International Journal of Epidemiology, 33*, 674–680.

Murray, C. J., & Lopez, A. (1996). Quantifying the burden of disease and injury to ten major risk factors. In C. J. Murray & A. Lopez (Eds.), *The global burden of disease: A comprehensive assessment of mortality and disability from diseases, injuries and risk factors in 1990 and projected to 2020* (pp. 295–327). Cambridge, MA: Harvard School of Public Health on behalf of the WHO.

Navarro, V. (2004). Commentary: Is social capital the solution or the problem? *International Journal of Epidemiology, 33*, 672–674.

Navarro, v., & Shi, L. (2001). The political context of social capital inequalities and health. *International Journal of Health services, 31*(1), 1–21.

Öhlander, E., Vikström, M., Lindström, M., & Sundquist, K. (2006). Neighbourhood non-employment and daily smoking: a population-based study of women and men in Sweden. *European Journal of Public Health, 16*(1), 78–84.

Pearce, N., & Davey Smith, G. (2003). Is social capital the key to inequalities in health? *American Journal of Public Health*, 93(1), 122–129.

Pinilla, J., Gonzalez, B., Barber, P., & Santana, Y. (2002). Smoking in young adiescents: an approach with multilevel discrete choice models. *Journal of Epidemiology and Community Health*, 56(3), 227–232.

Plotnikoff, R. C., McCargar, L. J., Wilson, P. M., & Loucaides, C. A. (2005). Efficacy of an E-mail intervention for the promotion of physical activity and nutrition behaviour in the workplace context. *American Journal of Health Promotion*, 19(6), 422–429.

Pollack, C. E., Cubbin, C., Ahn, D., & Winkleby, M. (2005). Neighbourhood deprivation and alcohol consumption: Does the availability of alcohol play a role? *International Journal of Epidemiology*, 34(4), 772–780.

Pomerleau, O. F., & Pomerleau, C. S. (1991). Research on stress and smoking, progress and problems. *British Journal of Addiction*, 86, 599–604.

Putnam, R. D. (1993). *Making democracy work. Civic traditions in modern Italy*. Princeton: Princeton University Press.

Putnam, R. D. (2000). *Bowling alone. The collapse and revival of American community*. New York, London: Simon and Schuster.

Rabin, D. L., & Barry, O. P. (1995). Community options for elderly patients. In W. Reichel (Ed.), *Care of the elderly. Clinical aspects of aging*. (4th edition, pp. 521–528). Baltimore, MD: Williams and Wilkins.

Rehm, J., Room, R., & Moneiro, M. (2004). Alcohol use. In M. Ezzati, A. D. Lopez, A. Rodgers, & C. Murray (Eds.), *Comparative quantification of health risks: Global and regional burden of disease attributable to selected major risk factors*, Vol. 1 (pp. 959–1108). Geneva: World Health Organization.

Reijneveld, S. A. (1998). The impact of individual and area characteristics on urban socioeconomic differences in health and smoking. *International Journal of Epidemiology*, 27(1), 33–40.

Resnicow, K., Futterman, R., Weston, R. E., Royce, J., Parms, C., Freeman, H. P., & Orlandi, M. A. (1996). Smoking prevalence in Harlem, NY. *American Journal of Health Promotion*, 10, 343–346.

Rice, N., Carr-Hill, R., Dixon, P., & Sutton, M. (1998). The influence of households on drinking behavior: A multilevel analysis. *Social Science and Medicine*, 46(8), 971–979.

Robertson, A., Brunner, E., & Sheiham, A. (2006). Food is a political issue. In M. Marmot & R. G. Wilkinson (Eds.), *Social determinants of health* (2nd edition, pp. 172–195). Oxford: Oxford University Press.

Rogers, E. (1983). *Diffusion of innovations*. New York: The Free Press.

Rose, G. (1992). *The strategy of preventive medicine*. New York: Oxford university Press.

Ross, C. E., Reynolds, J. R., & Geis, K. J. (2000). The contingent meaning of neighbourhood stability for residents' psychological well-being. *American Sociological Review*, 65, 581–597.

Schofield, G., Croteau, K., & McLean, G. (2005). Trust levels of physical activity information sources: a population study. *Health Promotion Journal of Australia*, 16(3), 221–224.

Smart, R. G., & Ogborne, A. C. (2000). Drug use and drinking among students in 36 countries. *Addictive Behavior*, 25, 455–460.

Sooman, A., MacIntyre, S., & Anderson, A. (1993). Scotland's health- a more difficult challenge for some? The price and availability of healthy foods in socially contrasting localities in the west of Scotland. *Health Bulletin (Edinburgh)*, 51, 276–284.

Sorensen, G., Emmons, K., Hunt, M. K., & Johnston, D. (1998). Implications of the results of community intervention trials. *Annual Review of Public Health, 19,* 379–416.

Subramanian, S. V., Nandy, S., Irving, M., Gordon, D., & Smith, G. (2005). Role of socioeconomic markers and state prohibition policy in predicting alcohol consumption among men and women in India: A multilevel statistical analysis. *Bulletin of the World Health Organization, 83*(11), 803.

Sampson, R. J., Raudenbush, S. W., & Earls, F. (1997). Neighborhoods and violent crime: a multilevel study of collective efficacy. *Science, 277*(5328), 918–924.

Svenson, G. R., & Hanson, B. S. (1996). Are peer and social influences important components to include in HIV-STD prevention models? Results of a survey on young people at Lund University, Sweden. *European Journal of Public Health, 6,* 203–211.

Szreter, S., & Woolcock, M. (2004). Health by association? Social capital, social theory, and the political economy of Public Health. *International Journal of Epidemiology, 33,* 650–667.

The World Health Report 2002. (2002). Geneva: World Health Organization.

Todd, M. (2004). Daily processes in stress and smoking: Effects of negative events, nicotine dependence, and gender. *Psychology of Addicictive Behaviors, 18*(1), 31–39.

US Department of Health and Human services. (1990). *Healthy people 2000: National health promotion and disease prevention objectives.* Washington, DC: US Government Printing Office.

van Lenthe, F. J., Brug, J., & Mackenbach, J. P. (2005). Neighbourhood inequalities in physical activity: the role of neighbourhood attractiveness, proximity to local facilities and safety in the Netherlands. *Social Science and Medicine, 60*(4), 763–775.

Weitzman, E. R., & Chen, Y. Y. (2005). Risk modifying effect of social capital on measures of heavy alcohol consumption, alcohol abuse, harms, and secondhand effects: national survey findings. *Journal of Epidemiology and Community Health, 59*(4), 303–309.

Weitzman, E. R., & Kawachi, I. (2000). Giving means receiving: the protective effect of social capital on binge drinking on college campuses. *American Journal of Public Health, 90,* 1936–1939.

Williams, M. V., Parker, R. M., Baker, D. W., Parikh, N. S., Pitkin, K., Coates, W. C., & Nurss, J. R. (1995). Inadequate functional health literacy among patients at two public hospitals. *Journal of the American Medical Association (JAMA), 274,* 1677–1682.

Wilson, D. K., Kirtland, K. A., Ainsworth, B. E., & Addy, C. L. (2004). Socioeconomic status and perceptions of access and safety for physical activity. *Annals of Behavioral Medicine, 28,* 20–28.

Woolcock, M. (1998). Social capital and economic development: toward a theoretical synthesis and policy framework. *Theory and Society, 27,* 151–208.

Woolcock, M. (2001). The place of social capital in understanding social and economic outcomes. *Canadian Journal of Policy Research, 15*(2), 225–249.

World Health Organization. (2000). *The first action plan for food and nutrition policy, WHO European Region 2000–2005.* (http://www.euro.who.int/nutrition/FoodandNutActPlan/20010906_2). Copenhagen, WHO.

11
Social Capital and Aging-Related Outcomes*

KATHLEEN A. CAGNEY AND MING WEN

Like other demographic characteristics, age introduces complexity into theoretical and empirical investigations of the relationship between social capital and health. Unlike its demographic counterparts, however, age is not fixed. Age and cohort differences in the reliance on social capital and perceptions of it indicate that models of the social capital-health relationship must be attentive to age. Arguably, no age group relies as much as older people do on the capacity of social connections or community resources to maintain health and community residence (Cannuscio, Block, & Kawachi, 2003). The social capital aspects of the lives of older adults, however, have not enjoyed the same attention as earlier stages of the life course (Sampson, Morenoff, & Earls, 1999; Settersten, 2005). In the social capital work of Coleman (1990), Lin (2001) and others (e.g., Portes, 1998), there is no explicit treatment of age or aging. Similarly, the most recent version of the *Handbook of Aging and the Social Sciences* (Binstock, George, Cutler, Hendricks, & Schulz, 2006) includes only a limited discussion of the term social capital. It appears that scholars of social capital are not currently considering age, and research on aging is not fully exploring social capital.

In this chapter, we review the research on social capital and the health of older adults with attention to the link between the gerontological health and sociological literatures. We focus on the community-level aspects of social capital, thus drawing on research related to neighborhood social context. We choose this approach because, as Wellman and Frank (2001) point out, the effects of individual, tie and network characteristics are interdependent and exist at multiple levels. The individual and tie aspects of older adult well-being are fairly well-developed (as in the social support, caregiving and long-term care literatures, e.g., Cornman, Goldman, Glei, Weinstein, & Chang, 2003) but the context in which they rest is less so. Thus, we draw out and discuss findings related to community-level social capital. For illustrative purposes we provide detailed accounts of recent findings from the Care after the Onset of Serious Illness project (COSI), the Chicago Health, Aging, and Social Relations Study (CHASR), the Neighborhood Organization, Aging and Health project (NOAH), and the Project on Human Development in Chicago Neighborhoods (PHDCN). We then conclude with an agenda for further research in community-level social capital for older adults. Our overarching goal is to address two key questions:

1. *What advancements in social capital theory and research are critical to the understanding of older adult well-being?*
2. *How could progress along both theoretical and methodological pathways help to enhance our knowledge of individual- and community-level social capital and inform policy related to the community context of aging?*

Elsewhere in this book scholars have defined social capital, described its features, and shared findings that delineate social capital's role in health and well-being. The reader is directed to these chapters for a fuller treatment of the origins of social capital and its implications for health more generally. For the purposes of our discussion we adhere most closely to the tenets outlined by Coleman (1990) and Bourdieu (1986) with attention to properties that emerge at the community level (Browning, 2002; Sampson, 2003; Sampson, Raudenbush, & Earls, 1997). In this way we are mindful of foundational work in social capital theory while also highlighting contemporary elaborations of it.

11.1. Forms of Social Capital in Aging-Related Research

11.1.1. Individual-Level Social Capital

We view individual social capital as the form of social capital that exists in the relational dyad. Gerontological studies of individual-level social capital are many, even though they may not be formally described as such (Barrett & Lynch, 1999; Feld, Dunkle, Schroepfer, & Shen, 2006; Krause, 1991; Kroenke, Kubzansky, Schernhammer, Holmes, & Kawachi, 2006). Research in gerontology has emphasized the critical importance of network ties and social support in the lives of older adults for decades (Coward & Dwyer, 1990; Lawton, 1970). The informal caregiving literature, for example, has focused on the type, quality, and setting of long-term care arrangements, often exploring the impact of kin networks and the implications of gender, age, and race for caregiving by adult children (Burton 1996; Cornman et al., 2003; Hibbard, Neufeld, & Harrison, 1996; Langa et al., 2001). The larger context in which such relationships operate is rarely discussed although recent work has examined the association between the propensity to provide intimate care and that of civic engagement (Burr, Choi, Mutchler, & Caro, 2005), theorizing that the capacity for care provision and community contribution may stem from the same underlying impulses.

Individual-level social capital is critical for the aged, who often rely on others to realize benefits to health (e.g., regular medical attention). In the general case, social relationships appear to be good for health whether or not instrumental assistance is an aspect (House, Landis, & Umberson, 1988; Strawbridge, Shema, Cohen, & Kaplan, 2001). Studies of the relationship between social connections and mortality suggest that these bonds are protective across a wide range of settings although the type and nature of the network might have some bearing on its effect (Litwin & Shiovitz-Ezra, 2006; Mendes de Leon et al., 1999). Litwin and Shiovitz-Ezra (2006), for instance, found that the association between network type and mortality was important primarily to persons 70 and older; those in diverse, friend-focused, and, to a lesser extent, community-clan networks experienced lower risk of all-cause mortality.

Individual-level social capital extends beyond conceptions of social support. Reciprocity, often assessed in family-based exchanges (Grundy, 2005; McGarry & Schoeni, 1997) is a critical feature of studies on individual-level social capital. Lack of reciprocity and civic mistrust are associated with poorer health (Pollack & von dem Knesebeck, 2004) and higher levels of individual- and community-level social capital with increased quality of life (Nilsson, Rana, & Kabir, 2006). Locher et al. (2005) found that indicators of social capital such as lack of regular church attendance, fear of being attacked, and perceived discrimination all were associated with nutritional risk for older African American men only (as compared to African American women and white men and women). Vehicles meant to increase the propensity for such exchanges, such as congregate housing, also have been explored (Moore, Shiell, Haines, Riley, & Collier, 2005).

Although social capital realized through social ties is typically theorized as a benefit to health several investigators have identified detrimental effects (Baum, 1999; Browning, Feinberg, & Dietz, 2004; Lynch, Due, Muntaner, & Smith, 2000; Portes, 1998). The downside of social capital, including its coercive aspects, may manifest itself in the inhibition of individual expression or the sanction of a group; the social capital of a group (e.g., criminal gangs) may provide resources for its members but meanwhile may be disruptive of the larger community's social cohesion (Crane, 1991; Kawachi & Berkman, 2000, 2001; Portes & Landolt, 1996; Portes, 1998; Woolcock, 1998). Another way in which social capital may have harmful effects is illustrated by the contagion model detailed and tested in Crane's highly cited work on neighborhood effects on dropout rates and teenage childbearing (Crane, 1991). Components of social capital also may be at odds with one another. Keating, Swindle, and Foster (2005) provide one example where small and intense care networks stave off nursing home entry, but, at the same time, lack the resources to create linkages to health-enhancing services outside the immediate care network.

The endogenous nature of social network formation and health status create challenges for developing causal claims. So too does disambiguating individual- from community-level effects. As Veenstra (2000) and Locher et al. (2005) note, social capital may indeed be a quality of social structure but the propensity to act rests at the individual level. Thus it may be difficult to tease out effects from both. For the purposes of our review we will attempt to distinguish levels of social capital. We now turn to that which rests in the community.

11.1.2. Community-Level Social Capital

Moore, Haines, Hawe, and Shiell (2006), examining the genesis of social capital investigations in public health, point to the dominance of what they describe as a "communitarian" approach to the measurement of social capital; one that relies primarily on measures of trust and civic participation at the cost of information on networks. They attribute much of this communitarian tack to the bonding and bridging principles of Putman (appealing to public health's advocacy bent). Not included in this description is the work of Sampson and colleagues (Sampson et al., 1997) who developed the concept of collective efficacy or the work of Wilson (1987) or Shaw and McKay (1969), which provided the basis for social disorganization theory. We draw from this literature to frame community-level social capital and its implications for elder health.

To distinguish collective efficacy from social capital we note that social capital is about relationships and collective efficacy is about converting those relationships into action that is beneficial to everyone. Communities where people not only feel attached to their neighborhood and trust one another, but are willing to intervene on each other's behalf, even when they do not know one another, can be described as having high collective efficacy. Sampson, et al.'s articulation of the collective efficacy concept emphasizes neighborhood social capital in the form of mutual trust and solidarity (social cohesion), and expectations for action (informal social control) in explaining the impact of neighborhood factors on residents' well-being. Focusing on crime rates in Chicago communities, for instance, Sampson, et al. found that collective efficacy had a significant beneficial impact on perceptions of crime, self-reported victimization, and homicide rates. Moreover, collective efficacy mediated a substantial proportion of the effects of poverty, residential instability, and ethnic heterogeneity on crime.

As applied to health, collective efficacy theory suggests that neighborhoods vary in the density and prevalence of community social networks and their associated levels of social cohesion and informal social control. The latter taps the community's capacity to mobilize existing social resources (network ties and community attachments) toward beneficial ends — including a healthy environment. Literature stemming from this and related theory indicates that neighborhood social and physical resources affect the lives of older adults (Cagney, Browning, & Wen, 2005; Glass & Balfour, 2003; Kawachi & Berkman, 2003; Krause, 1998; Robert & Lee, 2002; Wen, Cagney, & Christakis, 2005; Wen, Hawkley, & Cacioppo, 2006).

Older adults often age in place; approximately one-third have lived in their communities for 30 years or longer (Bryan & Morrison, 2004). As they age, they may become much more dependent on the context that their community provides. Neighborhood context may in large part make it feasible to take a walk, go shopping, or remain engaged in community-based activities such as church (Robert & Li, 2001; Ross & Jang, 2000). The circumference of social space may constrict as one ages, making the immediate environment all the more important. Balfour and Kaplan (2002) for instantly found that older adults who lived in neighborhoods with poorer quality environments (e.g., high crime, heavy traffic, excessive noise) experienced a greater risk of functional deterioration. In general, the antecedent literature examining the link between individual well-being and neighborhood criminal activity indicates that higher crime rates are associated with community withdrawal, stress, and fear of leaving older adult's one's home (Ferraro, 1995). This exposure may exacerbate an already compromised health state, and there may be few mechanisms in place to buffer these negative effects (Thompson & Krause, 1998).

Older adults may be more dependent upon the level of community social capital but they also may contribute more to it. Putnam's research (2000) indicates that a community with a disproportionate number of elderly residents is likely to have a more active neighborhood watch, better social services, and, in general, a community more engaged in civic affairs. Smith's analysis of the General Social Survey indicates that older adults, due to both age and cohort, are more trusting (Smith, 1997). Other research indicates that healthy older persons are well-integrated into community functions and that levels of volunteerism persist over the life course (Hendricks & Cutler, 2001; Liu & Besser, 2003). We have little evidence, however, about levels of participation for those whose health is failing or for those who are now required to care for them. We have some indication that people withdraw from community life when they are not feeling well (Wethington & Kavey, 2000). Health events likely to affect older persons (e.g., heart attacks, stokes, hip fractures), or a general decline in health status, may significantly reduce mobility or may require a prolonged hospital or nursing home stay. This withdrawal could mean that fewer persons are on the street, actively engaged in overseeing the community or contributing to community-level social capital.

11.2. Community Social Capital and the Health of Older Adults: Examples from the Literature

The relationship between community-level social capital and aging-related health outcomes is contingent upon the outcome of interest. We review select findings that shed light on the role of community-level social capital in morbidity and mortality. In keeping with the foundations of urban sociological study, we profile four projects that examine neighborhood structural context and social capital indicators and the extent to which they affect aging-related outcomes; Chicago is the laboratory in all cases. We note that this body of research is based on a social disorganization/ecological approach that views social capital as an emergent property. Figure 11.1 illustrates the connections between neighborhood structural resources, social processes, and health. It relies on collective efficacy theory, which, as discussed earlier, emphasizes neighborhood social resources in the form of mutual trust and solidarity (*social cohesion*), and expectations for action (*informal social control*) in explaining the impact of neighborhood structural factors on resident's well-being [see Sampson et al. (1997) and Sampson et al. (1999) for an extended discussion of the collective efficacy framework and its specific operationalization].

The first illustration stems from the work of Wen et al. (2005), who examined the effects of the urban social environment on mortality among Medicare beneficiaries who were 67 years old or older in 1993, lived in the City of Chicago, and were hospitalized for one of 13 serious diseases. Three data sources were used in this

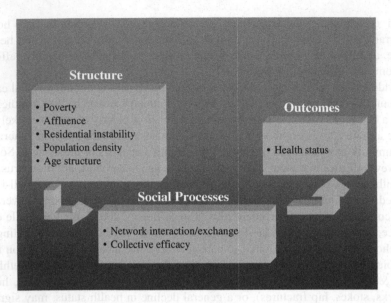

FIGURE 11.1. Social disorganization/ecological theory

study: the 1990 Decennial Census, the 1994–1995 Project on Human Development in Chicago Neighborhoods Community Survey (PHDCN-CS), and the Care after the Onset of Serious Illness (COSI) data set (1993–1999). Individual-level data were from the COSI data set (N=12,672). The core data of COSI were rooted in the 1993 inpatient hospitalization records from the Centers for Medicare and Medicaid Services. The COSI data set consisted of a cohort of patients newly diagnosed in 1993 with one of 13 serious illnesses and were followed for up to 6 years (Christakis, Iwashyna, & Zhang, 2002). Ecological measures of the economic and social context of local communities were obtained from the Census data and the PHDCN-CS. The PHDCN-CS is a probability sample of 8,782 residents of Chicago focusing on respondents' own assessments of the communities in which they live (Sampson et al., 1997). Individual assessments of community characteristics were aggregated to the community level using the *ecometric* method (Raudenbush & Sampson, 1999). ZIP code boundaries were used to define residential communities and to link the three data sources into one merged file. Survival analysis was performed to examine prospective and contextual effects of community characteristics on mortality following the onset of serious conditions in later life.

The study examined a range of community social capital indicators including collective efficacy, social support, social network density, prevalence of local organizations and voluntary associations, perceived violence, and personal victimization. As expected, collective efficacy was protective while violence and victimization were significant risk factors for mortality. That is, the data suggested that living in a cohesive community with effective social control enhanced older peoples' survival chances after the onset of serious diseases.

This result lends strong support for the hypothesis that community-level social capital promotes health over and above individual background.

However, the study also documented an intriguing relationship; community social network density (measured by the size of the social network and frequency of social interaction) was not beneficial, but detrimental. That is, living in communities characterized by high levels of social integration was a risk factor for diminished survival following serious medical conditions. Figure 11.2 illustrates predicted probabilities of death following the onset of serious conditions among Medicare beneficiaries living in Chicago corresponding to the increments of the 10th percentile of the social network density scale. The predicted probabilities were computed by a logistic regression model of mortality predicted by social network density and controlling for age and three years of comorbidity scores prior to the onset of the disease. A gradient relationship between social network density in the community and individual mortality risk is clearly shown in the figure with higher levels of network density predicting higher rates of mortality. Data from this research further suggest that areas with higher levels of social network density had more crime and violence and tended to have lower socioeconomic status (SES). Though appearing unexpected given evidence that social networks are largely salubrious (Berkman, Glass, Brissette, & Seeman, 2000), this finding resonates with Wilson's observation on neighborhood processes that many impoverished and dangerous neighborhoods share a relatively high degree of social integration and low levels of informal social control (Wilson, 1996).

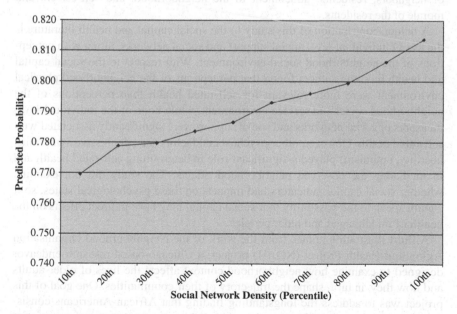

FIGURE 11.2. Predicted probability of mortality by social network density controlling for age and three years of comorbidity
(Source: COSI merged with PHDCN-CS)

The mixed results regarding community-level social capital and its effect on mortality of older patients suggest complex relationships between different dimensions of community social capital and health. They confirmed the contention that social capital is not a panacea but situational, with some aspects of social capital functional for specific kinds of outcomes while others not that beneficial in and of themselves (Berkman et al., 2000; Coleman, 1988; Keating et al., 2005; Portes, 1998; Stack, 1974).

A second illustration stems from the work of Wen et al. (2006), who conducted primary data collection on a population-based sample of 229 residents of Cook County, Illinois between the ages of 50 and 67 years in the Chicago Health, Aging, and Social Relations Study (CHASR) (Cacioppo, Hughes, Waite, Hawkley, & Thisted, 2006). Each respondent was then linked to the census tract to obtain information from the 2000 Census on local area SES. The key purpose of this study was to investigate the relationships among objectively assessed neighborhood SES, subjective perceptions of neighborhood environment, individual SES, psychosocial factors, and self-rated health among middle-aged and older adults. The authors took a novel approach to capturing local social capital. Rather than construct aggregate measures of neighborhood social environment from other sources of survey data, as done previously this research examined subjective perceptions of neighborhood quality, tapping physical, social, and service environments of local neighborhoods. The perceived social environment scale included important aspects of local social capital, such as friendliness/ helpfulness of neighbors, residents' attachment to the neighborhood, and self-esteem and morale of the residents.

A unique contribution of this study to the social capital and health literature is the test of individual-level social support and social networks, along with perceptions of the neighborhood social environment. With respect to the social capital and health link, the authors found that perceptions of the neighborhood physical environment were more relevant for self-rated health than perceptions of the neighborhood social and service environment, while none of the individual-level measures of social networks and social support were significantly associated with self-rated health. However, other psychosocial factors (i.e., depressive symptoms, hostility, optimism) played a significant role in determining self-rated health and in mediating the observed neighborhood effects. The study did not examine whether social capital indicators had impacts on these psychological states, so it cannot speak to the possibility that social capital may have indirect effects on the health of middle-aged and older people.

A third illustration comes from the work of the Neighbourhood Organisation Aging and Health Project (NOAH) project, a Chicago-based research endeavor designed to examine how neighborhood context affects the lives of older adults and how they, in turn, shape the trajectory of their communities. One goal of this project was to address the longstanding finding that African-Americans consistently report poorer health status than their White counterparts, even when controls are introduced for individual-level health and economic status. To our knowledge, this research is the first to examine the role of neighborhood-level factors in explaining the racial disparity in self-rated health (Cagney, Browning, & Wen, 2005) and to examine affluence as a critical covariate in health research. The authors theorized that affluence is not just the lack of poverty but rather an aspect of a community's socioeconomic profile that signals a resource-rich environment. Affluence may be the driving force behind the presence of health clinics, public parks, and responsive civic services.

Using the 1990 Decennial Census, the 1994–95 PHDCN-CS and selected years of the 1991–2000 Metropolitan Chicago Information Center Metro Survey, they examined the impact of neighborhood structure and social organization on self-rated health for a sample of Chicago residents 55 + (N=636). The authors used multi-level modeling techniques to examine both individual and neighborhood-level covariates. Consistent with previous research, they found that older urban African-Americans had a substantially higher likelihood of reporting low levels of health when compared to White respondents and that this relationship held even after controlling for a host of individual demographic, SES and heath factors.

Relying on collective efficacy theory to motivate the investigation the authors then considered the role of neighborhood social context in mediating the effect of race on health, examining the proportion of residents in both impoverished and affluent households as well as a latent indicator of residential stability. Consistent with expectations, neighborhood affluence exerted a strong and substantial effect on health, even after controlling for individual level SES and health background. Moreover, neighborhood affluence reduced the negative coefficient for African-American race and rendered it statistically insignificant. The proportional reduction in the race coefficient was nontrivial – older African-American residents may benefit substantially from the presence of economically advantaged neighbors with the capacity to mobilize on behalf of a health enhancing and health-protective environment.

At odds with theoretical expectations, however, residential stability was positively associated with poorer health. While inconsistent with collective efficacy theory, this result nevertheless parallels other recent findings that question the beneficial role of residential stability and the social processes with which it may be associated. Sampson et al. (1997), for instance, found that residential stability was positively associated with homicide rates in Chicago communities. Prior analyses (Browning & Cagney, 2003) also have offered evidence that the negative effect of residential stability on health holds for younger populations as well. The effect of residential stability may reflect processes described by Wilson, (1987) who suggests that, for some communities, stability may not produce or reflect social organization but, rather, economic and social isolation and constrained mobility (Ross, Reynolds, & Geis, 2001).

Finally, the operationalization of the collective efficacy concept—tapping social cohesion and health-related informal social control—did not predict self-rated health for older adults. Previous analyses indicate that collective efficacy is protective for a younger adult population (Browning & Cagney, 2002). Thus, collective efficacy, in its current conceptualization, may not be capturing the precise elements most important to the health of older persons.

A fourth illustration is derived from analyses of the July 1995 Chicago heat wave (Browning, Wallace, Feinberg, & Cagney, 2006). Evidence suggested that the distribution of heat-related mortality was concentrated in the most economically disadvantaged Chicago neighborhoods. Although age, race, socioeconomic status, and social isolation likely influenced the individual level capacity to cope with the excessive heat, the neighborhood-level absence of economic resources and other forms of disadvantage associated with local conditions may have independently contributed to excess mortality during the heat wave. The authors drew on Klinenberg's ethnography (2002) and recent neighborhood theory to explain community-level variation in mortality during the heat wave. They examined the impact of neighborhood structural disadvantage on heat wave mortality in 77 communities and considered three possible intervening mechanisms: social network interaction, collective efficacy, and commercial conditions. Combining 1990 Decennial Census and mortality data with the 1994–1995 PHDCN-CS and PHDCN Systematic Social Observation, the authors estimated hierarchical Poisson models of death rates both during the 1995 heat wave and comparable, temporally proximate July weeks (1990–94, 1996).

The authors found that declining commercial conditions contributed to differential heat wave vulnerability across neighborhoods. Although neighborhood social organization—represented by measures of social interaction/exchange and collective efficacy—was not a protective factor during the heat wave, they did find evidence of its beneficial effect under average conditions. Figure 11.3 illustrates the impact of collective efficacy and commercial decline for both heat wave and non-heat wave periods. The figure shows the percentage change in the mortality rate with a one-unit change in either collective efficacy or commercial decline. Collective efficacy, protective during regular time periods, may not have been able to be effectively activated during such an immediate crisis. Commercial decline, on the other hand, may have been particularly relevant for neighborhood residents who did not have access to other sources of information about neighborhood functioning. Older disabled individuals may be constrained in their ability to accumulate network-based information, some of which may take precedence over information provided by the condition of local businesses. As social sources of information constrict with age, visible cues regarding neighborhood functioning may be the only information that disabled older adults, confined to their households, are able to obtain. Even more mobile older adults may have felt uneasy traversing these areas to seek relief or may have been aware that few local establishments offered air conditioning or suitable indoor space. The research implies that enhancing local commercial venues would obviate the need for such mechanisms as cooling stations or other efforts that would require mobilization at the time of crisis. This research also extends the notion that older individuals may be isolated in isolated neighborhoods—the compounding nature of individual and neighborhood-level isolation may have repercussions during both crisis and non-crisis periods.

Commercial decline also accounted for a portion of the beneficial effect of the concentration of older residents within urban neighborhoods. This finding suggests

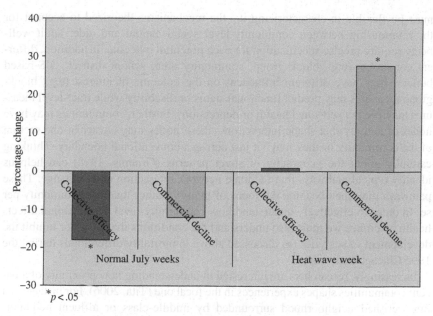

FIGURE 11.3. Percentage change in mortality rate with one-unit change in collective efficacy and commercial decline: Normal July and heat wave weeks.
(*Source:* Browning et al. 2006, *American Sociological Review*)

that high proportions of older residents may draw and sustain elder-relevant services, including businesses. Concentrations of older adults also may be able to more effectively resist the decline of local institutions and the shift toward potentially fear-inducing commercial enterprises such as liquor stores and bars.

11.3. Theoretical Challenges and Opportunities

In what follows we briefly discuss seven challenges to existing theory and potential next steps for innovation. We focus on factors that we believe need attention in order to advance theory and research in social capital, emphasizing community-level aspects salient for older adults.

11.3.1. Conceptualizing the Community

A critical and recurring issue in community-level research is the definition of "community." This is particularly important for research on the presence of community-level social capital; in order to identify trust and reciprocity we must be able to effectively situate respondents in a geographical space. Because much of the data used to characterize communities is census-based this leaves the construction of neighborhood boundaries at least partially dependent on these administrative units. Although clearly an empirical issue, the conceptual challenge precedes it. Theory must indicate the appropriate level of aggregation and must be flexible in characterizing it—the mechanisms theorized to account for the relationship between community-level social capital and older adult well-being require precise specification for each potential outcome. In addition, different constructs (e.g., block group, community area, school district, GIS-based buffers) may have different influences on the outcome of interest (e.g., block-group measures may predict functional status or disability while tract-level measures may predict self-rated health or depression). Further, communities may have nodes of activity that shape interaction—these nodes may cluster in one section of the community or they may sit just across a conventional boundary. Thinking carefully about the geography of street patterns (Grannis, 1998) can help us identify typical pathways that facilitate network interaction and exchange. These pathways may then become the focus of inquiry, rather than the community per se. In order to effectively understand how community-level social capital affects health outcomes we must also understand the conditions that foster or inhibit the development of such ties (as discussed above in mortality differentials during the 1995 Chicago heat wave).

Increasingly, researchers are interested in understanding how proximity of adjacent communities shapes experiences in the focal one (Tita, 2006). For instance, an impoverished neighborhood surrounded by middle-class or affluent neighborhoods may fare better than a neighborhood where all adjacent communities are impoverished (Pattillo-McCoy, 2000). Apart from immediate contiguity (Anselin, 1990), research focused on the effects of community-level social capital would benefit from an understanding of the networks of communitial not necessarily organized by space. Communities may form alliances based on such factors as political representation, ethnic allegiance, or economic profile. Individuals create their own set of networks, based on employment, routine activities, or family connections. For instance, the neighborhood where one family member resides in a nursing home becomes influential because it acts as a nexus for family interaction. As Lynch and colleagues (2000) assert, the ability to activate social capital is contingent, among other things, on the political and economic apparatus of the community. A more sophisticated understanding of boundaries could help us to isolate the distinct features of community-level social capital.

11.3.2. Dynamic Nature of the Community

Communities change by density, racial and ethnic composition, age distribution, and socioeconomic profile. The challenge is in tracking these changes, documenting their contemporaneous impact, and acknowledging that change may not be immediately discernable or may have a lagged effect. For instance, how long does a change in infrastructure (a new park, better lighting) take to change behavior? Does change itself have a positive or negative effect on well-being?

Consistent with a life course framework, research on community-level social capital could incorporate such notions as structural lag (i.e., policies and institutions have not kept pace with population change), tipping points, and the timing and sequencing of community change (Cagney, 2006; Riley, 1988). The dynamism applies both to the individuals and to the community—understanding their interaction is critical (O'Rand, 1996). Also important are analyses that take into account the specific age at which people entered or exited a community, or the age they were when the community experienced change.

11.3.3. Structural Characteristics beyond Composition

Poverty, affluence, education, residential stability and ethnic heterogeneity are commonly included as measures of neighborhood social structure (Browning & Cagney, 2003; Wen, & Browning, Cagney 2003). Critical to understanding the composition of communities, these factors alone do not capture context. In *The Death and Life of Great American Cities*, Jacobs (1961) describes how the physical structure of communities facilitates or discourages social interaction. This physical infrastructure—or "built environment"—can create opportunity for network development (Araya et al., 2006; Cannuscio et al., 2003; Clarke and George 2005; Gordon-Larsen, Nelson, Page, & Popkin, 2006; King et al., 2005). It can allow for the translation of social capital into street-level action, creating and reinforcing norms. If members of a community are predisposed to care for vulnerable populations, but no public space exists for them to meet, then that reservoir of assistance is never accessed. Technological innovations, such as satellite imaging, can provide precise information about the structural sources that facilitate or impede walking, social interaction, or the completion of routine activities.

11.3.4. Understanding When and Why People Move

Individuals may move from one community to another at key life turning points—marriage, childbearing, job change, illness and disability. Individuals may also move if they perceive that the new community will confer benefits, either immediately or over time (e.g., the Moving to Opportunity (MTO) demonstration, Goering, Feins and Richardson (2002). The motivations for why people move are varied. A better understanding of the decision to relocate would help the field to better describe and understand the role of neighborhood in residential stability. Further, the extent to which community context allows for "aging in place"(Golant & LaGreca, 1994) would inform our understanding of the choice set available to older adults as they contemplate options for a supportive residence.

11.3.5. Examining Age Structure and Integration

Studies of community context and health typically include individual-level controls, such as age, in their examination of neighborhood social processes. Much less common is the consideration of age at the neighborhood level, or the *age structure* of the community (Cagney, 2006). Inattention to age in empirical analyses is the result of inattention to age in the conceptualization of neighborhood context and neighborhood social processes. Theoretical developments related to social capital (Kawachi & Berkman, 2003; Portes, 1998) and contemporary elaborations of social disorganization theory (Sampson et al., 1997) have not incorporated the role of age structure. Analyses including the proportion of children (Coulton, Korbin, Su, & Chow, 1995) or the proportion of older adults (Cagney, Browning, & Wen, 2005) are helpful but do not incorporate the full age distribution. Age structure is important because it drives demand for services (e.g., health clinics), suggests a certain infrastructure (lighted sidewalks), and implies a set of expectations about interaction (informal monitoring of children) that could spill over into other forms of contact.

Age structure also indicates the level of age segregation or integration in the neighborhood. The implications of age segregation have not been fully examined—a disproportionate number of older adults has been cited for votes against tax increases for public schools or set-aside monies for public parks but evidence is mixed (Longino, 2001). The demand for age-based retirement communities indicates that some older adults desire a setting designed specifically for those in their age cohort.

11.3.6. Incorporating Reciprocal and Dynamic Processes

While considerable effort has been devoted to social capital and health, little research has examined the reverse causal process, i.e., the effect of aggregate neighborhood health status on community-level social capital (Cagney, Browning, & Wen, 2006). How, for instance, might poor health inhibit the ability of the community to maintain rich social networks or come together for the common good? Qualitative evidence indicates that people withdraw from community life when faced with health challenges (Wethington & Kavey, 2000). Compromised health status could attenuate the viability of local social networks, with indirect effects on a wide range of neighborhood outcomes. The relationship between health and community residence may assume a U-shape, where both the very sick and the very healthy are more likely to exit. This may help to explain, at least in part, why some apparently wealthier and resource-rich communities experience higher death rates (Waitzman & Smith, 1998). In general, we have little knowledge about how the presence of older persons in a neighborhood shapes social ties and community attachments.

11.3.7. Social Capital Across Multiple Social Domains

Although we have focused on the community as a key social domain in older people's lives, social capital can exist in other crucial life domains such as families, religious services, and volunteer work settings. How social capital of one ecological level interacts with that of another and/or with individual resources is largely unknown. Future work should examine these issues to determine which aspects of social capital—at which contextual level—confer protective effects for particular outcomes related to aging.

11.4. Conclusion

The importance of community context to the spread of disease and the health of a population has been a critical concern of public health since its inception (Koch & Denike, 2004; Paneth, 2004), and the study of its characteristics since the origin of urban sociology (Burgess, 1925; Park, 1925; Shaw & McKay, 1969). A resurgence in micro-level investigations of community life has led to a number of promising research trajectories that examine the role of community conditions in their own right. Vulnerable populations, such as young children and older adults, stand to benefit disproportionately from such investigations. Given both groups are more often tethered to their immediate surroundings the impact of the environment is likely greater. For older adults, the effect of social context has accrued over time. A life course perspective that incorporates early life information, key transition points, and the heterogeneity that exists at later ages could advance our understanding of the independent contribution of the immediate social environment.

Importantly, if research continues to demonstrate a relationship between community-level social capital and older adult well-being then future research should consider how best to create the form of social capital most likely to confer a benefit. Do we create and maintain public space, as Jacobs (1961) suggested, so we can draw older adults outdoors? Or, do we focus on programs that meet older adults in their own homes, facilitating social interaction within those confines? Can we tailor neighborhood-based initiatives such that they are available at, and applicable to, every stage of health and functional status? The community may be both a risk and a refuge—understanding how best to identify the beneficial features of community life motivates the next stage of inquiry.

Theory indicates that the social-structural influences on well-being are myriad and complex. Collecting and synthesizing data that reflect this complexity is a challenge. Combining data from multiple sources and developing innovative study designs are critical to testing hypotheses related to the points described above. These innovations are vital to neighborhood-based research in an older adult population—the dynamic nature of people and places can be observed in their life histories, and the community is a dominant feature of their daily lives.

References

Anselin, L. (1990). Spatial dependence and spatial structural instability in applied regression analysis. *Journal of Regional Science, 30*, 185–207.

Araya, R., Dunstan, F., Playle, R., Thomas, H., Palmer, S., & Lewis, G. (2006). Perceptions of social capital and the built environment and mental health. *Social Science & Medicine, 62*, 3072–3083.

Balfour, J. L., & Kaplan, G. A. (2002). Neighborhood environment and loss of physical function in older adults: Evidence from the Alameda County Study. *American Journal of Epidemiology, 155*, 507–515.

Barrett, A. E., & Lynch, S. M. (1999). Caregiving networks of elderly persons: Variation by marital status. *Gerontologist, 39*, 695–704.

Baum, F. (1999). Social capital: is it good for your health? Issues for a public health agenda. *Journal of Epidemiology and Community Health, 53,* 195–196.

Berkman, L.. F., Glass, T., Brissette, I., & Seeman, T. E. (2000). From social integration to health: Durkheim in the new millennium. *Social Science & Medicine, 51,* 843–857.

Binstock, R. H., George, L. K., Cutler, S. J., Hendricks, J., & Schulz, J. H. (2006). *Handbook of Aging and the Social Sciences.* Amsterdam, Boston: Academic Press an imprint of Elsevier.

Bourdieu, P. (1986). The forms of capital. In J. Richardson (Ed.), *Handbook of Theory and Research for the Sociology of Education* (pp. 241–258). New York: Macmillan.

Browning, C. R., & Cagney, K. A. (2002). Neighborhood structural disadvantage, collective efficacy, and self-rated physical health in an urban setting. *Journal of Health and Social Behavior, 43,* 383–399.

—. (2003). Moving beyond poverty: Neighborhood structure, social processes, and health. *Journal of Health Social Behaviour, 44* 552–571.

Browning, C. R., Feinberg, S. L., & Dietz, R. D. (2004). The paradox of social organization: Networks, collective efficacy, and violent crime in urban neighborhoods. *Social Forces, 83,* 503–534.

Browning, C. R., Wallace, D., Feinberg, S.L., & Cagney, K. A. (2006). Neighborhood social processes, physical conditions, and disaster-related mortality: The case of the 1995 Chicago heat wave. *American Sociological Review, 71,* 661–678.

Browning, C. R. (2002). The span of collective efficacy: Extending social disorganization theory to partner violence. *Journal of Marriage and the Family, 64,* 833–850.

Burgess, E. W. (1925). The Neighborhood. In R. E. Park & E. W. Burgess (Eds.), *The City* (pp. 142–155). Chicago: University of Chicago Press.

Burr, J. A., Choi, N. G., Mutchler, J. E., & Caro, F. G. (2005). Caregiving and volunteering: are private and public helping behaviors linked? *The Journals of Gerontology. Series B, Psychological Sciences and Social Sciences, 60,* S247–S256.

Burton, L. M. (1996). Age norms, the timing of family role transitions, and intergenerational caregiving among aging African American women. *Gerontologist, 36,* 199–208.

Cagney, K. A. (2006). Neighborhood age structure and its implications for health. *Journal of Urban Health, 83,* 827–834.

Cagney, K. A., Browning, C. R., & Wen, M. (2005). Racial disparities in self-rated health at older ages: What difference does the neighborhood make? *The Journals of Gerontology. Series B, Psychological Sciences and Social Sciences, 60,* S181–190.

Cagney, K. A., Browning, C. R., & Wen, M. (2006). *Death and decline:* The role of neighborhood-level mortality in the maintenance of social capital. The University of Chicago. Chicago, CL.

Cacioppo, J. T., Hughes, M. E., Waite, L. J., Hawkley, L. C., & Thisted, R. A. (2006). Loneliness as a specific risk factor for depressive symptoms: Cross sectional and longitudinal analyses. *Psychology and Aging, 21,* 140–151.

Cannuscio, C., Block, J., & Kawachi, I. (2003). Social capital and successful aging: The role of senior housing. *Annals of Internal Medicine, 139,* 395–399.

Clarke, P., & George, L. K. (2005). The role of the built environment in the disablement process. *American Journal of Public Health, 95,* 1933–1939.

Christakis, N. A., Iwashyna, T. J., & Zhang, J. X. (2002). "Care after the onset of serious illness (COSI): A novel claims-based data set exploiting substantial cross-set linkages to study end-of-life care. *Journal of Palliative Medicine, 5,* 515–529.

Coleman, J. S. (1990). *The Foundations of Social Theory.* Cambridge, Massachusetts: The Belknap Press of Harvard University Press.

Coleman, J. S. (1988). Social capital in the creation of human capital. *American Journal of Sociology, 94*, S95–S120.

Cornman, J. C., Goldman, N., Glei, D. A., Weinstein, M., & Chang, M. C. (2003). Social ties and perceived support: Two dimensions of social relationships and health among the elderly in Taiwan. *Journal of Aging and Health, 15*, 616–644.

Coulton, C. J., Korbin, J. E., Su, M., & Chow, J. (1995). Community-level factors and child maltreatment rates. *Child Development, 66*, 1262–1276.

Coward, R. T., & Dwyer, J. W. (1990). The association of gender, sibling network composition, and patterns of parent care by adult children. *Research on Aging, 12*, 158–181.

Crane, J. (1991). The epidemic theory of ghettos and neighborhood effects on dropping out and teenage childbearing. *American Journal of Sociology, 96*, 1226–1259.

Feld, S., Dunkle, R. E., Schroepfer, T., & Shen, H. W. (2006). Expansion of elderly couples' IADL caregiver networks beyond the marital dyad. *International Journal of Aging & Human Development, 63*, 95–113.

Ferraro, K. F. (1995). *Fear of Crime: Interpreting Victimization Risk.* Albany: State University of New York Press.

Glass, T. A., & Balfour, J. L. (2003). Neighborhoods, aging, and functional limitations. In I. Kawachi & L. F. Berkman (Eds.), *Neighborhoods and Health* (pp. 303–343). Oxford: Oxford University Press.

Goering, J., Feins, J. D., & Richardson, T. M. (2002). A cross-site analysis of initial moving to opportunity demonstration results. *Journal of Housing Research, 13*, 1–30.

Golant, S. M., & LaGreca, A. J. (1994). Housing quality of U.S. elderly households: Does aging in place matter? *Gerontologist, 34*, 803–814.

Gordon-Larsen, P., Nelson, M. C., Page, P., & Popkin, B. M. (2006). Inequality in the built environment underlies key health disparities in physical activity and obesity. *Pediatrics, 117*, 417–424.

Grannis, R. (1998). The importance of trivial streets: Residential streets and residential segregation. *American Journal of Sociology, 103*, 1530–1564.

Grundy, E. (2005). Reciprocity in relationships: socio-economic and health influences on intergenerational exchanges between third age parents and their adult children in Great Britain. *British Journal of Sociology, 56*, 233–255.

Hendricks, J., & Cutler, S. J. (2001). The effects of membership in church-related associations and labor unions on age differences in voluntary association affiliations. *Gerontologist, 41*, 250–256.

Hibbard, J., Neufeld, A., & Harrison, M. J. (1996). Gender differences in the support networks of caregivers. *Journal of Gerontology Nursing, 22*, 15–23.

House, J. S., Landis, K. R., & Umberson, D. (1988). Social relationships and health. *Science, 241*, 540–545.

Jacobs, J. (1961). *The Death and Life of Great American Cities.* New York: Vintage.

Kawachi, I., & Berkman, L. F. (2000). Social cohesion, social capital, and health. In L. F. Berkman, & I. Kawachi (Eds.), *Social Epidemiology.* Oxford: Oxford University Press.

Kawachi, I., & Berkman, L. F. (2001). Social ties and mental health. *Journal of Urban Health, 78*, 458–467.

Kawachi, I., & Berkman, L. (Eds.). (2003). *Neighborhoods and Health.* Oxford: Oxford University Press.

Keating, N., Swindle, J., & Foster, D. (2005). The role of social capital in aging well. In *Social Capital in Action: Thematic Policy Studies* (pp. 24–51). Canada: Policy Research Initiative.

Koch, T., & Denike, K. (2004). Medical mapping: The revolution in teaching—and using—maps for the analysis of medical issues. *Journal of Geography, 103*, 67–85.

Krause, N. (1991). Stress and isolation from close ties in later life. *Journal of Gerontology, Series B-Psychological Sciences and Social Sciences, 46*, S183–S194.

Krause, N. (1998). Neighborhood deterioration, religious coping, and changes in health during late life. *The Gerontologist, 38*, 653–664.

Kroenke, C. H., Kubzansky, L. D., Schernhammer, E. S., Holmes, M. D., & Kawachi, I. (2006). Social networks, social support, and survival after breast cancer diagnosis. *Journal of Clinical Oncology, 24*, 1105–1111.

Langa, K. M., Chernew, M. E., Kabeto, M. U., Herzog, A. R., Ofstedal, M. B., Willis, R. J. et al. (2001). National estimates of the quantity and cost of informal caregiving for the elderly with dementia. *Journal of General Internal Medicine, 16*, 770–778.

Lawton, M. P. (1970). Assessment, integration, and environments for older people. *Gerontologist, 10*, 38–46.

Lin, N. (2001). *Social capital : A Theory of Social Structure and Action.* Cambridge, New York: Cambridge University Press.

Litwin, H., & Shiovitz-Ezra, S. (2006). Network type and mortality risk in later life. *Gerontologist, 46*, 735–743.

Liu, A. Q. M., & Besser, T. (2003). Social capital and participation in community improvement activities by elderly residents in small towns and rural communities. *Rural Sociology, 68*, 343–365.

Locher, J. L., Ritchie, C. S., Roth, D. L., Baker, P. S., Bodner, E. V., & Allman, R. M. (2005). Social isolation, support, and capital and nutritional risk in an older sample: Ethnic and gender differences. *Social Science & Medicine, 60*, 747–761.

Lynch, J., Due, P., Muntaner, C., & Smith, G. D. (2000). Social capital—is it a good investment strategy for public health? *Journal of Epidemiology and Community Health, 54*, 404–408.

Longino, C. F. (2001). Geographical distribution and migration In R. H. Binstock, & L. K. George (Eds.), *Handbook of Aging and the Social Sciences* (pp. 103–124). San Diego: Academic Press.

McGarry, K., & Schoeni, R. F. (1997). Transfer behavior within the family: Results from the asset and health dynamics study. *Journals of Gerontology Series B-Psychological Sciences and Social Sciences, 52*, 82–92.

Mendes de Leon, C. F., Glass, T. A., Beckett, L. A., Seeman, T. E., Evans, D. A., & Berkman, L. F. (1999). Social networks and disability transitions across eight intervals of yearly data in the New Haven EPESE. *Journal of Gerontology Series B- Psychological Science and Social Sciences, 54*, S162—S172.

Moore, S., Haines, V., Hawe, P., & Shiell, A. (2006). Lost in translation: A genealogy of the "social capital" concept in public health. *Journal of Epidemiology and Community Health, 60*, 729–734.

Moore, S., Shiell, A., Haines, V., Riley, T., & Collier, C. (2005). Contextualizing and assessing the social capital of seniors in congregate housing residences: Study design and methods. *BMC Public Health, 5*, 38.

Nilsson, J., Rana, A. K. M. M., & Kabir, Z. N. (2006). Social capital and quality of life in old age – Results from a cross-sectional study in rural Bangladesh. *Journal of Aging and Health, 18*, 419–434.

O'Rand, A. M. (1996). The precious and the precocious: Understanding cumulative disadvantage and cumulative advantage over the life course. *Gerontologist, 36*, 230–238.

Paneth, N. (2004). Assessing the contributions of John Snow to epidemiology: 150 years after removal of the broad street pump handle. *Epidemiology, 15*, 514–516.

Park, R. E. (1916). *The City: Suggestions for the Investigation of Human Behavior in the Urban Environment.* American Journal of Sociology 20 (5): 577–60.

Pattillo-McCoy, M. (2000). *Black Picket Fences: Privilege and Peril among the Black Middle Class.* Chicago: University of Chicago Press.

Pollack, C. E., & von dem Knesebeck, O. (2004). Social capital and health among the aged: Comparisons between the United States and Germany. *Health Place, 10,* 383–391.

Portes, A. (1998). Social capital: Its origins and applications in modern sociology. *Annual Review of Sociology, 24,* 1–24.

Portes, A., Landolt, P. (1996). The downside of social capital. *American Prospect, 26,* 18–22.

Putnam, R. D. (2000). *Bowling Alone.* New York: Simon & Schuster.

Raudenbush, S. W., & Sampson, R. J. (1999). "Ecometrics": Toward a science of assessing ecological settings, with application to the systematic social observation of neighborhoods. *Sociological Methodology, 29,* 1–41.

Riley, M. W. (1988). On the significance of age in sociology. In M. W. Riley (Eds.), *Social Structure and Human Lives.* Newbury Park: Sage.

Robert, S., & Lee, K.Y. (2002). Explaining race differences in health among older adults. *Research on Aging, 24,* 654–683.

Robert, S. A., & Li, L. W. (2001). Age variation in the relationship between community socioeconomic status and adult health. *Research on Aging, 23,* 233–258.

Ross, C. E., & Jang, S. J. (2000). Neighborhood disorder, fear, and mistrust: The buffering role of social ties with neighbors. *American Journal of Community Psychology, 28,* 401–420.

Ross, C. E., Reynolds, J. R., & Geis, K. J. (2001). The contingent meaning of neighborhood stability for residents' psychological well-being. *American Sociological Review, 65,* 581–597.

Sampson, R. J., Morenoff, J. D., & Earls, F. (1999). Beyond social capital: Spatial dynamics of collective efficacy for children. *American Sociological Review, 64,* 633–659.

Sampson, R. J. (2003). Neighborhood-level context and health: Lessons from sociology. In I. Kawachi & L. F. Berkman (Eds.), *Neighborhoods and Health* (pp. 132–146). New York: Oxford University Press.

Sampson, R. J., Raudenbush, S. W., & Earls, F. (1997). Neighborhoods and violent crime: A multilevel study of collective efficacy. *Science, 227,* 918–923.

Settersten, R. A., Jr. (2005). Linking the two ends of life: What gerontology can learn from childhood studies. *The Journals of Gerontology. Series B, Psychological Sciences and Social Sciences, 60,* S173–S180.

Shaw, C. R., & McKay, H. D. (1969). *Juvenile Delinquency and Urban Areas:* Chicago: The University of Chicago Press.

Stack, C. (1974). *All Our Kin.* New York: Harper & Row.

Strawbridge, W. J., Shema, S. J., Cohen, R. D., & Kaplan, G. A. (2001). Religious attendance increases survival by improving and maintaining good health behaviors, mental health, and social relationships. *Annals of Behavioral Medicine, 23,* 68–74.

Thompson, E. E., & Krause, N. (1998). Living alone and neighborhood characteristics as predictors of social support in late life. *The Journals of Gerontology. Series B, Psychological Sciences and Social Sciences, 53,* S354—S364.

Tita, G. (2006). Neighborhoods as nodes: Combining social network analysis with spatial analysis to explore the spatial distribution of gang violence. University of California—Irvine.

Veenstra, G. (2000). Social capital, SES and health: An individual-level analysis. *Social Science & Medicine, 50*, 619–629.

Waitzman, N. J., & Smith, K. R. (1998). Phantom of the area: Poverty-area residence and mortality in the United States. *American Journal of Public Health, 88* 973–976.

Wellman, B., & Frank, K. (2001). Network capital in a multilevel world: Getting support from personal communities pp. 233–273. In Lin, N., Cook, K. S., & Burt, R. S. (Eds.), *Social capital: Theory and Research.* New York.

Wen, M., Hawkley, L. C., & Cacioppo, J. T. (2006). Objective and perceived neighborhood environment, individual SES and psychosocial factors, and self-rated health: An analysis of older adults in Cook County, Illinois. *Social Science & Medicine, 63*, 2575–2590.

Wen, M., Browning, C. R., & Cagney, K. A. (2003). Poverty, affluence and income inequality: Neighborhood economic structure and its implications for self-rated health. *Social Science & Medicine, 57*, 843–860.

Wen, M., Cagney, K. A., & Christakis, N. A. (2005). Effect of specific aspects of community social environment on the mortality of individuals diagnosed with serious illness. *Social Science & Medicine, 61*, 1119–1134.

Wethington, E., & Kavey, A. (2000). Neighboring as a form of social integration. In K. Pillemer, P. Moen, E. Wethington, & N. Glasgow (Eds.), *Social Integration in the Second Half of Life.* Baltimore: The Johns Hopkins University Press.

Wilson, W. J. (1987). *The Truly Disadvantaged: The Inner City, the Underclass, and Public Policy.* Chicago: The University of Chicago Press.

Wilson, W. J. (1996). *When Work Disappears.* Chicago: The University of Chicago Press.

Woolcock, M. (1998). Social capital and economic development: Toward a theoretical synthesis and policy framework. *Theory and Society, 27*, 151–208.

12
Social Capital and Health Communications

K. Viswanath

The concept of social capital has fired the imagination of scholars, policy makers and even activists engaged in the study and practice of social change, both planned and secular. Its popularity stems partly from a promise that its presence could lead to greater integration into the community, participation in civic affairs, better public health and overall comity and cohesion among disparate social groups (Hendryx, Ahern, Lovrich, & McCurdy, 2002; Kawachi & Berkman, 2000; Kawachi & Kennedy, 1997; Kawachi, Kennedy, Lochner, & Prothrow-Stith, 1997; Sampson, Raudenbush, & Earls, 1997; Scheufele & Shah, 2000; Subramanian, Kim, & Kawachi, 2002). This promise is partly responsible for its enormous popularity in a variety of fields including political science, sociology, communication and public health.

Yet, social capital is a "contested concept" with critics raising questions on its explication, measurement and even practice (Portes, 1998). This trenchant criticism and analysis not withstanding, its appeal remains unabated and continues to increase (Kawachi, Kim, Coutts, & Subramanian, 2004). In fact, Kawachi et al., drawing from their analysis of Pubmed, report a steady increase in the number of papers mentioning "social capital" from zero papers in 1992 to over 50 papers by 2002.

A question of empirical interest is the precise mechanism that connects social capital to outcomes of interest to us in public health. We posit that communication could potentially be one explanation that links social capital to public health outcomes.

Communication has been identified as playing a vital role in integrating people into their communities by helping to support and maintain their community ties and in promoting interpersonal trust (Cappella, Southwell, & Lee, 1997; Janowitz, 1952). Accordingly, the role of communication in social capital, at both mass and interpersonal levels, has attracted enormous attention from scholars for the purported reason that communication may lead to both an increase or in some cases a decrease in social capital, which in turn may affect public health. The relationship between communication and social capital, however, is not always direct and its association may often be with antecedents of social capital. A clearer delineation of the relationship between health communication and

259

social capital would not only be of academic interest but could be fruitful in the practice of social change in public health.

This essay focuses on the role of communication in social capital with specific relevance to public health. We will (a) define and identify some dimensions that have been commonly identified with social capital; (b) examine the relationship between mass media and social capital; (c) interpersonal communication and social capital; and (d) last, emerging issues such as communication inequality and how they may be related to social capital.

12.1. Social Capital: Definition and Characteristics

A precise definition of social capital, as averred earlier, has been elusive though there have been frequent efforts to capture it. There is, however, a broad agreement that social capital may be viewed as a resource (Loury, 1987) constituting the following dimensions: trust, norms of reciprocity, obligations, expectations, consensus and cohesion, and more germane to this chapter, information. Even though, possibly because of its seeming analogy to financial capital, some have proffered social capital as an individual property, a more appropriate characterization is that social capital is an emergent property that is constituted out of relations between two entities –person-person and person-organization. Thus even though it is considered an "individual asset" that one could draw upon to facilitate action, it "inheres in the structure of relations between and among persons" (Coleman, 1990). This later conception is critical since social relations are developed and maintained through communication thus giving it a centrality and the need for studying communication in social capital.

It is also worth noting the distinction offered by Szreter & Woolcock, (2004) who distinguished three forms of social capital: "bonding" social capital that is engendered by interactions with close groups and that could potentially result in social support. Bonding social capital could be affective or cognitive orienting people to their communities or community institutions. "Bridging" social capital among like minded social groups that could promote solidarity and fellowship, and "linking" social capital that ties individuals and groups with larger social institutions and that may be important in mobilization (Kawachi et al., 2004; Szreter & Woolcock, 2004). Bridging and linking social capital connect individuals and groups with community organizations (Lochner, Kawachi, Brennan, & Buka, 2003; McLeod et al., 1996; Poortinga, 2006).

12.2. Communication and Social Capital

The study of communication has been pursued at many levels: individual, interpersonal, organizational and social levels (Chaffee & Berger, 1987). A cogent understanding of a relationship between different dimensions of social capital and health communication warrants an appropriate focus on the level of analysis and in some cases, cross-level analyses. For example, watching a television program may engender discussions among co-workers, the so-called "water-cooler effect," cementing relationships between co-workers with a potential for trust and reciprocity. More often than not, the role of communication in social capital demands such cross-level analysis. We will next discuss the relationship between health communication and social capital at two levels: mass and interpersonal communications.

12.3. Mass Communication and Social Capital

12.3.1. Social Capital, Community Integration & Communication

Though the interest in social capital is relatively recent in its origin, social integration and cohesion have long been concerns of social theorists. Students of social change have sought to understand the factors that bind a society together and how societal changes can disrupt those ties. The concern with the effects of industrial society on communitarian life has been a running theme among social theorists (Durkheim, 1964/1933; Toennies, 1964) though they approached the issue from different points of view.

By extension, the recent resurgence in scholarly interest in the role of mass media in community integration has its origins in a concern about the alleged declining levels of civic engagement and social capital among the American public (For example, see (Putnam, 1993a, 1993b, 1995, 1996) among others) partially attributed to television. The connection between civic engagement and its impact on democracy, however, has long and deep roots in American intellectual discourse including de Tocqueville who in his *Democracy in America* was impressed with the American propensity for associational life, a feature of "bridging social capital" (Szreter & Woolcock, 2004). It is commonly believed that engagement with community institutions and neighbors promotes community solidarity and interpersonal trust, social capital in short.

Subsequently, concern about community integration emerged in an era of intense immigration to US cities early in this century. The primary concern of early researchers such as Park, Burgess, and Wirth was how millions of new residents would blend into American urban society to become productive citizens (Park, 1922; Wirth, 1964). Park first observed, for example, that immigrants with stronger ties to their communities made more use of ethnic newspapers than those with fewer ties. This was an important insight because it suggested a major mass media function in supporting processes of community integration. Park and his colleagues regarded community integration as a crucial factor in determining the health and welfare of democratic societies.

Morris Janowitz (1952) later continued to study the role of the mass media in promoting social integration. However, he expanded the perspective in three ways. He broadened the study to include citizens generally. He defined the concept of community integration as having affective dimensions that he called community "attachments." He also focused on the role of smaller local community newspapers. In this research, too, the more affective concept of "community attachments" (made operational as identification with, and participation in, community facilities and institutions) was strongly positive in its association with community newspaper use. Since Janowitz's initial study, others have continued to observe that community integration is related to use of local media especially community newspapers.

12.4. Mass Media Use and Social Capital

The association between media use and social capital in the context of health may occur through two mechanisms: the relationship between media use and community ties, and community ties and exposure to information on such topics as health.

12.4.1. Media Use and Community Ties

The relationship between ties to the community through such dimensions as membership in voluntary associations, local shopping, church attendance, homeownership, and length of residence, among others, and local mass media use (especially newspapers) has been one of the most enduring findings in the literature (McLeod, Scheufele, & Moy, 1999; Moy, McCluskey, McCoy, & Spratt, 2004; Viswanath, Finnegan, Rooney, & Potter, 1990). Reasons why this is so include Demers' (1996) finding that citizen interest in media information about the community is largely "primed" by social ties to the community. Moreover, recent studies have found that newspaper use is associated with membership in organizations including volunteer groups and churches (Finnegan & Viswanath, 1988; Rothenbuler, Mullen, DeLaurell, & Ryu, 1996; Stamm & Fortini-Campbell, 1983; Stamm & Weis, 1986; Viswanath et al., 1990) which act as contact networks. Another study found that even subscription to cable television was related to such membership (Finnegan & Viswanath, 1988). Others have reported that newspaper non-readers are less active in their communities (Sobal & Jackson-Beeck, 1981).

Studies using other dimensions of community ties such as residential stability, usage of local services and local employment have also showed a consistent relationship between community ties and local media use (Bogart & Orenstein, 1965; Kang & Kwak, 2003; Sobal & Jackson-Beeck, 1981; Stamm & Fortini-Campbell, 1983; Viswanath et al., 1990; Westley & Severin, 1964).

This well-established finding of local media use and community ties is important in understanding exposure to information of all kinds including health in the local media. Consistent use of media –reading the newspaper, watching television or listening to radio provides greater opportunities for exposure to content within those media. Some recent reports suggest that the amount of health information has been steadily increasing in the mass media consistent with interest in information on health among people (Viswanath et al., 2006). "Media effects" on audience awareness, knowledge, opinions, attitude about health, and such behaviors as purchasing healthy or unhealthy foods, physical activity or preventive behaviors, assume that such exposure to media content has taken place. In short, exposure is necessary for media to have an effect on people's health and local ties may enhance the opportunities for such exposure.

Another way community ties may influence media exposure is through social priming (Demers, 1996). Interaction with interpersonal networks and with members of local associations may "prime" audiences to attend to health information and as well as act as sources of information. In a recent study, (Viswanath, Randolph, & Finnegan, 2006) showed that members of communities who reported more ties with local voluntary associations were also most likely to have recalled a higher number of messages on cardiovascular health. In fact, those who reported active involvement in voluntary associations recalled more CVD messages than those who were less actively involved.

More recent research suggests that *how* media are used, may also matter to social capital. When media are used for "informational exchange," it is much more likely to contribute to social capital as opposed to using it for entertainment and "social recreation" (Besley, 2006; Brehm & Rahn, 1997; Newton, 1999; Shah, Kwak, & Holbert, 2001; Shah, McLeod, & Yoon, 2001). Broadly, use of news media (on television or through newspapers) has been positively associated with increased social capital, often in the form of group membership, civic engagement, and interpersonal trust (Beaudoin & Thorson, 2004) (Shah, Kwak et al., 2001). It is conceivable that news media provide greater opportunity for exposure to mobilizing information as well as arguments, opinions and frames that could promote engagement with civic affairs (Beaudoin, Thorson, & Hong, 2006; Shah, McLeod et al., 2001)

In summary, the role of mass media in social capital is possibly through an association between local community ties and local media use, which in turn provide the opportunity for greater exposure to media messages advocating or inhibiting healthy behaviors, and the exposure leading to either healthy or unhealthy outcomes.

12.5. Collective Action, Media Advocacy and Health

It is well documented that mass media are both agents of change and social control (Demers & Viswanath, 1999; Tichenor, Donohue, & Olien, 1980). Under certain circumstances, media may contribute to amplifying the agenda of organized social groups in support of social change, particularly when the advocated change is unlikely to threaten the fundamental power structure in the social system. Most organized efforts to promote public health such as public health communication campaigns work within the system and often use mass media as powerful advocates. One effort included using mass media campaigns to promote social capital including participation and positive perceptions towards youth, in essence, social capital (Beaudoin et al., 2006).

In sharp contrast, collective action to promote public health, often also called media advocacy, is not unheard of (Wallack & Dorfman, 1996). Radin (2006) offers the example of women suffering from breast cancer who organized "virtually" to support each other, for advocacy and to confront institutions and companies that may "penalize" women who are ill. Radin argues that the communication through the web started with trust before proceeding to collective action. Individuals who live in communities with high levels of social capital are able to work together and benefit from collective action, whether uniting to secure funding for police enforcement or through controlling the community in terms of domestic violence or alcohol abuse (Bracht & Tsouros, 1990; Kawachi & Berkman, 2000). When analyzing the community-level effects of social capital on individual health, Kawachi et al draw upon the research of Sampson et al (1997) to suggest that one of the mechanisms linking community-level social capital and individual health may be through the ability to mobilize to prevent loss of services from budget cuts, etc. and therefore have greater access to resources locally (Kawachi, Kennedy, & Glass, 1999; Sampson et al., 1997).

12.6. Community Characteristics, Social Capital and Health Communication

Drawing on the reports on the role of social capital in saving lives during the Chicago city heat wave in 1995, Kawachi et al. (2004), posited that residents in communities with higher levels of social capital –"richer social interactions" – were more likely to have been saved even if they were "socially isolated." This hypothesis draws attention to a factor that has not always received adequate attention in the literature–the characteristics of the community and how they may play out in promoting or inhibiting social capital.

Within communication, the structure of the community – its size, economic base, ethnic, racial and social class diversity, and centralization or decentralization of power among others—influence the availability of information, how media cover information, diversity of media choices and how people use the mass media. For example, Olien and her colleagues (Olien, Donohue, & Tichenor, 1985) studied whether diversity of community, termed "community pluralism" modified the relationship between newspaper reading and feeling "close" to the community and other community attachments. They reported that the relationship was stronger in more pluralistic communities but were virtually non-existent in the less pluralistic communities. They indicated that a reason for the finding was that news media serve a different function in more pluralistic compared to less pluralistic communities. Specifically, residents of large pluralistic communities rely more on the mass media than interpersonal communication to support and maintain their community ties and attachments. In contrast, Olien and her colleagues also implied, residents of smaller, less pluralistic communities depend less on the mass media and more on interpersonal communication to support and maintain their community ties and attachments.

Rothenbuler et al. (1996) also used a structural variable, population density, to examine its influence on community attachment and involvement. In their study they took the view that media exposure is a necessary intervening variable that led to community attachment and identification. They distinguished the two dimensions proposing that community attachment is an affective feeling with the community giving them the sense that they belong to the community. On the other hand, community involvement is a measure of more active and cognitive interaction with the community.

Rothenbuler et al. (1996) found that population density was negatively associated with involvement but was not related to attachment. They reported that local newspaper readership promoted involvement and attachment while local television was not related to attachment or involvement although it was influenced by population density. The denser the community, the greater the reliance on television to stay current with community affairs. Density was not related to newspaper readership. In our view, population density is another indicator of pluralism and supports the argument that the nature of the interaction between media exposure and community ties varies by community social structure.

We argue that residents of more pluralistic communities enjoy ties to a diverse range of community organizations, groups, and institutions unlike residents of less pluralistic communities. However, despite a narrower range, it is also possible that residents of smaller, less pluralistic communities enjoy stronger ties while their counterparts in larger communities have weaker ties to a greater diversity of community organizations, groups, and institutions. It is therefore possible that the strength of "weak ties" (Granovetter, 1973) in larger communities facilitates greater exposure to media messages both in quantity and content diversity such as health.

We also argue that the diversity of organizations, groups, and institutions in larger, more pluralistic communities (subsystem specialization), influences the information environment. Those residents who belong to, and participate in, such organizations, groups, and institutions should be more likely to be exposed to a range of information, especially on topics such as health.

In the study on the recall of CVD messages discussed earlier, Viswanath et al. (2006) examined if the number of messages recalled by the respondents was associated with the number of associational ties and if this relationship varied by the size and pluralism of the community. The data were drawn from people living in three different communities: small cities, larger independent regional cities and large exurban cities proximal to a metropolitan area. The number of CVD messages recalled not only increased with number of ties to different voluntary associations, but the relationship differed by the nature of the community. Residents from larger cities recalled more message than residents from smaller cities but more interesting, residents who reported most associational ties in the larger cities recalled greatest number of CVD messages compared to residents who reported no ties in the smaller cities. Viswanath et al argue that holding fewer ties *and* residing in a health information-poor environment "may result in a sort of double-dose of media isolation. This doubled impediment to media exposure may be a major source of gaps in health knowledge."

12.7. The Emergence of the Internet and its Role in Social Capital and Health

It is too early to predict the impact of the Internet and the World Wide Web (WWW) on interpersonal communications, social capital and health. Nonetheless, its unique characteristics are likely to heavily impact the nature of social interactions and consequently, trust, reciprocity, and dimensions of health communication. These characteristics of the Internet that are particularly relevant to health include:

- Its aynchronous nature that tempers or even eliminates the constraints of time and space;
- The ability to store and transfer large amounts of information quickly across geographical boundaries;
- Its characteristics that allow for one-to-one as well as one-to-many communications facilitating social interaction as well mobilization.

Given its recency, it is difficult to predict how Internet may promote social capital. Some recent studies suggest that

- Informational uses of Internet may potentially enhance social capital while recreational uses may deter social capital (Shah, Kwak et al., 2001). The effects are more pronounced among the "Generation X" rather than among baby boomers.
- Internet is also increasingly being used to promote collective action to mobilize patients to advocate for their rights (Radin, 2006).
- Internet has emerged among patients as a forum to seek social support and information. Discussion groups and chat rooms are widely visited for social support and to obtain additional information (Lamburg, 1997).

While these findings are intriguing, the future trajectory of Internet in social capital and communication in so far as it is relevant to health requires more empirical work.

12.8. Interpersonal Communication and Social Capital

Interpersonal communication, that is communication among dyads, triads, small groups—in short, social networks, has been of abiding concern to the students of social capital. Most of the dimensions of social capital such as trust, reciprocity, expectations and information exchange are generated and sustained among social networks through interpersonal communications. Interpersonal communications may also reinforce, moderate and contradict information people are exposed to in mass media. The relationship between interpersonal communication, social capital and health may be discussed in two broad areas: patient-provider communication and social support.

12.8.1. Provider-Patient Communication and Social Capital

The relationship and communication between physicians or providers and patients is usually been characterized by a degree of asymmetry with controlled exchange of information between the two parties. Physicians, by virtue of specialized knowledge, training and experience, have enjoyed power and control over this relationship and their ability to resolve immediate problems of patients allowing them to enjoy status and the perceived obligations of the patients. There was an inherent degree of trust between the two despite the asymmetry. Ahern and Hendryx (2003) find that community social capital is a significant predictor of trust in physicians and thereby impacts access of primary care providers. Trust and collaboration may very well be related to health care quality and access, Ahern and Hendryx contend (Ahern & Hendryx, 2003).

This sense of obligation and trust between the provider and patient, social capital, a singular characteristic in this relationship has come under severe strain over time because of information revolution. For example, over time, the monopoly over knowledge enjoyed by the physicians has been facing increasing challenge with widespread dissemination of health and medical information through mass media, and lately over the Internet.

The Direct to Consumer Advertising (DTCA), an effort by drug companies to aggressively market their brand named drugs, is having the effect of patients seeking advertised brand names again challenging the monopoly of the doctors.

12.8.2. Health Communication and Social Support

There is some confusion and even disagreement whether social support is legitimately considered as an aspect of social capital (Kawachi et al., 2004). Without taking a position on that issue, it is nevertheless worth pointing out that support is unlikely to be countenanced without trust and a degree of expectations of reciprocity. Networks built through Internet, for example, were used to widen access to surgery for a chest deformity through provision of information and communication (Thakur et al., 2002). Demonstrations of concerns, aid and information could decrease stress and improve well-being (Duggan, 2006). Most of the work on interpersonal communication so far has focused on social support by understanding how interactions and relationships affect support. More work on how interpersonal interactions influence social capital and health remains to be investigated.

12.9. Communication Inequality and Social Capital

Communication inequality may be defined as differences among social classes in the generation, manipulation, and distribution of information at the group level and differences in access to and ability to take advantage of information at the individual level (Viswanath, 2006). One potential reason for the emergence of inequalities in communication could be because of (a) the nature of one's social networks and (b) engagement with the networks themselves.

People who participate in voluntary associations are, in general, come from a higher socioeconomic position compared to those who do not. Such ties may potentially provide an opportunity to learn more about health (Viswanath et al., 2006) thus leading to inequalities in communication. The nature of association and the network itself may also matter. For example, Viswanath et al. show that networks may also provide specialized information in health allowing members to learn more about health. Heterogeneous networks facilitate the distribution and dissemination of new information –bridging social capital, and collective mobilization (linking social capital) compared to more closely aligned networks of family and friends (bonding social capital).

In short, it is intriguing to explore if the nature of social capital may influence what people may learn or do not learn from communications and if that varies by social class exacerbating inequalities.

12.10. Conclusions

Despite its controversy, social capital as a construct, is intuitively and intellectually appealing and has heuristic value. Its precise meaning remains elusive, yet the dimensions that constitute social capital –trust, reciprocity, engagement, provide a useful explanation for linkage among social groups and the larger society. It could be very well be the glue that holds the society together. Communication, we argue is a critical ingredient that sustains the links and plays a different role in different types of social capital–bridging, bonding and linking-and health. From the point of view of health, communication facilitates diffusion of new information, reinforces social norms, mobilizes people for collective action and creates social support thus providing the base for understanding how social capital may impact public health. And communication may also be used to explain how different variants of social capital–bonding, bridging and linking–may be related to each other. A more rigorous, systematic and through understanding of the relationship between health communication and social capital could be valuable in improving public health and reducing inequities among different social classes.

References

Ahern, M. M., & Hendryx, M. S. (2003). Social capital and trust in providers. *Social Science Medicine, 57*(7), 1195–1203.

Beaudoin, C. E., & Thorson, E. (2004). Social capital in rural and urban communities: Testing differences in media effects and models. *Journalism & Mass Communication Quarterly, 81*(2), 378–399.

Beaudoin, C. E., Thorson, E., & Hong, T. (2006). Promoting youth health by social empowerment: A media campaign targeting social capital. *Health Communication, 19*(2), 175–182.

Besley, J. C. (2006). The role of entertainment television and its interactions with individual values in explaining political participation. *Harvard International Journal of Press-Politics, 11*(2), 41–63.

Bogart, L., & Orenstein, F. E. (1965). Mass-Media and Community Identity in an Interurban Setting. *Journalism Quarterly, 42*(2), 179–188.

Bracht, N., & Tsouros, A. (1990). Principles and strategies of effective community participation. *Health Promotion International, 5,* 199–208.

Brehm, J., & Rahn, W. (1997). Individual-level evidence for the causes and consequences of social capital. *American Journal of Political Science, 41*(3), 999–1023.

Cappella, J., Southwell, B., & Lee, G. (1997). *The demise of interpersonal trust and civic capital: why is it happening.* Paper presented at the Mass Communication and Interpersonal Divisions of the International Communication Association, Montreal, Canada.

Chaffee, S. H., & Berger, C. R. (1987). What Communication Scientists Do. In C. R. Berger & S. H. Chaffee (Eds.), *Handbook of Communication Science* (pp. 99–122). Newbury Park: Sage Publications.

Coleman, J. S. (1990). Commentary: Social institutions and social theory. *American Sociological Review, 55*(3), 333–339.

Demers, D., & Viswanath, K. (1999). What promotes or hinders the role of mass media as an agent of social control or social change? In D. Demers & K. Viswanath (Eds.), *Mass Media, Social Control and Social Change: A Macrosocial Perspective*. Ames IA: Iowa State University Press.

Demers, D. P. (1996). Does personal experience in a community increase or decrease newspaper reading? *Journalism & Mass Communication Quarterly, 73*(2), 304–318.

Duggan, A. (2006). Understanding interpersonal communication processes across health contexts: Advances in the last decade and challenges for the next decade. *Journal of Health Communication, 11*(1), 93–108.

Durkheim, E. (1964/1933). *The division of labor in society*. Translate by G. Simpson. New York: Free Press.

Finnegan, J., & Viswanath, K. (1988). Community ties and use of cable television and newspapers in a Midwest suburb. *Journalism Quarterly, 65*(2), 456–463.

Granovetter, M. S. (1973). Strength of Weak Ties. *American Journal of Sociology, 78*(6), 1360–1380.

Hendryx, M. S., Ahern, M. M., Lovrich, N. P., & McCurdy, A. H. (2002). Access to health care and community social capital. *Health Services Research, 37*(1), 87–103.

Janowitz, M. (1952). *The Community Press in an Urban Setting*. Chicago: University of Chicago Press.

Kang, N., & Kwak, N. (2003). A multilevel approach to civic participation – Individual length of residence, neighborhood residential stability, and their interactive effects with media use. *Communication Research, 30*(1), 80–106.

Kawachi, I., & Berkman, L. (2000). Social cohesion, social capital, and health. In L. Berkman & I. Kawachi (Eds.), *Social Epidemiology* (pp. 174–190). New York: Oxford University Press.

Kawachi, I., & Kennedy, B. P. (1997). Socioeconomic determinants of health .2. Health and social cohesion: Why care about income inequality? *British Medical Journal, 314*(7086), 1037–1040.

Kawachi, I., Kennedy, B. P., & Glass, R. (1999). Social capital and self-rated health: a contextual analysis. *American Journal of Public Health, 89*(8), 1187–1193.

Kawachi, I., Kennedy, B. P., Lochner, K., & Prothrow-Stith, D. (1997). Social capital, income inequality, and mortality. *American Journal of Public Health, 87*(9), 1491–1498.

Kawachi, I., Kim, D., Coutts, A., & Subramanian, S. V. (2004). Commentary: Reconciling the three accounts of social capital. *International Journal of Epidemiology, 33*(4), 682–690; discussion 700–684.

Lamberg, L. (1997). Online support group helps patients live with, learn more about the rare skin cancer CTCL-MF. JAMA. 14; 277 (18): 1422–1423

Lochner, K. A., Kawachi, I., Brennan, R. T., & Buka, S. L. (2003). Social capital and neighborhood mortality rates in Chicago. *Soc Sci Med, 56*(8), 1797–1805.

Loury, G. (1987). Why should we care about group inequality? *Social Philosophy and Policy, 5*, 249–271.

McLeod, J. M., Daily, K., Guo, G. S., Eveland, W. P., Bayer, J., & Yan, S., et al. (1996). Community integration, local media use, and democratic processes. *Communication Research, 23*(2), 179–209.

McLeod, J. M., Scheufele, D. A., & Moy, P. (1999). Community, communication, and participation: The role of mass media in interpersonal discussion in local political participation. *Political Communication, 16*, 315–336.

Moy, P., McCluskey, M. R., McCoy, K., & Spratt, M. A. (2004). Political correlates of local news media use. *Journal of Communication, 54*(3), 532–546.

Newton, K. (1999). Mass media effects: Mobilization or media malaise? *British Journal of Political Science, 29*, 577–599.

Olien, C. N., Donohue, G. A., & Tichenor, P. J. (1985). *Community structure, newspaper use and community attachment.* Paper presented at the annual conference of the American Association for Public Opinion Research, McAfee, NJ.

Park, R. E. (1922). *The city.* Chicago, IL: University of Chicago Press.

Poortinga, W. (2006). Social relations or social capital? Individual and community health effects of bonding social capital. *Social Science & Medicine, 63*(1), 255–270.

Portes, A. (1998). Social capital: Its origins and applications in modern sociology. *Annual Review of Sociology, 24*, 1–24.

Putnam, R. D. (1993a). *Making Democracy work: Civic traditions in Modern Italy.* Princeton, NJ: Princeton University Press.

Putnam, R. D. (1993b). The prosperous community: Social capital and public life. *The American Prospect, Spring*, 35–42.

Putnam, R. D. (1995). Tuning in, tuning out: the strange disappearance of social capital in America. *PS: Political Science & Politics, 28*(4), 664–683.

Putnam, R. D. (1996). The strange disappearance of Civic America. *The American Prospect, 24*, 65–78.

Radin, P. (2006). "To me, it's my life": Medical communication, trust, and activism in cyberspace. *Social Science & Medicine, 62*(3), 591–601.

Rothenbuler, E. W., Mullen, L. J., DeLaurell, R., & Ryu, C. R. (1996). Communication, community attachment, and involvement. *Journalism & Mass Communication Quarterly, 73*, 445–466.

Sampson, R. J., Raudenbush, S. W., & Earls, F. (1997). Neighborhoods and violent crime: A multilevel study of collective efficacy. *Science, 277*(5328), 918–924.

Scheufele, D. A., & Shah, D. V. (2000). Personality strength and social capital – The role of dispositional and informational variables in the production of civic participation. *Communication Research, 27*(2), 107–131.

Shah, D. V., Kwak, N., & Holbert, R. L. (2001). "Connecting" and "disconnecting" with civic life: Patterns of Internet use and the production of social capital. *Political Communication, 18*(2), 141–162.

Shah, D. V., McLeod, J. M., & Yoon, S. H. (2001). Communication, context, and community – An exploration of print, broadcast, and Internet influences. *Communication Research, 28*(4), 464–506.

Sobal, J., & Jackson-Beeck, M. (1981). Newspaper Non-readers: A national Profile. *Journalism Quarterly, Spring*(58), 9–14.

Stamm, K. R., & Fortini-Campbell, L. (1983). The relationship of community ties to newspaper use. *Journalism Monographs, 84*(August).

Stamm, K. R., & Weis, R. (1986). The newspaper and community integration – a study of ties to a local church community. *Communication Research, 13*(1), 125–137.

Subramanian, S. V., Kim, D. J., & Kawachi, I. (2002). Social trust and self-rated health in US communities: a multilevel analysis. *Journal of Urban Health, 79*(4 Suppl 1), S21–34.

Szreter, S., & Woolcock, M. (2004). Health by association? Social capital, social theory, and the political economy of public health. *International Journal of Epidemiology, 33*, 650–667.

Thakur, A., Yang, I., Lee, M. Y., Goel, A., Ashok, A., & Fonkalsrud, E. W. (2002). Increasing social capital via local networks: Analysis in the context of a surgical practice. *American Surgeon, 68*(9), 776–779.

Tichenor, P. J., Donohue, G. A., & Olien, C. N. (1980). *Community Conflict and the Press.* Newbury Park, CA: Sage Publications.

Toennies, F. (1964). Community and Society: Gemeinscharft und Gesellschaft. In A. Etzionio & E. Etzionio (Eds.), *Social Change.* New York: Basic Books.

Viswanth K. (2006) Public communications and its role in reducing and eliminating health disparties . In: Thomson GE, Mitchell F, Williams MB, eds. Examining the Health Disparities Research Plan of the National Institutes of Health: Unfinished Business. Washington, D.C.: Institue of Medicine, 215‑253.

Viswanath, K., Breen, N., Meissner, H., Moser, R. P., Hesse, B., & Steele, W. R., et al. (2006). Cancer knowledge and disparties in the information age. *Journal of Health Communication, 11*(Suppl 1), 1–17.

Viswanath, K., Finnegan, J. R., Rooney, B., & Potter, J. (1990). Community ties and the use of newspapers and cable TV in a rural Midwestern community. *Journalism Quarterly, 67*, 899–911.

Viswanath, K., Randolph, W., & Finnegan, J. R. (2006). Social capital and health: civic engagement, community size,and recall of health messages. *American Journal of Public Health, 96*(8): 1456–1461.

Wallack, L., & Dorfman, L. (1996). Media advocacy: a strategy for advancing policy and promoting health. *Health Education Quarterly, 23*(3), 293–317.

Westley, B., & Severin, W. (1964). A Profile of the Daily Newspaper Non-reader. *Journalism Quarterly, Winter*(41), 45–50.

Wirth, L. (1964). *On Cities and Social Life: Selected Papers.* Chicago, IL: University of Chicago Press.

13
Disaster Preparedness and Social Capital

HOWARD K. KOH AND REBECCA O. CADIGAN

The first decade of the 21st century has pushed the field of disaster preparedness to the forefront of public health. In a few short years, the world has witnessed the far–ranging ramifications of 9/11 and anthrax (2001), SARS (2003), the Indian Ocean tsunami (2004), Hurricane Katrina (2005) and the looming threat of pandemic influenza. Societies everywhere are responding to these developments with new policies that commit added resources for protection against future disasters.

Concepts of social capital have major salience to these growing efforts. While other fields have previously explored social capital as a dimension of community integration, public health can find particular value in applying such concepts to disaster preparedness. A growing body of literature supports the integral role of social capital in all phases of disaster management i.e., preparedness, mitigation, response, and recovery. Though traditional disaster management emphasizes the value of physical, economic, and human capital, increasing research supports the notion that dimensions such as social cohesion and social networks particularly apply to preparedness work (Dynes, 2006).

In this chapter, we first comment on how social capital concepts can apply to the evolving public health world of disaster preparedness, with contributions of both bonding and bridging capital. We also explore how social capital relates not only to response and recovery phases after disasters, but just as importantly, to preparedness and planning before a disaster even occurs. While all these concepts are relevant to a broad range of disasters and emergencies, we will focus much of our attention on the current worldwide threat of pandemic influenza.

13.1. Applying Social Capital to Disasters

Disasters and emergencies can be characterized as natural and man-made. Medical attention to humanitarian relief has often centered on response and recovery efforts after hurricanes, floods, heat waves, earthquakes, tsunamis and other catastrophic events. Man-made disasters have received heightened public health attention since the unprecedented anthrax attacks of Fall, 2001 which affected 22 people and left 5 dead. This abrupt entrance of bioterrorism and

273

preparedness as critical priorities has fundamentally reshaped public health in the new 21st century. Moreover, the emergence of H5N1 avian influenza has triggered renewed concerns about a possible global pandemic. Currently, much of the world is directing renewed energy and resources toward pandemic planning.

In this context, social capital concepts offer a rich public health lens for analysis. Whether the focus is groups or individuals, social cohesion or social networks, or bonding or bridging, social capital themes drive to the heart of much of this current public health work. Furthermore, distinguishing between applying existing social capital and building new social capital offers another useful perspective for policy makers and the public alike.

In Chapter 1 of this volume, authors Kawachi, Subramanian, and Kim note that concepts of social capital have attributes related both to groups and to individuals. With respect to disasters and emergencies, such groups could include businesses, schools, religious organizations, community organizations and a host of government agencies, such as emergency management, health departments, fire departments or police departments, just to name a few. Such groups can improve disaster preparedness through collective socialization, preparation, and efficacy, e.g., formal joint training, drills and exercises, and practice of implementation of incident command systems. Individuals could range from vulnerable persons at risk in local communities to major leaders and officials in the groups noted above. At-risk individuals need to access resources through social engagement and support. Government agency leaders need to reach across to colleagues in other areas to ensure the highest levels of communication and coordination before, during and after a crisis.

Kawachi and colleagues further note that social capital can be conceptualized to include both broad social cohesion and individuals' access to resources through social networks. Once again, such concepts have special relevance to disasters and emergencies. A community with social cohesion may be better able to prepare for, and recover from, a flood than one less unified. Also individuals with ready access to support from family members and others in their community may be better able to cope with, or even avoid, the consequences of a disaster, compared to those without such networks. As one major example, Hurricane Katrina focused worldwide attention on the tragic outcomes of those without networks and resources. No doubt dimensions of social capital can influence emergency preparedness outcomes at the level of the individual, the community, the state, the country or indeed, the entire globe.

Also, both bonding and bridging social capital have complementary relevance in these contexts. As noted by others, bonding capital refers to resources accessed within social groups consisting of members alike with respect to social features such as class and race (Gittell & Vidal, 1998). With respect to emergencies and disaster preparedness, examples include strengthening local communities through better information channels and mobilization of volunteers. Meanwhile, bridging capital refers to resources built through connections made across social identity boundaries. In preparedness, such examples could include creating connections between local communities and official agencies and building trust between local residents and authorities.

13.2. Utilizing Existing Social Capital to Enhance Mitigation & Recovery

To date, literature relevant to social capital has focused largely on the value of *existing* social capital in disaster mitigation and recovery. For example, among environmental scientists, there is growing interest in the role of social capital and global climate change (Adger, 2001; Pelling & High, 2005). In light of the causal link between global climate change and the increasing incidence of natural disasters such as hurricanes, tsunamis and floods, researchers have identified social capital as an important tool in disaster mitigation. For example, Semenza, et al. (1996) found that during the 1995 heat wave in Chicago, in addition to location (i.e., living on the top floor of building) and access to air conditioning, variables related to social contact and networks were also strong predictors of mortality. Specifically, the authors found that individuals who participated in church or social groups had a significantly lower risk of death during the heat wave. It is clear from these findings that social networks and social capital are important tools in community coping with stresses, and serve to mitigate adverse outcomes of disasters and other events associated with climate change.

Similarly, existing social capital has served as a vital instrument in the recovery and rebuilding efforts following numerous natural disasters. Nakagawa and Shaw (2004) hypothesized that differing rates of post-disaster recovery following major earthquakes in Kobe, Japan and Gujarat, India could be attributed to disparate levels of existing social capital in the two cities. In the immediate aftermath of the 1995 Kobe earthquake, neighborhood groups (previously formed in the 1960s to protest polluting factories) quickly reconvened to assist with school evacuation, establish community kitchens, and help protect against looting. These actions accelerated response efforts and served to initiate rebuilding.

Following Hurricane Katrina in 2005, a number of observers (Garreau, 2005; Turner & Zedlewski, 2006) attributed many of the barriers to rebuilding New Orleans to the previously documented low social capital there (Putnam, 2000). Nevertheless, exceptions were notable. For example, within a matter of weeks, select tight-knit groups such as the Vietnamese enclave in East New Orleans were already engaged in rebuilding efforts (Hauser, 2005; Shaftel, 2006). Many of the 20,000 Vietnamese in New Orleans had previously emigrated to the U.S. in the 1970–1980s and have since maintained strong social and cultural networks. Using a church as headquarters, the Vietnamese residents of East New Orleans formed neighborhood teams to rebuild, repair, and decontaminate houses, prepare meals for families visiting to check on their property, and drive one another to work, church, and temporary housing.

13.3. Building New Social Capital through Preparedness & Response

For the preparedness and response phases of preparedness, much of the current efforts are focusing on the process of creating *new* social capital. One poignant illustration is the dramatic volunteer convergence on New York City following the terrorist attacks on September 11th, 2001, documented to include over 15,000 individuals within two and a half weeks. A qualitative study conducted by Lowe and Fothergill (2003) found that the primary motivation for volunteering was a need "to contribute something positive and find something meaningful in the midst of a disaster characterized by cruelty and terror" (p. 298). The authors characterized the impact of such spontaneous volunteerism on both the community and the volunteers themselves, i.e., affecting both groups and individuals. One volunteer described the work as "honoring our commitment to the American public" (p. 303), implying a broad national community. Individual impact was noted when "the volunteers found that by working with new groups of people. . . . . they experienced a sense of solidarity with different community members" (p. 303). In another example outside of the United States, an estimated 2 million volunteers responded to assist with search and rescue, medical aid, transportation, and provision of shelter following the 1985 earthquake in Mexico City (Dynes & Quarantelli, 1990).

A major benefit of preparedness planning would be to strengthen local public health infrastructure which has been traditionally fragmented and severely underfunded. Over a few short years, nascent efforts on preparedness have broadened the initial focus on training federal and state government leaders to include local officials and indeed all members of society. Lessons from SARS and Hurricane Katrina have underscored the message that every person has an opportunity and responsibility to protect themselves, their families and their communities.

As a result, in the world of public health, emergency preparedness training now extends deeply to the local level with respect to planning, communication and training. In many parts of the United States, efforts have focused attention to regionalization of local public health, surge capacity planning, vulnerable populations, risk communication, and training through exercises and drills. All these efforts have the potential to boost local public health infrastructure and build a legacy of social capital and social networks in local communities.

The remainder of this chapter will explain in greater detail how such preparedness efforts apply to dimensions of social capital at the local level, particularly with respect to pandemic influenza preparedness.

13.4. Building Social Capital through Pandemic Influenza Preparedness

13.4.1. Planning

The threat of pandemic influenza has sparked heightened planning worldwide. The World Health Organization (WHO) urges that each country and community develop and regularly update a pandemic preparedness plan. WHO guidance centers on issues such as surveillance, communications and prioritization of scarce resources. As of December 2005, 40 countries have completed such plans

(Uscher-Pines, Omer, Barnett, Burke & Balicer, 2006). The United States unveiled its National Pandemic Influenza Plan in November, 2005, addressing areas such as domestic and international surveillance, vaccine development and production, antiviral therapeutics, communications and state/local preparedness. Moreover, each of the 50 states has developed and publicized plans, as summarized on www.pandemicflu.gov. All nations understand the importance of priority setting in preparedness planning, although such plans currently vary by rationale of prioritization of antiviral agents, vaccines and other scarce resources (Uscher-Pines, Omer, Barnett, Burke, & Balicer, 2006). As "all preparedness is local" however, such plans can only come alive through full engagement at the local level. Both bonding and bridging social capital apply throughout such plans.

13.4.1.1. Local/Regional Planning

The current fragmented status of local public health in the United States has left few cities or towns (aside from the major metropolitan areas) capable of responding on their own. For the most part, local health departments lack the personnel, resources or capacity to respond to mass casualties without the support of surrounding communities.

To address this challenge, many states have turned to regionalization of resources and services to build emergency preparedness capacity at the local level. A study of state public health preparedness programs conducted in Fall, 2004 by the Association of State and Territorial Health Officials (ASTHO) found that most states tended to subdivide their organizations into regions for preparedness purposes, with more than half of such regions created post-9/11 (Beitsch et al., 2006). Massachusetts, Nebraska, Illinois, Kansas and the Northern Capital Region (greater metropolitan Washington DC) are among the states that have done so. For example, Massachusetts, a state of 6.3 M, traditionally had a highly decentralized local public health system with 351 autonomous cities and towns. Nevertheless, after 9/11 the state reorganized into seven emergency preparedness regions and 15 subregions (Koh, Elqura, Judge, & Stoto, 2008). In another example, the primarily rural state of Nebraska of 1.7 M people has developed 16 regions in efforts to improve capacity.

Preliminary qualitative information suggests that regionalization has built social capital for groups and individuals. The National Association of County and City Health Officials (NACCHO) notes that regionalization has promoted *coordination* (of local public health and partners in public safety and emergency medical services), *standardization* (of resources and emergency plans) and *centralization* of local emergency response capability (Bashir, Lafronza, Fraser, Brown, & Cope, 2003; Hajat, Brown, & Fraser, 2001). In so doing, improved collective efficacy can be realized. Analyses have noted that regionalization has served as a foundation for sharing resources, coordinating planning, conducting trainings and improving capacity. For example, in Massachusetts, regionalization led to emergency local capacity essential for pandemics and mass casualties, such as establishment of 24/7 emergency on-call capacity for all local public health officials in the state (when none previously existed) and mutual aid agreements for over 60% of local public health departments (compared to none previously). In fact, in the few short years of its existence, regionalization has facilitated the efficient organization of Hepatitis A immunization clinics in the face of food borne outbreaks, and coordination of seasonal flu vaccine distribution during the shortages of the 2004–2005 season (Koh, Shei, Judge et al., 2006). Such examples reflect enhanced social capital within groups (e.g., nurses and allied health professionals) and bridging between groups (local health groups and state public health officials).

Most notably, regionalization has fostered communication and connections between multiple groups: public health and public safety, interested parties in neighboring towns, local and state leaders, and volunteers across the state. Multiple parties that rarely worked together prior to 9/11 are now meeting regularly to plan joint responses and clarify roles and responsibilities.

13.4.1.2. Coordination of Health Care Assets and Surge Capacity

Planning for pandemics and mass casualties requires ramping up the current national health care system to care for thousands of extra ill patients. Building surge capacity in this way can generate bonding and bridging capital, mobilizing and unifying a vast array of societal resources. Based on past pandemics, the U.S. Department of Health and Human Services (DHHS) has modeled its pandemic planning on scenarios ranging from moderate (such as the 1957 and 1968 pandemics) to severe (such as the 1918 pandemic). Current models project as many as 90 M cases nationally, 50% of cases requiring outpatient medical care, and up to 9.9 M requiring hospitalization (Hamburg et al., 2005). The U.S. Centers for Disease Control and Prevention (CDC) has developed the software program FluSurge, which provides hospital administrators and public health officials local estimates of the surge in demand for hospital-based services during the next influenza pandemic.

The challenge of surge capacity remains enormous, as national trends over the past several decades reflect declining, not increasing, capacity. In fact from 1993 to 2003, the number of hospitals in the U.S. decreased by 703, with the number of hospital beds declining by 198,000. This drop in capacity has only added to the tremendous strain on emergency departments in the country, where visits have increased from 90.3 M to 114 M in the same time period (Institute of Medicine Committee on the Future of Emergency Care in the United States Health System, 2006).

With this daunting backdrop, the United States is working toward increasing surge capacity, explicitly defined by the U.S. Agency for Healthcare Research and Quality (2004a) as "a health care system's ability to expand quickly beyond normal services to meet an increased demand for medical care in the event of bioterrorism or other large-scale public health emergencies" (p. 1). The U.S. Health Resources and Services Administration (HRSA) has offered surge capacity benchmarks with respect to staff, space and supplies, as shown in Table 13.1 (Agency for Healthcare Research and Quality, 2004b).

Building staff can be viewed as an exercise in creating bonding capital, i.e., within the community of health care providers. Additional personnel needed for

TABLE 13.1. Health care surge capacity benchmarks per the U.S. Health Resources and Services Administration.

Staff	
Health Care Personnel	Response system that allows immediate deployment of:
	250 additional personnel per million population in urban areas
	125 additional personnel per million population in rural areas
Space	
Hospital Beds	500 additional acute care beds per million population
Decontamination Facility	Adequate portable or fixed decontamination system for 500 patients & workers per million population
Isolation Facility	At least one negative pressure, HEPA-filtered isolation facility capable of supporting 10 patients per health system
Supplies	
Personal Protective Equipment	Adequate equipment for all health care providers, including additional personnel per above benchmark

deployment in a crisis would include, in addition to physicians (approximately 800,000 in the U.S.) and nurses (approximately 2.2 M in the U.S.), veterinarians, pharmacists, mental health professionals and a host of other allied health professionals. Such providers would not only administer direct care to those who are sick but could also aid with mass prophylaxis efforts to the many more who may be exposed or at risk. To augment this national network, communities across the U.S. are engaging volunteers in emergency response. For example, in 2002, the U.S. Office of the Surgeon General founded the Medical Reserve Corps (MRC), a network of community-based teams of local volunteer medical and public health professionals, which now includes approximately 100,000 volunteers in over 500 MRC units (U.S. Office of the Surgeon General, 2006). Additionally, in 2002, HRSA established the Emergency System for the Advanced Registration of Volunteer Health Professionals (ESAR-VHP) whereby states are funded to establish pre-registration systems for emergency volunteer health professionals. Through both initiatives, volunteers are prospectively identified, trained, and credentialed to respond during an emergency.

With respect to space, all hospitals have been charged by HRSA and other organizations to identify additional beds for use in pandemics and emergencies. In addition to staffed beds (beds that are licensed, staffed, and physically available), all acute care hospitals are ascertaining surge capacity by identifying other beds that: are licensed but not staffed, can be made available within 24 hours (by discharging patients and canceling elective procedures) or within 72 hours (through use of non-traditional locations such as hospital cafeterias, chapels, etc.). In the event that hospital capacity is still overwhelmed, professionals across the country are currently identifying other health care facilities such as community health centers (Koh, Shei, Bataringaya et al., 2006) or even non-medical sites such schools, gymnasiums, armories, and convention centers. Considerations for such facilities include dimensions such as bed capacity, sanitary facilities, food services, and security.

The shortage of medical supplies has also prompted bridging outside the medical world to other parts of government and society to generate sufficient resources. Many have argued that preparing for pandemic influenza first entails mastering the proper coordination of national vaccination efforts for annual seasonal influenza, which yearly leads to 36,000 deaths and 200,000 hospitalizations (Thompson, Shay, & Weintraub, 2003, 2004). In particular, the fragmented nature of the national seasonal influenza vaccine supply became starkly apparent during 2004–2005, when a national low of 61 M doses led to prioritization of risk groups for immunization for the first time. Production for 2006–2007 is now estimated to reach a high of 115 – 120M doses, however (Fauci, 2006). Shortages of antibiotics and antiviral agents may require interaction with the federal Strategic National Stockpile (SNS), managed by the CDC and DHHS. The SNS contains prepackaged pharmaceutical agents that can be deployed to states at the governor's request. All states have prepared preliminary plans for the receipt and management of stockpile materials, and many have initiated planning for emergency dispensing at the local level.

Acquiring such resources and even determining the resources needed are a tremendous source of activity and controversy. One area involves personal protective equipment (PPE) where, for example, experts differ about recommendations regarding proper use of surgical masks, N 95 respirators and other equipment (Institute of Medicine Board on Health Sciences Policy, 2006). Additionally, ventilators represent a critical limiting physical resource. There are approximately 105,000 ventilators in the U.S., with as many as 80,000 in use at any given time for medical care; and more that 100,000 required during a typical influenza season (Osterholm, 2005). In the event of a pandemic, the number of patients requiring mechanical ventilation would likely exceed this capacity in excess of 500% (Hamburg et al., 2005).

13.4.1.3. Attention to Special Populations

All disasters expose disparities. As mentioned previously, Hurricane Katrina has been a recent disaster that has graphically highlighted vulnerabilities of special populations, the varying levels of social capital within those populations, and the need to ensure equity in preparedness. A survey revealed that 38% of those who did not evacuate before Hurricane Katrina were either physically unable to do so or had to care for someone who was physically unable to leave. 52% of evacuees reported having no health insurance coverage at the time of the hurricane (Brodie, Weltzien, Altman, Blendon, & Benson, 2006).

National groups have redoubled efforts to address the needs of special populations, defined by the CDC (2006) as "groups whose needs are not fully addressed by traditional service providers or who feel they cannot comfortably or safely access and use the standard resources offered in disaster preparedness, relief, and recovery" (p. 4). They include, but are not limited to: 1) those who are physically or mentally disabled (blind, deaf, hard-of-hearing, cognitive disorders, mobility limitations); 2) limited or non-English speaking; 3) geographically or culturally isolated; 4) medically or chemically dependent; 5) homeless; 6) frail/elderly and children. Such groups would need to bridge to resources currently not available to them. Issues of trust in, and trustworthiness of, authorities charged to protect them further complicate this issue.

Planning for special populations has increased recently. Such planning may differ dramatically for densely populated urban settings as opposed to more sparsely populated rural settings; each community with its own profile of risks and assets. Examples of special populations planning include evacuation planning for elderly immobile populations in nursing homes, targeted risk communication strategies for non-English speaking populations, and coordination of services for people who are homeless, homebound, or medically or chemically dependent. Such populations are particularly vulnerable to broader social forces affecting their communities. Overcoming social isolation in these instances remains a daunting societal challenge.

13.4.2. Communication of Risk

In a time of crisis, all members of society expect and deserve accurate information that is conveyed simply, clearly, and in a timely fashion. Such information is critical not only for all to understand roles and responsibilities in times of crisis but also for how and when to access resources. In this regard, the WHO, CDC and other organizations have afforded considerable attention and resources to upgrading media plans, training of communicators, and message preparation and delivery.

To a great extent, the responsibility for such risk communication will fall on government public health authorities through broad use of the media. This presents special challenges in the U.S., where recent surveys show that less than 50% of the general public trust government public health authorities "a lot" as a source of useful and accurate information about an outbreak, compared to significantly higher levels in other parts of the world, such as Taiwan, Hong Kong and Singapore (Blendon et al., 2006).

In particular, it is unclear exactly how much the public understands the concept of "pandemic influenza" and how it differs from the term "avian influenza". Also, there are many other subtleties in communicating relevant information to the public and the press. For example, the uncertain efficacy of antiviral agents for pandemic influenza may not be well known. In Chapter 12 of this book, Viswanath explores the information disparities affecting populations in society. Building public awareness now through regular communication can enhance trust and confidence in advance of any future pandemic.

13.4.3. Training Emphasizing Exercises & Drills

In preparing for a disaster, professionals and the public need continuous education and training. Groups such as the federally funded Academic Centers for Public Health Preparedness have been charged with exploring many such educational avenues, including face-to-face teaching, train-the-trainer initiatives (Orfaly et al., 2005), distance learning initiatives (Moore, Perlow, Judge, & Koh, 2006) and other modalities.

Recently, the public health community has moved aggressively into exercises and drills as a favored educational modality (Cadigan, Biddinger, & Koh, 2006). Mounting a rapid, coordinated, integrated local response to mass casualty events such as pandemic influenza necessitates tight collaboration among a host of participants, including emergency management, public health, law enforcement, fire, emergency medical services, health care providers, public works, municipal government, and community-based organizations. Exercises, defined as any event beyond the planning process that gathers people to test or improve preparedness (U.S. Department of Homeland Security, 2004), both teach and test such coordination for individuals and organizations. Involving representatives from multiple agencies to exercise together in a regular fashion facilitates an iterative cycle of developing plans, training personnel, testing preparedness, and improving plans even further to clarify specific roles and responsibilities.

Both bonding and bridging capital can be enhanced in this way. For example, tabletop exercises are often organized around multiple tables, with each table representing one local municipality. Key government officials from across various agencies work together at each table, while being forced to interact with other towns/tables as well as state agencies. Resources can be enhanced by building bonding capital within each professional group, each agency, each town, as well as bridging capital across agencies, communities and between local and state officials.

Furthermore, since public health disasters are critical but rare, exercises serve the vital function of testing plans in a concrete and memorable fashion. Use of local tailored scenarios provides exercise participants with a sense of urgency as well as concrete opportunities to understand the complex coordination involved in local emergency response. Furthermore, respondents can test their understanding of the National Incident Management System and the Incident Command System. Such active, experiential learning appears to have greater educational impact than more conventional, didactic lectures, particularly for rare events (Streichert et al., 2005).

These exercises build social networks of responders. Qualitative studies suggest that exercises improve communications with colleagues from other agencies, force participants to address inadequacies in communications systems and protocols, and promote strategies to ensure presentation of consistent messages. By convening with local/regional partners, participants realize potential opportunities to increase capacity by sharing resources with neighboring communities. Bringing together participants from a range of disciplines enhances opportunity to learn about the unique services, skills, and expertise offered by others. An ongoing area of research is to quantify these outcomes in a standardized way that demonstrates enhanced preparedness.

13.5. Conclusion

While we offer our ideas here on the ramifications of social capital on evolving public health preparedness work, much of this information is qualitative and/or preliminary. Many observations noted here need verification and validation.

Furthermore, the intense current focus on community disaster preparedness is still relatively new. Academic investigation should verify and extend these concepts, offer more quantitative assessments of social capital as applied to disasters, demonstrate their utility through more rigorous analyses, and ascertain whether initial societal changes found in qualitative studies will be enduring and sustained. Moreover, we have presented concepts of social capital as being overwhelmingly positive in their nature when in fact research in other areas has documented possible negative ramifications noted elsewhere in this book.

Nevertheless, much of the current work regarding public health preparedness can enhance social capital through stabilization and growth of the current fragile public health infrastructure, i.e., workforce capacity and competency, information and data systems, and organizational capacity (CDC, 2001). Disaster planning has undoubtedly revived and accelerated community discussions about societal planning, obligations, and expectations in a time of crisis. Regionalization of local health has generated new local capacity. Attention to special populations has renewed emphasis on commitments to equity and raises key questions about obligations of community members to one another. Efforts to enroll volunteers through MRC and other initiatives have revitalized discussions on expectations of service in a community. Attention to surge capacity, resource shortages and the prospect of alternate sites of care during a mass casualty event has raised explicit discussions about obligations and expectations. Agencies have advanced bridging in the common mission of protecting the public. Inherent in all planning has been the importance of trust building, particularly in information sharing and risk communication.

Moreover, such investments may well be helping to build a more cohesive, integrated, prepared national and global community where all understand their interdependence in the midst of a crisis. In a time of social isolation where many are "bowling alone", disaster preparedness efforts may serve as a force that reverses this trend and contributes to a legacy of stronger local public health and a more revitalized society for the future.

References

Adger, W. N. (2001). Social Capital and Climate Change. Tyndall Centre for Climate Change Research – Working Paper No. 8.
   http://www.tyndall.ac.uk/publications/working_papers/wp8.pdf (accessed Jan. 23, 2007).
Agency for Healthcare Research and Quality. (2004a). Surge Capacity–Education and Training for a Qualified Workforce. Issue Brief No. 7.
   http://www.ahrq.gov/news/ulp/btbriefs/btbrief7.pdf (accessed Nov. 21, 2006).
Agency for Healthcare Research and Quality. (2004b). Optimizing Surge Capacity–Regional Efforts in Bioterrorism Readiness. Issue Brief No. 4.
   http://www.ahrq.gov/news/ulp/btbriefs/btbrief4.pdf (accessed Nov. 21, 2006).
Bashir, Z., Lafronza, V., Fraser, M. R., Brown, C. K., & Cope, J. R. (2003). Local and state collaboration for effective preparedness planning. *Journal of Public Health Management Practice, 9*(5), 344–351.

Beitsch, L. M., Kodolikar, S., Stephens, T., Shodell, D., Clawson, A., Menachemi, N. et al. (2006). A state-based analysis of public health preparedness programs in the United States. *Public Health Report, 121,* 737–745.

Blendon, R. J., DesRoches, C. M., Cetron, M. S., Benson, J. M., Meinhardt, T., & Pollard, W. (2006). Attitudes toward the use of quarantine in a public health emergency in four countries. *Health Affair, 25,* 15–25.

Brodie, M., Weltzien, E., Altman, D., Blendon, R. J., & Benson, J. M. (2006). Experiences of hurricane Katrina evacuees in Houston shelters: Implications for future planning. *American Journal of Public Health, 96*(8), 1402–1408.

Cadigan, R. O., Biddinger, P. D., & Koh, H. (2006). Using regional multi-agency exercises to enhance public health preparedness. Abstract presented at the 134th Annual Meeting of the *American Public Health Association.*

Dynes, R. R. (2006). Social capital: Dealing with community emergencies. *Homeland Security Affairs, 2*(2), 1–26.

Dynes, R., Quarantelli, E. L., & Wenger, D. (1990). *Individual and organizational response to the 1985 earthquake in Mexico City.* Newark, DE: Disaster Research Center, University of Delaware.

Fauci, A. S. (2006). Seasonal and pandemic influenza preparedness: Science and counter-measures. *Journal of Infectious Diseases, 194*(Suppl 2), 73–76.

Garreau, J. (2005). A sad truth: Cities aren't forever. *The Washington Post,* p. B01.

Gittell, R., & Vidal, R. (1998). *Community organizing: Building social capital as a development strategy.* Thousand Oaks, CA: Sage Books.

Hamburg, M. A., Hearne, S. A., Levi, J., Elliott, K., Segal, L. M., & Earls, M. J. (2005). *A killer flu.* Trust for America's Health, Issue Report. http://healthyamericans.org/reports/flu/Flu2005.pdf (accessed Jan. 22, 2007)

Hauser, C. (2005) Sustained by close ties, vietnamese toil to rebuild. *The New York Times,* p. 22.

Institute of Medicine Committee on the Future of Emergency Care in the United States Health System. (2006). *The future of emergency care in the United States health system.* Washington, DC: The National Academies Press.

Institute of Medicine Board on Health Sciences Policy. (2006). *Reusability of facemasks during an influenza pandemic.* Washington, DC: The National Academies Press.

Koh, H., Elqura, L., Judge, C., & Stoto, M. (2008). Regionalization of local public health systems in the era of preparedness. *Annual Review of Public Health, 29* (In Press).

Koh, H. K., Shei, A., Bataringaya, J. A., Burstein, J. L., Biddinger, P. B., Crowther, S. et al. (2006). Building community-based surge capacity through a public health and academic collaboration: The role of community health centers. *Public Health Report, 121,* 211–216.

Koh, H., Shei, A., Judge, C., Stoto, M., Elqura, L., Cox, H., et al. (2006). Emergency preparedness as a catalyst for regionalizing local public health. Abstract presented at the 134th Annual Meeting of the *American Public Health Association.*

Lowe, S., & Fothergill, A. (2003). A need to help: Emergent volunteer behavior after september 11th. In J. L. Monday (Ed.). *Beyond september 11th: An account of post-disaster research.* Boulder, CO: Natural Hazards Center.

Moore, G. S., Perlow, A., Judge, C., & Koh, H. (2006). Using blended learning in training the public health workforce in emergency preparedness. *Public Health Report, 121,* 217–221.

Nakagawa, Y., & Shaw, R. (2004). Social capital: A missing link to disaster recovery. *International Journal of Mass Emergencies and Disasters, 22*(1), 5–34.

Hajat, A., Brown, C. K., & Fraser, M. R. (2001). *Local public health agency infrastructure: A chartbook.* Washington, DC: National Association of County and City Officials.

Orfaly, R. A., Frances, J. C., Campbell, P., Whittemore, B., Joly, B., & Koh, H. (2005). Train-the-Trainer as an educational model in public health preparedness. *Journal of Public Health Management Practice, 11*(6 Suppl), S123–S127.

Osterholm, M. T. (2005). Preparing for the next pandemic. *New England Journal of Medicine, 352*(18), 1839–1842.

Pelling, M. & High, C. (2005). Understanding adaptation: What can social capital offer assessments of adaptive capacity? *Global Environmental Change, 15*(4), 308–319.

Putnam, R. D. (2000). *Bowling alone. The collapse and revival of American community.* New York: Simon & Schuster.

Semenza, J. C., Rubin, C. H., Falter, K. H., Selanikio, J. D., Flanders, W. D., & Howe, H. L. (1996). Heat related deaths during the July 1995 heat wave in Chicago. *New England Journal of Medicine, 335*(2), 84–90.

Shaftel, D. (2006). The ninth reward: The Vietnamese community in New Orleans East rebuilds after katrina. *The Village Voice.*

Streichert, L. C., O'Carroll, P. W., Gordon, P. R., Stevermer, A. C., Turner, A. M., & Nicola, R. M. (2005). Using problem-based learning as a strategy for cross-discipline emergency preparedness training. *Journal of Public Health Management Practice, 11*(6 Suppl), S95–S99.

The Office of the U.S. Surgeon General (2006). *MRC Reaches 500 MRC Unit Milestone.* http://www.medicalreservecorps.gov/NewsEvents/2006/MRCUnitMilestone (accessed Nov. 21, 2006)

Thompson, W. W., Shay, D. K., Weintraub, E., Brammer, L., Bridger, C. B. Cox, M. J., & Fukuda, K. (2004). Influenza-associated hospitalizations in the United States. *JAMA, 292,* 1333–1340.

Thompson, W. W., Shay, D. K, Weintraub, E., Brammer, L., Cox, M., Anderson, L. J., & Fukuda, K. (2003). Mortality associated with influenza and respiratory syncytial virus in the United States. *JAMA, 289,* 179–186.

Turner, M. A., & Zedlewski, S. R. (2006). *After Katrina: Rebuilding opportunity and equity in New Orleans.* Washington, DC: The Urban Institute. http://www.urban.org/UploadedPDF/311406_after_katrina.pdf (accessed Jan. 23, 2007).

Uscher-Pines, L., Omer, S. B., Barnett, D. J., Burke, T. A., & Balicer, R. D. (2006). Priority setting for pandemic influenza: An analysis of national preparedness plans. *PLoS Medicine, 3*(10), e436.

U.S. Centers for Disease Control and Prevention. (2006). *Public health workbook to define, locate, and reach special, vulnerable, and at-risk populations in an emergency.* http://www.bt.cdc.gov/workbook/ (accessed Nov. 27, 2006).

U.S. Centers for Disease Control and Prevention. (2001). *Public health's infrastructure: A status report.* http://www.phppo.cdc.gov/documents/phireport2_16.pdf (accessed Nov. 21, 2006).

U.S. Department of Homeland Security, Office for Domestic Preparedness. (2004). *Homeland security exercise and evaluation program,* Volume I: Overview and Doctrine. http://www.ojp.usdoj.gov/odp/docs/HSEEPv1.pdf (accessed Nov. 23, 2006).

World Health Organization. (2005). *Avian influenza frequently asked questions.* http://www.who.int/csr/disease/avian_influenza/avian_faqs/en/index.html (accessed Nov. 27, 2006).

Index